Consider This:

Many women of color will go to church all day Sunday, choir rehearsals, bible study, missionary meetings, and cakewalks every week of every year, *but won't take* one *day out of the year to get their Pap test and mammogram done.*

Obesity is a leading cause of life-threatening heart disease, diabetes, and stroke. More than 60 percent of African-American women are overweight and over 40 percent are obese, more than any other ethnic population.

Stress causes the release of stress hormones in the body. Prolonged stress severely affects the immune system, diminishing its ability to protect one from life-threatening cardiovascular disease, cancers, and infections. A strong prayer life and spiritual base have been shown to decrease stress.

Black American women are still dying from diseases that many other women are being cured of.

Learn how you can guard your health.

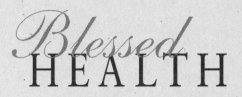

Blessed HEALTH

**The African-American Woman's Guide
to Physical and Spiritual Well-Being**

Melody T. McCloud, M.D.,
and Angela Ebron

A FIRESIDE BOOK
Published by Simon & Schuster
New York · London · Toronto · Sydney · Singapore

FIRESIDE
Rockefeller Center
1230 Avenue of the Americas
New York, NY 10020

For information about special discounts for bulk purchases,
please contact Simon & Schuster Special Sales:
1-800-456-6798 or business@simonandschuster.com

Designed by Lisa Stokes

Illustrations by John Del Gaizo

Manufactured in the United States of America

Library of Congress Cataloging-in-Publication Data
McCloud, Melody Theresa.
    Blessed health : the African-American woman's guide to physical and spiritual
well-being / by Melody T. McCloud and Angela Ebron.
      p.   cm.
    1. African-American women—Health and hygiene—Religious aspects.
I. Ebron, Angela.   II. Title.
RA778.4.A36 M385   2003
613'.04244'08996073—dc21   2002030678

10 9 8 7 6 5 4 3 2

ISBN 0-7434-1042-4

This publication contains the opinions and ideas of its authors. It is intended to provide
helpful and informative material on the subjects addressed in the publication. It is sold
with the understanding that the authors and publisher are not engaged in rendering medical, health, or any other kind of personal professional services in the book. The reader
should consult his or her medical, health, or other competent professional before adopting any of the suggestions in this book or drawing inferences from it.

The authors and publisher specifically disclaim all responsibility for any liability,
loss, or risk, personal or otherwise, which is incurred as a consequence, directly or indi-
rectly, of the use and application of any of the contents of this book.

Contents

. . . .

Introduction

. . . .

$\mathcal{A}$RE YOU one of the millions of sisters out there who never has time for herself? If it's not the kids, it's your man. If it's not your man, it's the job. If it's not the job, it's your relatives. The list could go on and on. You find yourself tending to so many other people that you never have time to tend to yourself. You constantly think, *I need some balance in my life,* but sister-friend, it goes much deeper than that. Sure, leading a hectic life is a juggling act. But, truth be told, the dozens of balls you're trying to keep in the air are just the surface of the problem. Forget those deadlines, the dishes in the sink, the laundry piling up in the hamper. What about *you*? Are you at peace with yourself? Do you feel energetic and full of life? Are you in touch with your inner spirit? Are you in good health? These are the things we're talking about. The sad fact is that too many sisters never take stock of their lives, never stop long enough to truly reflect on their own well-being.

If this is you, *Blessed Health* is here to help. Far too many of us never give our physical or spiritual well-being the attention each deserves. What you may not realize is that one nourishes the other. When your spiritual self is cared for and nurtured, it helps to replenish, rejuvenate, and safeguard your physical self. And when it comes to health, we sisters can use all the help we can get. Just consider these alarming statistics:

- African-American women are 38 percent more likely to suffer a fatal heart attack than white women.

- One in four black women age 55 and older has diabetes, and we are more likely to develop complications from it than are our white counterparts.

- Sisters have the fastest-rising rate of increase for contracting HIV, and we are dying of AIDS at a rate ten times that of white women.

- Nearly a third of all African-American women have high blood pressure.

- Sisters are three times more likely to die of a stroke than are Caucasian women.

- Black women have the highest mortality and lowest survival rates for breast cancer. In fact, we are twice as likely to die from it as are white women.

- Black women are more likely to give birth prematurely than are Caucasian, Asian, Hispanic, and Native American women. Worse still, our infant mortality rate is more than twice that of white women.

When it comes to health, sisters fare very poorly. In practically every medical category we carry the worst prognosis for conditions that are often curable or manageable. Clearly, our lives are not in balance, and we are suffering because of it. Something is out of sync, and it goes far beyond putting off that doctor's appointment or not paying attention to your body's aches and pains. Yes, these factors are certainly part of the reason why too many of us are in poor health, as are heredity and, often, insufficient medical coverage. But two other factors play just as important a role: lack of information and lack of spirituality.

Many sisters may ignore their body's creaks and twinges out of fear. None of us wants to hear bad news about our health. But the more likely reason is lack of knowledge. We don't mean that as a slight, but the fact remains that many sisters simply don't know how to read their body's messages. A little pain in the chest? Some of us are quick to chalk it up to heartburn. A recurring headache? How often have you attributed it to pressure at work? Feeling tired and run-down? Many black women would blame it on a busy schedule and leave it at that. While all of these explanations may be valid, there's a chance that a more serious health condition is the real culprit. You simply may not know how to recognize the symptoms, or are finding it more convenient to ignore them. Arming yourself with knowledge is the first step, and *Blessed Health* will give you the tools to do so.

The second step is resolving to do in-depth spiritual work on a daily basis in order to boost your overall health, and *Blessed Health* will act as your guide on that journey as well. Some may scoff at the connection between spirituality and physical well-being, but studies show a solid link between the two. In fact, as part of their ongoing health and spirituality research at the Center for the Study of Religion/Spirituality & Health, under the direction of Dr. Harold G. Koenig, Duke University recently studied 4,000 people age 64 and older, black and white, and found that those who attend religious services every week tend to live longer. According to the researchers, churchgoers have a healthier immune system than those who don't attend services regularly, and women appear to benefit even more than men. In another study at the Mind/Body Medical Institute in Boston, founder Herbert Benson, a Harvard researcher, found that patients who practiced the technique of repeating a prayer many times and disregarding all other thoughts that came to mind saw significant improvements in a host of ailments, from insomnia and PMS to migraine headaches and cancer.

Although the evidence of spirituality's positive effect on health is clear, many sisters don't always use their faith as a means to better health. Yes, we are a deeply religious people who have a history of relying on inner work to see us through difficult times. But do we really use it to bless our health on a daily basis? African-American women recognize and rejoice in the power of prayer, calling upon God when a serious illness strikes. But you don't have to wait for a health emergency to occur before turning to your faith. Do spiritual work in the name of good health every day, and you will be witness to all kinds of "mini miracles." You will feel better than you have in years. Why? Because spirituality not only improves your immune system, enabling your body to better fight disease, but it also acts as a buffer against the ill effects of stress.

If you don't make time for yourself each day, to do inner work, to care for your soul, this can adversely affect your equilibrium and cause physical and biochemical changes that may result in illness. *Blessed Health* will show you how to keep such damage from happening. Within these pages you will learn how to achieve optimal health by combining solid medical information with increased spirituality. By the time you turn the last page you will truly understand the connection between how you feel physically and how you feel spiritually. And you will be empowered to make that relationship stronger, richer, and more life-affirming. All the tools you need are right here, and we're not just talking about learning facts and figures, although you'll find those here, too. Girlfriend, within these pages you will also discover how to find the right doctor, one who ministers to both your physical and emotional needs. You'll learn how to successfully cope with illnesses from a faith-based perspective. You will gain wisdom about preparing yourself spiritually for motherhood, menopause, and other health milestones. You'll learn important information about breast care, medications, and what to expect if you ever need surgery—all coupled with soul-nourishing guidance that will enable you to shore up your health for the long run.

The Bible tells us "I would that ye prosper and be in health even as your soul prospers." It's time for sisters to heed that message. God has made us stewards, or caretakers, of our physical selves, and we need to protect that temple. We can't afford to be complacent. After all, your physical self is the only true thing you possess. Material goods may be lost, people may come in and out of your life, but your body and soul are with you always. Without your health and a spiritual foundation, what do you really have? Resolve to nurture both, and each will fortify the other. Everything you need to live a healthy, spiritually fulfilling life is right here. So take this time for yourself. Turn the page and discover enlightenment, empowerment, and total well-being. It's all within your hands. For once you experience good health, you will feel truly blessed.

What Makes Sisters Unique?

· · · · · · · · · · ·

An African-American proverb correctly asserts that you can't know where you're going if you don't know where you've been. But let history and past experiences instruct rather than determine your destination.

—Johnnetta B. Cole, president of Bennett College, president emeritus of Spelman College, and author of *Dream the Boldest Dreams*

NEWS YOU CAN USE

· Black women carry the highest risk for heart disease, diabetes, certain cancers, stroke, hypertension, fibroid tumors, and HIV/AIDS.

· Health care facilities in many African-American communities are understaffed, underfunded, and overwhelmed.

· Research shows that African Americans feel more of a participatory role in decision making when receiving health care from black doctors.

· Many black women fall prey to a "superwoman" mentality, which prevents them from making their health a priority.

WE ARE a resilient people. One need only look at history to see just how true this is. When our African foremothers were brought to this country in shackles, who could have imagined that generations later the women who share their strong characters, their beautiful features, and their spirited hearts would have risen so high? From the brutality and back-breaking hardship of slavery, to the continued struggle and persistent fear of freemen following emancipation, to the indignity and cruelty of Jim Crow, to the powerful battle cry of the civil rights movement, to the dissemination of affirmative action—through all of this we have persevered. As sister-poet Maya Angelou proclaims, "And still I rise!" That we do. Sisters, we have really come into our own over the years. Black women are more highly educated. Many of us own our own businesses or successfully compete in corporate America. We are doctors, judges, elected officials, dot-com entrepreneurs. We are bringing up our youngsters, caring for our elders, nurturing our men, tending our communities. We are carving out lives our great-great-grandmothers may have only dreamed about. Yet amid all of these strides, we are still miles behind in one very crucial area: our health.

As a physician, I am constantly reviewing medical literature and the most current studies, taking continuing medical education courses, and attending medical conferences and seminars. What I have found is that, in general, sister-patients are usually the ones in poorest health. Statistics bear this out. Black women carry the highest risk for heart disease, diabetes, certain cancers, stroke, HIV/AIDS, hypertension, and fibroid tumors, just to name a few. Though I risk sounding like Brother Job, this harsh and painful reality often makes me question God. *Lord, what is going on? Why do my sisters suffer so?*

Unlike Job, who had done everything perfectly right, African-American women often fail to do the right thing, namely taking the necessary steps to safeguard their health. Sadly, sisters are not alone in their lapse of responsibility. Statistically, many women of color fall victim to poor health, most notably Hispanic, Native American, and some Asian women. But black women fare the worst by far.

The question often arises: Is it nature or nurture? Is there some genetic predisposition to certain illnesses that causes African-

American women to always pull up the rear when it comes to health? Are black female infants destined from conception to be burdened with an unhealthy life?

Or is it lifestyle? Diet? Apathy? Fear? What is it? Is there some definite anatomical or physiological difference in black women's bodies? Do certain conditions truly "run in the family," or is it that certain lifestyles are passed down from generation to generation—lifestyles that lead to obesity, diabetes, hypertension, and the like?

HEALTH CONCERNS

As a physician and surgeon specializing in obstetrics and gynecology, I have counseled, examined, treated, and operated on thousands of women of many colors—African-American, Hispanic, Caucasian, and every ethnicity in between. As a result of my experience, I can say with reasonable certainty that the normal human female—regardless of race—is the same anatomically (structure) and physiologically (function). Her hair may be a different texture, her skin may be a different tone, but the inner workings are the same, when normal.

So, if structure and function are the same, why is the outcome terribly different in many cases? Why are sisters still carrying a poorer prognosis and higher mortality rate for many conditions that others are readily cured of, in astounding numbers? Take a look at some numbers from the U.S. Department of Health and Human Services' Office on Women's Health and I think you'll start to see just how alarming the state of black female health really is (see page 4).

Obviously, all women need to be concerned about their health. But as the statistics make clear, heeding that message is especially important for African-American women. The big question is, why don't more of us do it? Why don't we make our health our top pri-

	Black	White	Hispanic	Native American	Asian
Life expectancy	**74.2**	79.7	77.1	74.4	82.9
Rate of premature birth	**13%**	6.3%	7%	6.5%	7.1%
Infant mortality (# of deaths per every 1,000 live births)	**14.7**	6.1	6.1	10.0	5.2
Heart disease (# of deaths per 100,000 women)	**156**	94	66	92	55
Stroke (# of deaths per 100,000 women)	**39.6**	22.9	17.3	25.1	21.4
Hypertension	**34%**	19%	22%	—	—
HIV/AIDS (# of deaths per 100,000 population)	**12.2**	0.8	2.8	too few to count	too few to count
Breast cancer (# of deaths per 100,000 women)	**27**	18.9	12.7	9.2	9.2
Lung cancer (# of deaths per 100,000 women)	**28.3**	28	8.9	58.3	11.5
Diabetes	**25%**	15%	30%	50%	3.8%
Gonorrhea (rate per 100,000 women)	**426**	18	40	49	less than 1
Syphilis (rate per 100,000 women)	**55**	less than 1	3	2	less than 1
Overweight	**66.6%**	48%	67%	—	13–26%
Violence against women (rate per 1,000)	**56**	42	52	98	21

Source: U.S. Department of Health and Human Services Office on Women's Health, 2000.

ority? There are various reasons, some rooted in the history of our society, others spurred by our own fears and traditions, and still others linked to our lackadaisical consideration of our health.

REASON #1—DISTRUST OF HEALTH CARE PROFESSIONALS

Whenever you hear a story on the news about an unnecessary surgery or a mistake made on the operating table, a chill runs up your spine. This is true of anyone. All of us fear surgery; it's human nature. We imagine something going wrong and it leaves us nervous and afraid. So is it any wonder that stories of mistakes that actually happened cause that much more anxiety? When you can see and hear folks on *Dateline* and 20/20 talking about their frightful experiences, it's not imagination anymore. It's reality. It doesn't matter that these sorts of incidents are rarities. When you can put a face on it, it becomes 100 times more scary and feeds our distrust of our nation's health care system and health care professionals.

For African Americans, this sort of public distrust is coupled with a more deeply imbedded personal distrust, the origins of which span scores of prior generations. When hundreds of thousands of slaves arrived on these shores, an African woman's body was no longer her possession. It belonged to her master, and as such, its care was in his hands, not hers. If her temple was broken, beaten, and abused, if it was plagued by illness and disease, its tending was at her master's discretion. Yes, our people did what they could to tenderly nurture one another's physical selves back to health, relying on the spirituality and root-based remedies used in our Motherland. But access to medical care was tendered as necessary maintenance of valued labor, not as a protection of life itself. We, as black women, were viewed as commodities, not as human beings.

After slavery, this inferiority mentality continued and affected every aspect of life, including health care, especially in the South.

Many hospitals refused to admit us. Those that did housed us in segregated wards with lower standards of care. We would have eagerly turned to black physicians, but we would have been hard-pressed to find one in those days. Since African Americans were denied access to medical training through the trajectory of medical school and residency until the 1840s, most black women had to rely upon white male doctors for their health care services.

While many white doctors of the time upheld the Hippocratic oath, some freely violated that oath by performing numerous unnecessary procedures, including countless hysterectomies, on African-American women. Only later, often after many years had passed, would a black woman come to know that she had received a procedure that she may never have actually needed.

As blacks migrated to the North and West, they took with them a belief system shaped by years of medical mistreatment, disrespect, and indifference. As a result of this long history of distrust, many African Americans still don't seek the medical care they need, even if they can't really articulate why. The legacy of our ancestors speaks volumes.

REASON #2—POVERTY AND LACK OF INSURANCE

It's no surprise that financial security equals better health care. We all know that the more money you have, the more health care options you have. However, for those of us who are struggling to make ends meet, quality health care is often a luxury we can't afford. In fact, the U.S. Department of Health and Human Services' Office on Women's Health has found that low income is strongly associated with decreased use of health services and poor health outcomes. And as government research shows, minority women are more likely to have lower incomes and to live in poverty than white women. Even when sisters have levels of education similar to their Caucasian counterparts, they still earn less money and have fewer assets, according to the Office on Women's Health.

In many respects, it all comes down to employment—not just having a job, but having a job with good benefits. If your workplace offers comprehensive medical insurance, you can at least feel secure in knowing that you are covered. But if you are underinsured, work at a job with no medical benefits, or are unemployed and cannot afford private insurance, then you are at risk. Often, sisters in this situation do not get routine preventive care. If they do fall ill, they wait until the symptoms are severe before seeking medical attention. And then it's usually at the emergency room rather than with a private primary care physician.

What's worse, the health care facilities serving African Americans in many of our country's inner cities and rural outposts are understaffed, underfunded, and overwhelmed—when they are available at all. And many sisters who are eligible for Medicaid can look forward to long waits at crowded public clinics. Not the most reassuring setting, to be sure.

Poverty also forces far too many sisters to choose between paying for regular routine tests such as Pap smears, breast exams, and annual physicals, or paying the rent and putting food on the table. If black women are feeling well—and sometimes even if they are not—the necessities of life (like food and shelter) will take priority.

Even when sisters are well insured and can afford the best care, we are less likely to receive "quality" treatment than our white counterparts. According to studies conducted at Johns Hopkins University in Baltimore, race and gender significantly affect the quality of doctor/patient relationships. Their study found that (1) African-American patients rated their visits to doctors as significantly less participatory than whites, (2) black patients felt they had more participation in decision making when receiving care from African-American doctors and health professionals, and (3) patients of female physicians had more participation in their visits than those with male doctors.

REASON #3—LACK OF KNOWLEDGE

As a patient, it is your responsibility to understand fully any medical procedure or course of medical action suggested by your doctor. Seems like common sense, doesn't it? It's your body; you need to know what's going on with it. But too many of us don't. Worse still, we don't ask. When I see patients, I routinely ask about prior care. Of course, I can get this information from their medical records, and I do. But I find it helpful to talk to my patients about their health as well—to get their take on things, to hear about it from their perspective. Also, a one-on-one conversation will often tell me so much more than what's written down on a medical record. Talking to patients in depth helps me fill in the gaps. I want to know all about any operations they may have had, any medications they may have taken (or are still taking), anything at all—and I want to know why. Why were you on that medication? Why did you have that procedure? I'll tell you, I am often surprised, pained, and frustrated when sisters say they don't know. They never asked their doctor probing questions. Now, I know you may feel a bit uneasy about quizzing your doctor in order to clearly understand your illness and treatment. After all, this is a person who has gone through years of schooling and medical training. You don't want to appear ignorant or rude by asking a barrage of questions. *Who am I to give a doctor the third degree?* you might think to yourself. You're the patient, that's who, and you have every right to fully understand your condition and your doctor's prescribed treatment, even if it means having him or her explain it to you three times. Without having all the facts, how can you make an informed decision about your health?

REASON #4—FAMILY TRADITIONS

Because ours is a history steeped in self-healing, spiritual practices, and reliance upon the herbal cures of our African ancestors, when we are feeling sick, we often try the home remedies that have been passed down from our mothers, grandmothers, and great-grandmothers. Certainly, many of these therapies work wonders, but they should not be implemented to the exclusion of traditional medical care.

Sometimes what may seem like a simple cough, a slight fever, or a bit of fatigue may actually be a symptom of a more serious problem. Relying solely on home remedies that ease the symptoms may make you feel better in the short term, but if something else is going on with your health, you might not realize it until later—a delay that could do you great harm.

REASON #5—THE HEALTH CARE SYSTEM ITSELF

As much as personal barriers such as fear, lack of knowledge, family traditions, and poverty play a part in sisters not making good health a priority, some of the blame also rests with the health care system itself. The U.S. Department of Health and Human Services pinpoints several key issues within the health care system that limit access and adversely affect black women.

One is problematic medical practices. As government research makes clear, there are an inadequate number of primary care physicians serving African-American women. Doctors tend not to practice in the poor, rural, and low-income urban areas in which many sisters live. What's more, because sisters are apt to receive care in community health centers, clinics, and other high-volume facilities, they are not able to spend as much time with the physician and thus receive less preventive care counseling than is common in other medical practices.

Another failing of the health care system, according to government research, is the lack of cultural training physicians receive during their medical education. A doctor who possesses cultural understanding and sensitivity is more prepared to treat patients of diverse backgrounds, not just in terms of bedside manner, but also regarding communication, diagnosis, and treatment. As Dr. Gary C. Dennis, former president of the National Medical Association, an organization of African-American physicians, points out, doctors must know enough about the culture and lifestyle of their patients, as well as about the disease itself, in order to provide competent diagnoses and treatment. Simply put, having a wide breadth of knowledge about different cultures makes for a better physician.

The state of medical research also poses problems for black women. Few minority women take part in research studies, which translates to inadequate or inaccurate medical data on these populations.

Finally, a lack of female and minority physicians and health care professionals is yet another issue that negatively impacts sisters. This shortage leaves many health providers insensitive to the needs and preferences of minority women, according to the Office on Women's Health. Just as we like to see ourselves reflected in the movies and television shows we watch, so it is with our doctors. Sometimes it takes a sister to understand a sister. At the very least, black women deserve not to have their choices limited.

IT'S TIME FOR A CHANGE

Certainly, our legacy colors the way we view the health care system today. On the one hand, we don't always trust our doctors, but on the other, we don't feel we have the right to question their recommendations. Too many of us lack sufficient medical coverage, and we don't always have access to the best facilities. Worst of all, we allow our strength, tenacity, and endurance—all blessings of character that have seen our people through unbelievably difficult times—to compromise our health. How can that be? Think about it. Every time you shrug off a cold, or work right through a blinding headache, or keep on keeping on when your body feels as if it's running on empty, you put your health at risk.

It is time for sisters to become truly empowered. Letting go of the "superwoman" mentality is the first step. African-American women have historically carried a heavy load, often at the expense of our own well-being. No more, my sisters. Your strength, tenacity, and endurance—those magnificent attributes that keep you on course in the face of racism, sexism, and every other "ism"—will multiply tenfold if you simply start taking better care of yourself. You don't have to forge on if you're feeling ill; doing so will only adversely affect your long-term health. Take the time to tend to you. Still not convinced? Then consider the statistics we told you about earlier. Compared to white, Hispanic, Asian, and Native-American women, you, my sister, are at the highest risk for everything from high blood pressure to diabetes to heart attack—and even death. The time is now. Black women need to implement a new plan of action if we are to safeguard our health. Keep reading and you will learn everything you need to do just that.

RX: A PRESCRIPTION FOR YOUR SOUL

As women, we have long had to rely on our faith to see us through unimaginable hardships. From the shores of Africa to the Atlantic coast of the United States, from the slave plantations to the streets of Selma, from washboards to boardrooms, our belief in a higher power has sustained us.

Sisters' belief in faith is evidenced by our commitment to the church. Over the past fifty years, the number of African-American men in congregational life has decreased. In fact, churchgoing sisters generally tend to outnumber the brothers. Just look around your own congregation. What's the ratio of women to men in your church? It's not unusual to find a black woman in church on Sunday, at choir rehearsal on Tuesday, bible study on Wednesday, night service on Friday, and the missionary board meeting on Saturday— all while maintaining a home and a job. Each of us knows sisters like this; it might even be you. And even if we are not quite so diligent in our divine service, we still make it a priority to praise His name come Sunday. Indeed, 43 percent of all African Americans in this country attend church on Sunday, according to a 2001 study by the Barna Research Group, a marketing research company that provides information and analysis on cultural trends and the Christian Church. What's more, a whopping 93 percent of blacks pray every week, and 52 percent read the Bible weekly.

Today, as we make our way in the new millenium, our faith will continue to help us face any challenge and any trial head-on. It is what keeps us moving forward while always remembering our past. It is what gives us strength when we feel our most fragile and vulnerable. It is what lets us know that we are never alone. It empowers us. But sisters must realize that the grace that assists us in daily living is not one-dimensional. Our spirituality is not used solely as a means of successfully coping with external problems and pitfalls. It is also a method of *internal* healing, a salve that can soothe us physically. We simply have to begin viewing it that way on a daily basis. And it all starts from within, from our relationship with God.

How Can We Know God?

Easily, for He is everywhere at all times. He lives within each and every one of us. Knowing God does not mean you must follow the same path as everyone else. The souls of black women traverse every faith: Baptist, Muslim, Protestant, Catholic, Jehovah's Witness, and many more. Some sisters view God as Spirit, or Allah, or Creator, or their Maker. Some of us think of Him as a Higher Power or Higher Being. Some of us attend regular religious services, while others find divinity in less formalized settings. Some of us find the spirit of God in shared worship, and others are blessed through solitary ritual. And some sisters simply invoke spirit anytime, anyplace—whenever they feel the need for guidance, serenity, strength, comfort, validation, or love. That's the beautiful thing about spirituality. No one can dictate your relationship with it. Your spirituality is truly a unique experience.

For our people, however, spirituality does flow from a common ancestral source. When our forebears brought ancient religions from the Motherland, the sharing of that faith through our oral tradition during enslavement—mingled with American Christianity—helped form the concept that we now call the Black Church. Despite the different denominations, the collective Black Church continues to be the mainstay of the African-American community. It is from this collective experience that we find our faith, whatever our current individual incarnations of it happen to be. The belief systems of old have trickled down and shaped our lives, touched our souls, and given us a sense of spirituality that manifests in each of us today. As the Reverend Dr. Wyatt Tee Walker, senior pastor of New York City's Canaan Baptist Church, so eloquently affirms, the Black Church is the American fruit of an African root. History truly is a powerful thing. Those centuries-old ancestral influences have passed from one generation to the next to the next. How can we not be visited by spirit in some way, shape, or form? It is inherent in us as a people. How we choose to bring spirituality into our lives is up to us. It may lie dormant for years, but it is within us nonetheless.

Isn't that a comforting thought—to know that you can tap your inner divinity whenever you need to? Let us put it to good use, sisters. Maintaining our unique spiritual connection and making it a priority in our lives helps us stay grounded, focused, and strong for any battles that lie ahead. Our faith enables us to encourage one another to remain on course as we deal with the daily issues of Black life. But my sisters, let us rely upon our faith as more than a source of strength during difficulty. Let us call upon it to shore up our physical selves as well, to protect our health, to strengthen and sustain us inside and out.

The Unique Healing Power of Spirituality

Whenever you are out of touch with your spiritual side, it can adversely affect your equilibrium, leading to physical and biochemical changes that may result in poorer health. A little skeptical? Then think about this: Research shows that being stressed out can wreak havoc on your health, suppressing your immune system and leaving you susceptible to a whole host of ills, including heart disease, hypertension, stroke, and ulcers, to name a few. But faith, spirituality, and prayer can act as a buffer, boosting your immunity and enabling your body to better protect itself.

And Lord knows, black women are nothing if not vulnerable to stress. We have so much on our plates, it's a wonder we get half of it done. Many sisters feel overworked, overwhelmed, and overloaded. It's so easy to let the demands of life take control. We feel we have to do so much for everyone else, we never have time to do for ourselves. There's no room for inner work and meditative pause in this superwoman scenario. Why do you think you hear so many stories of people leaving the fast track for a simpler way of life? The pressure becomes too much to bear, and rather than continue to feel stressed, harried, and sick, these folks choose to walk a less congested path. But African-American women aren't apt to go that route; the truth is, many of us simply can't afford to. We have too many responsibilities and too little help.

Racism adds yet another layer of stress. The day-to-day slights we encounter simply because we are black can build up a seething anger. It makes us feel powerless, and therein lies the problem. Experts agree that people who feel that they have control over their lives experience less stress. However, if you feel you have little or no control, then your stress level rises. Suppressed anger contributes not only to stress but also to high blood pressure and heart disease. Consider all of this as a whole, and you can see why sisters are in desperate need of relief.

The good news is that you don't have to look far to find peace of mind—and better health. That's what's so wonderful about getting in touch with your spirituality. Inner work can be done anytime, anywhere. As I've said before, God is within you. You simply have to call Him forth to receive His healing grace. However, inner work should be done every day, not just when serious illness strikes or a personal crisis develops. This is where so many sisters stumble. We fail to realize the true power of our faith 24/7. We don't do spiritual work to bless our physical health as a daily ritual, as routine. If we did, we'd be so much more successful at keeping illness at bay.

Our ancestors knew the healing power of spirituality well. They understood that the mind, body, and spirit work in tandem as one, and that environment plays a crucial role in poor health. When illness occurred, our African kin believed some "force" was at work and they used ritual dance and conjuring of spirits to help get rid of it. Our ancestors considered the physical symptoms to be only one piece of the puzzle; to truly uncover the cause of poor health they looked at every aspect of a person's being and beliefs. Simply put, this history lesson implies that illness is never just about illness. How we live our lives plays a vital role. Unfortunately, as we have come to rely on the advances of modern medicine, we have lost touch with that age-old link between spirituality and health, even as religion and faith continue to be driving forces in our lives. Our foremothers used whatever they had to improve their health. Today, we have so much more available to us, yet we won't take advantage of the blessings we've been granted. To truly be at our best, we need both modern medicine and spirituality. They go hand in hand, involving caring, knowledgeable medical professionals who can administer the regular tests and screenings we need to stay healthy, and a strong sense of faith and spirituality to bolster our overall well-being.

It's a balance black folks want to achieve. A recent study by the Barna Research Group found that 94 percent of African Americans want "a sound spiritual life" and 93 percent want "good health." Obviously, we recognize the importance of each in our lives. However, as George Barna, founder of the Barna Research Group, notes, people seem to be less concerned with the means than with the ends. In other words, sisters *say* they want deep spirituality *and* good health, but are they really willing to do what it takes to get there?

The key is to attain both in balance. The first step to achieving this equilibrium is having the right outlook. Make good health a priority: Don't put off doctor's appointments, pay attention to your body's aches and pains, get regular checkups, take a personal health inventory, do inner work every day, reconnect with faith's unique healing properties, allow spirituality to bless you physically and emotionally. Read on for step-by-step guidelines on how to do all of this and more. In the end, you will be so much better off because you will have achieved true total health—body, mind, and spirit.

Understanding Your Body and Soul

· · · · · · · · · · · ·

*I couldn't care less whether people remember me as an
athlete. I just want them to remember me as a genuinely
good person.*

—Marion Jones, Olympic gold medalist

NEWS YOU CAN USE

· Your brain and your internal systems are inexorably linked. They
work in concert to keep the female body functioning smoothly.

· Just as your physical self relies on the circuitry between your brain
and your internal functions, your spiritual self relies on the circuitry
between you and God.

WHAT MAKES you marvel? For me, it's the wonder of nature and
the brilliance of technology. How the stars, moon, and sun hang in
the sky. How the petals of a flower unfold to reveal such delicate
and perfect beauty. How cruise ships keep from sinking to the
depths of the oceans. How the click of a computer mouse can in-
stantly connect me to the other side of the world. All of these
things, whether created by God or by man, hold me in awe.

But, to my mind, nothing will ever surpass the wonderment of
God's greatest creation: the human body. Especially the female
body. If ever there was a true marvel, this is it. With our temple we
give nourishment. We give sustenance. We give life. My sisters, if
we marvel at anything, let us marvel at God's majesty in us, because the female body—its form and its function—is truly a work

of art. The more you appreciate and understand it, the better you'll care for it.

Imagine a masterful orchestra. Every musician performs in perfect combination with the others, blending and melding to create a wonderful fusion of sound. A woman's body functions in much the same way. Its internal passages and movements work together to form a beautiful symphony in motion. Some may say that's overstating the case, but the reproductive system is a lot more amazing and hardworking than people might think.

A BRIEF OVERVIEW OF THE FEMALE REPRODUCTIVE SYSTEM

Exactly how does the female body work? What are the basic structures and functions? What are its rhythms? Let's take a closer look.

The Vulva

The *vulva* refers to the outer genitals. The first part of the vulva is the *mons pubis*. This is the fat pad, or the plump outer folds, that covers the pubic bone and leads to the outer lips, known as the *labia majora*. The mons pubis and the labia majora are both covered with pubic hair. Beneath the labia majora is the *labia minora*, the inner lips. These flaps of hairless skin directly cover the vagina.

The Vagina

The *vagina* is a long, tubular part of the female reproductive tract that has a great capacity to expand. The vaginal opening is separated from the internal reproductive organs by a thin circular membrane called the *hymen*. Once a woman has intercourse, the

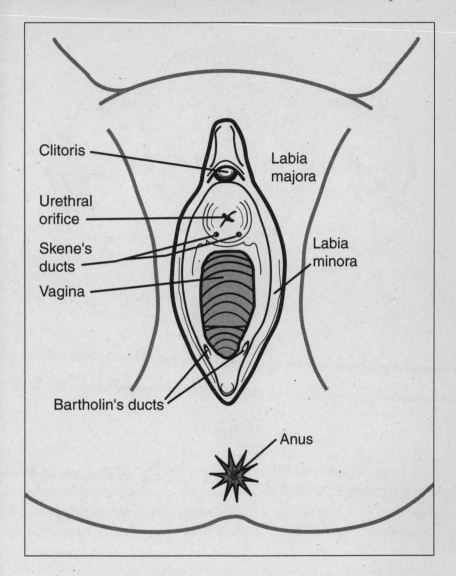

Clitoris

Labia majora

Urethral orifice

Skene's ducts

Vagina

Labia minora

Bartholin's ducts

Anus

hymen is broken. However, the hymen may also be torn by other sexual activities or by strenuous activities such as horseback riding.

The vaginal walls are muscular and are lined with glands that secrete lubricating fluids during sexual excitement and intercourse.

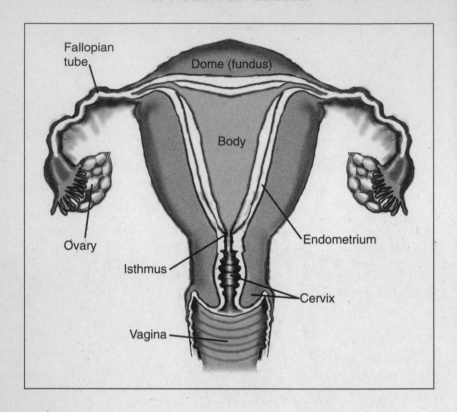

Fallopian tube

Dome (fundus)

Body

Ovary

Endometrium

Isthmus

Cervix

Vagina

The Uterus

Also referred to as the womb, the *uterus* is the centerpiece of the internal female reproductive system. It is located behind the bladder and is shaped like an upside-down pear. It has two parts: the body (the wider upper section that opens into the fallopian tubes), and the *cervix* (the narrower lower section, also known as the neck of the uterus, which opens into the vagina).

Normally, the uterus is only three to four inches in length and weighs about two to three ounces. But once a woman becomes pregnant, it expands in size to accommodate the growing baby.

The outer surface of the uterus, called the *serosa*, is shiny and smooth, similar to the inside of your mouth but thicker. The middle layer of the uterus, the *myometrium,* is all muscle. Finally, the innermost layer of the uterus is the *endometrium,* a lining of cells that sheds each month unless conception occurs. This shedding process is called *menstruation.*

The Fallopian Tubes

The two fallopian tubes, also called *oviducts,* are connected to either side of the uterus at its uppermost corners. Fertilization takes place in the fallopian tubes. Each tube extends from the uterus to the ovaries. After an egg is expelled from an ovary it is swept up by the fingerlike projections (the *fimbria*) at the end of the fallopian tube, drawn into the tube, and propelled toward the uterus. After intercourse, sperm swim up the fallopian tubes from the uterus. If the egg connects with a sperm in the fallopian tube and is fertilized, it will travel to the uterus, where it attaches to the womb's lining and develops into an embryo. If fertilization does not occur, the egg is expelled during menstruation.

The Ovaries

The two *ovaries* are situated on either side of the uterus. They are relatively small, each one about half the size of a small strawberry, yet they house numerous egg-producing follicles. During various stages of a woman's menstrual cycle, the ovaries may undergo a slight enlargement. In menopausal women, the ovaries shrink in size.

In addition to producing eggs, the ovaries also produce the female sex hormones estrogen and progesterone.

The Breasts

Because our society is so preoccupied with breast size, some women seek implants for purely cosmetic reasons. But our breasts' real purpose has nothing to do with physical appearance. Their function is to provide nourishment for our babies. Breasts are made up mostly of fatty tissue, with milk ducts and glands coursing through them. The milk ducts come together at the nipples. After birth, your hormones activate these milk glands, allowing you to nurse your child.

THE BRAIN/BODY CONNECTION

As amazing as your reproductive system is, it does not work solely by its own impulses. Much of the stimuli that get the ball rolling, so to speak, come from the brain, which houses the glands that produce, secrete, store, or respond to chemical messages called hormones. For many of us, making sense of how hormones work (a field of study called *endocrinology*) is confusing. While some of it is indeed intricate and complex, it really isn't that hard to understand the basics. Perhaps the best way to get a handle on how hormones, your brain, and your reproductive system all link together and work in concert is by taking a step-by-step look at your menstrual cycle. Before we begin, it's important that you keep three points in mind:

1. From the time menstruation begins (menarche) until the time it ends (menopause), your body prepares itself for pregnancy every month.

2. Always refer to the first day of your menstrual bleeding as "day one" of your cycle.

FEMALE REPRODUCTIVE ORGANS

STRUCTURE	FUNCTION
Vulva	protective covering for the vagina
Vagina	passageway for infants; portal for intercourse; menstruation outlet; secretes lubricating fluids to aid in intercourse
Uterus (cervix)	passageway for sperm from the vagina to the uterus; dilates during labor to allow a baby to be delivered; secretion of lubricating fluids
Uterus (body)	storage place for the developing fetus; builds the lining to prepare for implantation each month
Fallopian tubes (oviducts)	place where sperm fertilizes the egg; ends of a tube grasp an egg from near the ovary to make it available to the sperm
Ovaries	secrete and produce hormones; grow and release an egg for fertilization
Breasts	organs that produce and secrete milk to nurse infants

3. The number of days from the beginning of one period to the beginning of the next is generally twenty-eight. However, the number can vary from woman to woman, from as few as twenty days to as many as thirty-five.

Days 1 to 4

You may think that your "period" signals the end of your reproductive cycle, but the truth is that monthly bleeding is actually the beginning of the cycle. Here's how it works:

The lining of the uterus (the endometrium) thickens during the menstrual cycle in preparation for a fertilized egg. However, if no pregnancy occurs, your levels of the hormones estrogen and progesterone decrease, and the endometrium breaks its hold from the wall of the uterus and begins to shed, producing the menstrual flow.

While all of this is going on, your brain gets the message that hormone levels are low and that more follicle-stimulating hormone (FSH) is needed to promote the growth of egg follicles.

Days 5 to 13

Menstrual bleeding comes to an end by approximately day five as the endometrium completes its shedding and is at its thinnest. (Although five days is the average length of a woman's period, it can be a few days shorter or longer, depending on the woman.) Having received the signal to produce more FSH, the pituitary gland, located at the base of the brain, springs into action and releases the follicle-stimulating hormone. FSH levels increase, causing the development of many follicles in the ovaries. Each follicle not only contains an egg but also produces estrogen. As the follicles grow and mature, more and more estrogen is made and secreted.

The lining of the womb—the endometrium—begins to grow again as well, thickening in anticipation of a fertilized egg; this is called the proliferative phase of the cycle.

The increase in estrogen eventually signals the brain that the egg follicles are mature, estrogen levels are high again, and FSH is no longer needed. What is needed, though, is the hormone that will cause the egg to emerge from the ovary—*luteinizing hormone* (LH). The pituitary gland in the brain responds by sending a surge of LH, which causes an egg to be released from one of the ovaries and travel to the fallopian tubes. This process is called ovulation.

Days 14 to 28

After an egg is released, its follicle—now called the *corpus luteum*—produces the hormone progesterone, which helps the endometrium thicken even more. If the egg has not been fertilized by the time it reaches the uterus, LH levels drop and the endometrium breaks down and sheds, along with the unfertilized egg, through menstrual bleeding. And so begins day one of the next cycle.

RX: A PRESCRIPTION FOR YOUR SOUL

As you've just learned, the connection between your brain and your reproductive system is truly remarkable. The brain receives and sends out certain signals and messages to different parts of your body, and suddenly hormones are flowing and internal functions are activated. The circuitry that keeps our physical selves humming really is amazing.

The same holds true for the "circuitry" between you and God. The connection you have with Him needs to be just as strong. When your spiritual self isn't as it should be, the circuit linking you and God is disconnected. Messages do not flow and are not received. The result? A life out of balance.

Sisters not only need to do all that they can to keep their mind/body connection strong, they must maintain their spiritual circuitry as well. Begin to think of the mind/body link in a broader sense. It really is a threefold connection: mind, body, and spirit. We shouldn't focus only on one or two parts and neglect the other. All three work together. The goal here is enlightenment. You've gained a better understanding of how your body works. Isn't understanding your soul just as important? Fine-tuning and maintaining your spiritual circuitry will give you strength and a sense of empowerment. You will feel at ease knowing that the signals and messages that flow between you and God will always come through loud and clear.

Sisters need that sense of ease and assurance, given all the demands we juggle. Stress knocks on our door daily, and without divinity we'd be hard-pressed to face it down. I talked a bit about the pressure put upon black women in Chapter 1, but it's a message that bears repeating. Some people say that life is hard. Others say it's only as hard as you make it. As Jack Kornfield notes in *Buddha's Little Instruction Book*, most of the sorrows of the earth humans cause for themselves. When you combine that truth with the fact that we as human beings are not perfect, that trouble and turmoil can come our way, that bad things sometimes do happen to good people, that a kind heart may be met with a harsh word, then it becomes clear that daily living can, at times, take a toll on our souls.

For African-American women, the added burden of racism can chip away at the psyche even more. Thankfully, many of us have a respite, a place to turn to for solace, fortification, and renewal: our faith. It is what helps us proclaim, "I am strong!" even when we are at our weakest. It is what keeps us going. Knowing that a Higher Power dwells within your heart empowers you to dig deep and come up with a heaping scoop of fertile soil for your life.

The Blessings of Spirituality

When sister-diva Patti LaBelle advised, "Don't block the blessings," she was right on target. We must allow God's love to wash over us if we are to truly rejoice in our lives. We need to recognize that He touches us in many ways, not just when we're sitting in the pew on Sunday. You know the saying "God is in the details"? Well, it's true. Don't just give praise for the big events that fill your heart with joy; relish the small moments as well. Take time to outwardly cherish the people in your life. Are there folks you might be taking for granted? Tell them you love them. Do it every day. Look around and see all of the ways in which you are blessed. Give thanks and resolve to strengthen your connection with God. Deepen it. Enrich it. Fine-tune your spiritual circuitry.

Doing so allows you to walk by the word of God—that is, to walk by principles, not by popular behavior or pop culture. It's easy to get caught up in what we see on television, or hear on the radio, or witness in others. It's easy to be turned around by what other folks are doing, how they are behaving, and what they are thinking. If your conduct is based on what you see or how you feel in the heat of the moment, you may take a wrong path. But if you base your activities on the word of God, you will be victorious in all that you set out to do, be it making career choices, building a stable and happy home with your spouse, being a wonderful parent, being a good friend, or being physically healthy.

A strong spiritual base and constant spiritual circuitry to God also enable you to recognize and find security in the fact that God always has your best interests at heart. You are His child and He loves you beyond compare. So even when you are faced with difficult times, it is by His permissive will. He will give you only as much as you can bear. Rely on your faith, your trust in Him, and your knowledge of His innate love and goodness, and you will overcome hardship. Look upon life's trials as an opportunity to see God—not literally, but figuratively. By virtue of your navigating life's rough waters with faith, He reveals Himself to you and proves His power to see you through anything.

The most wondrous gift God has given us is life itself. To be able to rise each morning and draw breath each day is the greatest blessing of all. We owe it to God—and to ourselves—to take care of that divine gift. To honor and safeguard our health. And God has blessed others with the gift of knowledge to help us in our quest for good health—doctors, nurses, and various health care professionals. With their skills, your own spirituality, and a commitment to do right by your health, you can rise above the devastating statistics about African-American women and disease. Does that mean you'll never get sick or face a health crisis? Of course not. But you can make sure that you are well equipped to fight back should illness strike. That means having a bolstered immune system, getting regular medical tests so that you can catch any abnormalities early, and knowing what symptoms may be indicators of disease. Forewarned is forearmed, as they say. And as long as you are here on this earth, each day offers you a new beginning. It's not too late to do better, to make a new start, to change your approach to your health and well-being. Having a strong spiritual foundation and healthy circuit to God will help you take those necessary steps.

Maintain Spiritual Stability

In early 2000, an Alaska Airlines jet crashed, killing everyone on board. The National Transportation and Safety Board and the FAA determined the cause of the crash to be a faulty "stabilizer."

Everyone who knows me knows that, in general, I like to fly, but I still get a bit anxious about it. Before every trip, I always say, "Well, if the plane doesn't crash, I'll see you when I get back." It's sort of my little public mantra (in addition to a definite preflight private prayer). I say it with a smile and some humor, but deep down I'm thinking, *You never know.*

Recently, I flew from my home in Atlanta to San Diego to attend a medical conference, and for some reason, I didn't say my mantra before leaving. The plane was cruising along nicely at 33,000 feet and the cabin service was halfway done when the FASTEN SEAT BELT sign flashed on. Then I heard the pilot's voice. There was "rough air" ahead and, "just as a precaution," all passengers and flight attendants should return to their seats. He didn't expect the rough air to last long. Nonetheless, cabin service was suspended.

For most frequent fliers, such comments and actions are fairly common and unalarming. A little turbulence, a few bumps and rumbles, then it's over. No big deal, right? Not this time. This was the worst turbulence I've ever experienced in many years of travel. The plane was losing altitude. Every time the pilot gained a bit of incline, the air pockets would beat us back down, jolting and tilting the plane like a roller coaster. With each sudden descent and thrash, people would gasp and whisper or cry out pleas to God. In between, there was absolute silence; no one said a word.

The pilot informed us that he was getting clearance for a higher altitude in an effort to rise above the turbulence. But as we climbed to 39,000 feet it was no better. Minutes later we heard the pilot's voice again, this time telling us that we'd reached a maximum height and we'd have to descend in order to try to find a smoother altitude. After twenty-two minutes of sheer terror, we were eventually able to continue the flight relatively smoothly at an altitude of 24,000 feet. Thankfully, we landed safely in San Diego three hours later.

What would have happened, however, if the stabilizer for that plane had not been working properly, as was the case on the Alaska Airlines flight? We almost certainly would have crashed. But because the stabilizer was in sound condition, we were able to weather the turbulence and make it through just fine.

The purpose of this anecdote? To drive home the point that, just as on that plane, your internal stabilizer must be in order at all times because you never know when life will throw severe turbulence in your path. But if your stabilizing force, namely your faith and spirituality, is intact, you can weather the storm as well. Always remember, when your spiritual life is out of balance and the depths of your soul are lacking, it can leave you depressed, distressed, and oppressed—basically, in a mess.

Nurturing a Neglected Soul

Perhaps your circuitry to God has a disconnect, a spiritual "short." Perhaps your soul *isn't* as perfect as you'd like it to be. Maybe you have neglected it, or only looked within during times of crisis. Or it may be that you simply had no idea your soul needed any tending at all. Don't fret, sister. You can restore your soul, bring more spirituality into your life, and reestablish your connection to God. Each upcoming chapter will show you a variety of ways, both obvious and subtle, to do just that. The first thing you should do right now, however, is to rejoice in the fact that there is a Higher Power greater than yourself. This is your first step on the path to increased spirituality. Remove "self" from your thinking at this very moment. What realization are you left with? Remember when I talked about the things that make me marvel? High on my list is the wonder of nature. If we truly ponder our glorious environment we can't help but realize that we are but a small part of God's magnificent creation. How is the earth held in the sky? What keeps the planets aligned? How is it that our hearts continue to beat second after second? It is God. When you can see beyond yourself, you can see Him in everything.

The next step you can take to restore your soul and prepare it anew for more spirituality is to find time to appreciate God's creations. Run your fingers through the rich, fertile soil. Breathe deeply and take in the air that gives you life. Sit by the ocean or a lake or a pond and revel in the power and glory of the water. Appreciate the beauty and divine workings of nature. Becoming one with nature brings you so much closer to God.

The third step on your journey to heightened spirituality is reflection. Sit quietly, still your mind, and think of the many times God has given you assistance, shown you His love, cleared the right path. Remind yourself that He will always be there for you, no matter the situation. Keep in mind, too, that "normal" to God is a state of wellness, wholeness, and holiness—not just spiritually, but physically. If you want to lead a normal, balanced life, your spiritual *and* physical selves must always be attuned. Your journey to attaining both is just beginning. As you read on you will uncover more methods by which you can rejuvenate your body, your mind, and your spirit. The key to successfully utilizing these methods is to be in touch with God and with yourself. In the next chapter, you will delve more deeply into reflection, examination, and evaluation, learning avenues that lead to better knowledge of yourself and of God. You will come away truly knowing yourself physically and spiritually.

3

Take Time to Take Stock

· · · · · · · · · · ·

There are spiritual parts of ourselves that play a critical role in health and healing. Listen to your heart, for it's in your heart where that feeling tells you, "I'm not quite complete, not quite where I want to be." Once you hear that, honor it. Then you can begin to do something.

—Dr. Marcellus A. Walker, founder of the Center for Lifelong Health, and medical director of Wayne Woodland Manor

NEWS YOU CAN USE

· Taking a "health inventory" on a periodic basis helps you stay in tune with your body.

· Make regular checkups, tests, and screenings a consistent part of your life. These should include pelvic exams, Pap smears, breast exams, vaccination updates, and bone density tests, to name a few.

· For total and complete well-being, your physical self and your spiritual self need to be in balance.

· Stress, anxiety, depression, and anger can all stem from spiritual deficiency.

· When you are under constant stress it can wreak havoc with your health. Stress lowers immunity, making your body less able to fend off illness.

ARE YOU, like so many sisters, caught up in a routine that never seems to stop? Imagine this typical day: Early to rise, rouse the kids for school, give your husband a quick kiss good-bye as you both head off to work, commute for an hour (each way) in heavy traffic, chauffeur the kids (yours and others) to various activities after work, get dinner going, help with homework, ready the kids for bed, straighten up the house, spend time with your man (if you can). Now, if you're active in church or in your community, you'll need to squeeze a few choir practices, committee meetings, and bible study classes into the mix. Sound familiar? I bet it does. Many of us are leading lives filled to the brim with responsibilities and demands. With this type of schedule, it's amazing that women keep standing, let alone get it all done. And they call *us* the weaker sex. Ha!

We get it done, all right—because we have to. Sisters seem to live life by the motto *If I don't do it, who will?* But the sad truth is, that's a health- and spirit-sapping maxim to live your life by. We have no problem taking stock of what or who needs tending to, then stepping up to the plate. But amid all this rippin' and runnin', have you ever stopped to take stock of yourself? The needy people in your life, the poor state of your house, the projects piled up on your desk—all of those things are peripheral. They are not *you*. You don't define yourself by those things, do you? If you do, you shouldn't. Girlfriend, the true essence of you has to do with your health—spiritual, physical, and emotional—the vital aspects that make up the core of your being. That's what I'm talking about. So let me ask again. Have you stopped to take stock of you? Have you asked yourself *Have I tended to me?* As Janet Jackson might say, what have you done for you lately?

Too often we put others first and ourselves last. We don't feel entitled to self-care. We feel guilty about self-nourishment. But the truth is, all of the other stuff we spend so much time worrying about and taking care of is secondary. You—your essence—comes first. It has to. That's not being selfish; it's not indulgent. It's self-preserving. Whatever your schedule, lifestyle, religious commitments, or personal obligations to other folks, the reality is that you won't be able to do anyone any good if you're in poor or failing health.

So right now I want you to honestly ask yourself, *What have I done for me lately? Have I taken care of myself?* Ponder beyond the occasional hot bath or precious moments spent alone reading a juicy book or catching a nap. Those are worthwhile pursuits, to be sure. But I want you to really focus your mind on your health. As a physician, I see your health as my number one concern. So my question to you is, Are you taking time to care for your health? In fact, when was the last time you really thought about your health in a serious, deliberate, and comprehensive way?

If it's been a while (or never!) you may feel inclined to beat yourself up about it. *I know I should take better care of myself,* you might say. Or maybe you feel as though you should just give up on the notion of getting started. *Well, it's been so long, why start worrying about it now,* you may think to yourself. Sister, please run those negative thoughts right out of your mind. They serve no purpose other than to distract you from the real goal, one that is worth pursuing and definitely possible to achieve: the goal of good health. In *Buddha's Little Instruction Book,* Jack Kornfield wisely reminds us that "each morning we are born again and what we do today is what matters most." Truer words were never written. Kornfield goes on to tell us that "if compassion does not include one's self, it is incomplete." So rejoice! With each new sunrise you are blessed with another opportunity for self-care. Look at each morning anew. See the possibility of the day that lies ahead. And resolve to make your compassion whole by having some for yourself. The fact that you are reading this book shows excellent promise. It proves that you are now motivated and moving in the right direction.

GET IN TOUCH WITH *YOU*—A HEALTH INVENTORY

Rather than continually taking stock of what needs to be done at home or at work, start taking stock of your health. By that I mean take a "health inventory." Think of it this way: Before you go grocery shopping you spend a few minutes taking inventory, right? You check the fridge and the cupboards to see what needs replenishing. Then you make a handy checklist. A health inventory follows the same basic principle. Because you use your body every day, you also need to take time to make a checklist. Then go about the business of replenishing your physical stores by stocking up on healthy habits.

Taking a health inventory is easy. First, find time to be alone for at least an hour. No kids, no husband. Just you. Next, create a calm, relaxing mood. Light a few aromatherapy candles, put on your favorite soothing CD, and take a warm, spirit-easing bath. After drying off, begin your head-to-toe personal checklist while you are still nude. Have a mirror on hand for close examination (preferably a full-length mirror) and a pen to jot things down. As you answer the following simple questions, check the appropriate line. Be sure to answer honestly.

Skin

Your skin system includes your hair and nails, too. Look at all three carefully. Check for thinning hair and for any changes in your skin. Don't forget to also check your back, in any skin creases and folds, and the skin of your feet.

	Yes	No
Is your hair thinning?	____	____
Are there any new or changing moles?	____	____

	Yes	No
If so, do they bleed?	_____	_____
Do you sweat under your breasts?	_____	_____
Do you have any rashes, scaliness, unusual itching?	_____	_____
Does your abdomen hang low, near your pubic hair?	_____	_____
If so, do you sweat beneath your belly? Do you have sweat marks?	_____	_____
Do you have any scars that won't heal?	_____	_____
Any new skin discoloration?	_____	_____

Head and Neck

	Yes	No
Have you been to the eye doctor in the last year to have your eyes examined?	_____	_____
Do you need a new eye prescription?	_____	_____
If you wear contact lenses, check the expiration date on your contact lens solution bottle. Has it expired?	_____	_____
Do you visit the dentist every six months for cleanings and X rays?	_____	_____
Do you have trouble keeping your balance?	_____	_____
Do you get dizzy frequently?	_____	_____
Is your hearing seemingly normal?	_____	_____

Breasts

	Yes	No
All women should perform monthly breast self-examinations. Do you do monthly breast self-exams?	_____	_____
Have you had a professional breast exam and a mammogram in the last year?	_____	_____
Have you noticed any lumps or bumps in either breast?	_____	_____
Any indentations or puckering in the skin overlying your breasts?	_____	_____

Any discharge from either nipple? If so, state the color, and other characteristics: _____

Lungs

	Yes	No
Have you ever smoked?	_____	_____
Do you currently smoke?	_____	_____
Do you have asthma or other lung conditions?	_____	_____
If you take medication for a respiratory condition, check your prescription bottle. Is your medication current and stocked?	_____	_____
Have you had any unusual coughing?	_____	_____
Are you coughing up blood?	_____	_____
Do you have any shortness of breath?	_____	_____
Do you live in a city with frequent smog alerts?	_____	_____

Heart

	Yes	No

As we age, heart disease becomes more of a factor. Heart disease can kill—both men and women. Are you having any unusual chest discomforts?

If so, do you tend to think it's gas?

Have you ever had an EKG (electrocardiogram) or other cardiovascular tests?

Is there a history of heart disease in your family?

Do you have chest pain either on exertion or at rest?

Do you often feel rapid flutters in your chest?

Do you experience chest pain, shortness of breath, and pain down your left arm?

Blood

You should have your cholesterol, sodium, sugar, and other blood levels checked regularly. Do you bruise easily?

If you cut or scratch yourself, does the blood clot quickly?

Nutrition/Weight

	Yes	No
Are you overweight?	_____	_____
If yes, have you been overweight since childhood?	_____	_____
Are you underweight?	_____	_____
Do you exercise for thirty minutes or more at least three to four times a week?	_____	_____
Do you eat a balanced diet high in whole grains, vegetables, fruit, fish, skinless poultry, lean meat, and low-fat dairy products?	_____	_____
Do you often eat "junk food"?	_____	_____
Are several members of your family overweight?	_____	_____
When you eat, do you tend to have large portions or more than one helping?	_____	_____
Is your work physical or sedentary?	_____	_____
Are you a yo-yo dieter, constantly losing weight then gaining it back?	_____	_____

Stomach/Intestines

	Yes	No
Have you had any change in your daily bowel habits?	_____	_____
Is there any change in the color, texture, or shape of your stool?	_____	_____

	Yes	No
Is there any blood in or on the stool?	_____	_____
Do you notice fat globules floating in the water when you stool?	_____	_____
Is your stool much darker than usual?	_____	_____
If you are over age 50, or have a family history of bowel problems, have you ever had a colonoscopy?	_____	_____

Urinary System

	Yes	No
Have there been any changes in your urinary habits?	_____	_____
Are you having problems with incontinence (you leak urine)?	_____	_____
Do you suffer with *urgency* (the need to go right away; you can't wait)?	_____	_____
Do you see any blood in your urine?	_____	_____
What about bladder pressure—have you noticed any?	_____	_____
Do you drink eight glasses of water a day?	_____	_____
Have you ever had any type of kidney disease?	_____	_____

Pelvic/Reproductive System

	Yes	No
Did you have a pelvic exam this year?	_____	_____
If so, did it include a Pap smear?	_____	_____

	Yes	No
Did it include testing for sexually transmitted diseases?	_____	_____
Do you have any bumps or abscesses in your pubic hair?	_____	_____
Do you have any open blisters on your genitals?	_____	_____
Are your menstrual cycles regular?	_____	_____
If menopausal, any bleeding since?	_____	_____
If you are trying to get pregnant, are you having trouble conceiving?	_____	_____
Is your sex drive normal?	_____	_____
Can you have orgasms?	_____	_____
Do you commonly get vaginal infections like yeast or trichomoniasis?	_____	_____
Any history of sexually transmitted diseases?	_____	_____
Do you currently have fibroid tumors?	_____	_____
Have you ever had fibroid tumors?	_____	_____

Extremities (Arms and Legs)

	Yes	No
Carefully examine your arms and legs. Do you notice any skin changes?	_____	_____
Have you had any swollen joints?	_____	_____
What about decreased mobility of any joints?	_____	_____
Do you notice any creaking in your joints, such as your knees?	_____	_____

	Yes	No
Are your arms and legs usually warm to the touch?	_____	_____
Or, are they cold?	_____	_____
Do your thighs rub together when you walk?	_____	_____

Feet

We can't forget about the feet. They get us from one place to another. Inspect them all over, not just on the tops. Examine the soles of both feet. Do they look normal?	_____	_____
Check for corns, calluses, and bunions. Do you have any?	_____	_____
Look between your toes and under your toenails (especially the big toe). Do you see any signs of fungus or other infection?	_____	_____
Do you have ingrown nails?	_____	_____
Are your nail beds changing color?	_____	_____

Mind/Emotions

Would you describe yourself as generally happy?	_____	_____
Or generally sad?	_____	_____
Are you a "giver," someone who is always doing for others?	_____	_____
If yes, do you think you need to pull back from being so giving?	_____	_____

	Yes	No
Or, are you more "self" oriented, rarely sharing yourself with others?	___	___
If you are married, is your marriage happy and strong?	___	___
Are you both still deeply in love with each other?	___	___
Do you "put up a front" about your marriage, telling others it's fine when deep down inside you know it is not?	___	___
Do you surround yourself with good people?	___	___
Do you have people in your life who are "toxic" to your well-being?	___	___
Is it important to you to "keep up with the Joneses"?	___	___
If you have children, do you spend as much time with them as you would like?	___	___
Do you ever spend time alone relaxing or engaged in an activity you love?	___	___

ASSESSING YOUR ANSWERS

Now look back at your answers. They can reveal a lot about the state of your health. Of course, performing a health inventory should only be considered a first step. If any of your answers seem troubling and point to potential problems, you should follow up with your doctor. Let her or him know that your answers to certain questions raised a red flag and you want to discuss it. There might not be a problem at all. The point, though, is self-awareness. Just because you are experiencing a symptom or sign of disease or illness *does not* mean you have that disease or illness. The bottom line is that it's better to be in tune with your body, raise any concerns with your physician, and be certain about the state of your health than never to perform a personal health inventory at all. Remember, knowledge is power. That said, let's take a look at what certain answers to certain questions *may* indicate.

Skin

• Thinning hair may be a sign of poor diet and vitamin deficiencies, a scalp infection, or thyroid or nervous disorders.

• It's important to check moles regularly because bleeding or a change in their appearance (such as growing larger than the head of a pencil eraser, developing irregular borders, or changing color, to name a few) could indicate skin cancer.

• When you sweat underneath your breasts, you risk skin infections or the development of sores.

• Rashes, scaliness, or unusual itching may be a sign of infection or, in some cases, possibly cancer.

• A low-hanging belly indicates obesity and increases your risk of heart disease.

• As with breasts, sweating beneath a low-hanging stomach puts you at risk for skin infections.

• Scars that won't heal are one symptom of diabetes.

• New skin discoloration could be a sign of tumors or cancers.

Head and Neck

- Not having regular eye exams, which can detect glaucoma and other vision problems, puts your sight at risk. And on a more basic level, uncorrected (through glasses or contact lenses) poor vision seriously impairs driving and a myriad of other day-to-day activities.

- If you use contact lens solution that has expired, you risk infection.

- Regular dental visits help prevent cavities, periodontal disease, and a host of other tooth and gum problems.

- Balance problems may be a sign of ear infection, poor circulation, neurological disease, or heart disease.

- Frequent dizziness may point to the same potential maladies as balance problems, especially poor circulation.

Breasts

- Lumps, bumps, indentations, puckering, and nipple discharge are all signs of possible breast tumors or cancer.

Lungs

- Smoking has been linked to cancer, emphysema, heart disease, and bronchitis. The longer you continue to smoke, the more you increase your risk.

• Asthma and other lung conditions are potentially lethal if you don't care for them properly. That's why it's so important to make sure any medications you take are current and well stocked at all times.

• Unusual coughing may indicate lung disease, tumors, or asthma. And coughing up blood could mean the possibility of cancer.

• Shortness of breath may be symptomatic of asthma or other lung disease, or it could be a forewarning of a heart attack.

Heart

• Unusual chest discomfort could be a sign of heart attack. Don't always assume it's gas.

• Having chest pain when you exert yourself or when you are at rest, having a family history of heart disease, and never having taken an EKG or other cardiovascular tests are all factors that put you at risk for heart disease, heart attack, stroke, and high blood pressure.

• Rapid flutters in your chest could be a red flag for abnormal heart valve structure.

• Chest pain, shortness of breath, coughing, nausea, sweating, and left arm pain are signs of a heart attack.

Blood

- If you bruise easily or your blood doesn't clot quickly when you cut or scratch yourself, you could have low platelets—a condition called *thrombocytopenia*. Because platelets play a major role in blood clotting, having a deficiency of them can cause bleeding disorders.

Nutrition/Weight

- Being overweight, not eating a well-balanced diet, and leading a sedentary lifestyle put you at risk for developing high blood pressure, diabetes, heart disease, and certain forms of cancer. What's more, the heavier you are, the more pressure you place on your heart and lungs. Digestive diseases, reproductive problems, and obstetrical complications can also be related to obesity.

Stomach/Intestines

- A change in daily bowel habits, changes in the appearance of stool, and blood in the stool are all signs of colon cancer.

- If you notice fat globules floating in the water after you defecate, it could point to gallbladder disease or a very serious intestinal disorder called Crohn's disease.

- Stool that looks much darker than usual might indicate intestinal bleeding.

Urinary System

- Incontinence, bladder pressure, and a sense of urgency to urinate could all indicate that there is a mass, such as fibroids, in your pelvis.

- Blood in the urine may be a sign of infection, kidney disease, or cancer.

Pelvic/Reproductive System

- By not having an annual pelvic exam that includes a Pap smear and tests for sexually transmitted disease (STDs), you are leaving yourself at risk for developing undetected, potentially fertility-threatening, and even life-threatening problems, including STDs, infections, and cancer.

- Bumps or abscesses in your pubic hair indicate that you may have an infection.

- Open blisters on your genitals can be a sign of herpes or other very serious infection.

- Irregular menstrual cycles could be symptomatic of hormone problems, undiagnosed pregnancy, tumors, or cysts.

- If you are menopausal but still experience any vaginal bleeding, it could simply be vaginitis caused by estrogen deficiency. But such abnormal bleeding at this stage of life more strongly suggests endometrial cancer.

- Difficulty getting pregnant could be caused by any number of factors, such as hormone problems, an obstructed cervix or uterus, the existence of fibroid tumors, the possibility of blocked fallopian tubes or adhesions on the tubes, or less viable eggs (depending on your age); or your partner may have a low sperm count.

- A good sex drive is part of overall good health. If your libido is below par, you may have a hormone deficiency, you might just be under a lot of stress, or you may be grappling with psychological issues that are affecting you physically.

- The inability to reach orgasm, similarly, may be linked to emotional issues that are manifesting themselves in the bedroom. The neurological effects of diabetes could also be the culprit. Or you may simply need to have a little talk with your man, girlfriend. (Often a bit of honest, sexy "guidance" will do the trick.)

- Suffering from vaginal infections such as yeast or trichomoniasis on a regular basis is a signal that either your partner is infected, your diet and/or hygiene habits aren't as good as they should be, or it's even possible that you have developed diabetes (which is sometimes linked to recurrent vaginal infections).

- If you have a history of sexually transmitted diseases, you need to have follow-up exams regularly to make sure no other related problems have developed.

Extremities (Arms and Legs)

- Unusual changes in your skin's appearance may indicate poor circulation, varicose veins, or diabetes.

- Swollen joints are a sign of arthritis or infection.

- If you have experienced a decrease in mobility in any of your joints it could mean arthritis or lupus.

- Creaking joints, such as those in your knees, might point to arthritis or degenerative joint disease.

- If your arms and legs are cold to the touch it could be symptomatic of poor circulation caused by diabetes or vascular disease.

- If your thighs rub together when you walk it means you are carrying too much weight, a serious condition since obesity is linked to osteoarthritis, hypertension, stroke, diabetes, heart disease, certain cancers, and other health problems.

Feet

- You need to check whether the soles of your feet look normal, because one trait of syphilis is the appearance of spots on the soles of the feet.

- Painful corns, calluses, and bunions are the price you pay for wearing ill-fitting shoes.

- Fungus between the toes or under toenails means the area is infected.

- Ingrown toenails, which are quite painful, can lead to infection of, and damage to, the nail and nail bed.

- If your nail beds are changing color, it might be a sign of infection or of diabetes.

Mind/Emotions

• Whether you are generally happy or sad, upbeat or pessimistic, overly self-sacrificing or somewhat selfish, it all plays a role in your health. That's because total well-being encompasses body, mind, and spirit. And when one is out of balance, it can throw everything else off-kilter as well.

• The same holds true when it comes to the folks in your life. An unhappy, strained marriage, coupled with too few good friends and loving relatives means that your support network is sorely lacking. Not having that solid base of support in your corner leaves you susceptible to stress, illness, and general poor health.

So how did you fare? As you can see, making time to perform a personal health inventory is a crucial step on your journey to wellness.

CHECKUPS AND TESTS

The next step on this all-important journey is resolving to have the regular checkups, tests, and screenings every sister needs. Make a pact with yourself to do it—starting now. Think of it as your personal blessed health vow. I know what you're thinking: *That's all well and good, doc. But I have no idea what sorts of exams and procedures I need, much less when I need them. I want to make a blessed health vow, but I don't know where to begin or what to expect.*

No problem, my sister. That's what I'm here for, to break it down for you. What follows is a brief description of the basic tests and procedures you should undergo, and a table listing the age at which you should have them. As we grow older, we definitely need to be on the lookout for certain problems.

Pelvic Exams

Any woman who is age 18 or older, and younger women who are (or have ever been) sexually active, should have a pelvic exam every year. Gynecological exams are extremely important because they enable your doctor to detect sexually transmitted diseases, cervical cancer, and other problems early. Chances are your visit to the gynecologist will turn out just fine. Nothing will be wrong with you. But early detection is the key to successful treatment, so it's always better to have your annual pelvic exams and be on the safe side.

During a pelvic exam you will lie on your back with your legs apart and your feet up in stirrups—little foot holders located at the end of the examining table. First, your doctor will likely place her stethoscope against your abdominal area to listen to your bowel sounds. Surprisingly, the different rumblings can reveal a lot about your intestinal function. Just by listening, your doctor can tell if your bowels are sluggish or normal, and if there might be a serious blockage or obstruction in the bowel.

Next, your doctor will palpate (examine by touching) your abdomen, usually with the balls of her fingers, in a slightly circular motion. Feeling the abdomen in this way allows your doctor to check for any abnormal masses, tumors, growths, and protrusions, such as fibroids, cysts, or other conditions. She can also check the bottom edge of the liver for normal size and for tenderness, which could indicate growths. You might notice your doctor also pressing into your abdomen, then quickly letting go. This is called a "rebound" test. She is looking to see if that mild press and release action causes a sharp reaction or pain. Patients with an internal infection in their fallopian tubes—or with a ruptured appendix, or ruptured tubal pregnancy—usually have "rebound tenderness," which means the pus or blood is irritating the inner lining of the abdominal wall.

Next up is the part of the pelvic exam that causes many women a bit of unease. But there really is no need to be uncomfortable. You should rest easy in the knowledge that you are taking A+ care of yourself by getting an exam that you need. The key thing to remember at this point is to try to relax. In order for your doctor to make an accurate assessment of your pelvis, she needs for you to be as calm and at ease as possible. Try not to tense up. Just let your legs and your pelvis relax. Now the pelvic exam truly starts.

A good doctor will talk to you continuously as she begins the exam, telling you what she's getting ready to do each step of the way. Wearing rubber gloves, your doctor will begin to feel and visually inspect the pubic hair and mons pubis (the outer surface of the vulva), checking the shape and thickness of the hair, and looking for any infection, boils, or discoloration surrounding the mons pubis. She will also inspect the vaginal lips (labia). During this part of the exam, your doctor will be able to detect such conditions as Bartholin's cysts, abscesses, or other labial abnormalities.

Next, as your doctor prepares to insert a speculum, she will gently spread your vaginal lips with her fingers. You will feel her fingertip at the very base of your vagina, and she may tell you to relax "this muscle," the perineal muscle. You'll probably be tensing it without even realizing. Don't worry; every woman does that. But the more you can relax your vaginal muscles, the easier the whole process will be for you. As you release the tension in your perineal muscle, your doctor will gently insert the speculum into your vagina, open the instrument's two sides, then "lock" it so that it stays open, thus freeing her hands. (A quick word on speculums:

These instruments are either plastic or metal and come in different sizes. Generally, a medium one is used. This size works very well for most women. Women who have had many children, have excess vaginal tissue, or who are overweight may need a large speculum. There are even special speculums used for women who are still virgins or who have structural abnormalities that won't permit entry of a regular speculum.)

Once the speculum is in place, your doctor will check your vaginal walls for lesions, infection, and other abnormalities, and your cervix for infection and a condition called "cervical motion tenderness," commonly seen in the presence of internal pelvic infection, gonorrhea, internal bleeding, and other problems.

With the speculum still inserted, your doctor will move on to the Pap smear. She will swab the cervix with a wooden Pap stick, a plastic brush, or a combination of the two. A Pap checks for two types of cells: the cells inside the cervical canal and the cells on the actual surface of the cervix. Though both types of cells can be used to determine the existence of cancer or precancer, the cells inside the canal usually give the earliest and best signs. So make sure your doctor is testing both the surface of the cervix and inside the cervical canal.

Once the Pap smear is done, a cotton swab (similar to a Q-Tip) may be used to swab for sexually transmitted diseases (STDs), such as gonorrhea and chlamydia. Herpes, if present and active, may also be detected. Syphilis is detected by blood, not through vaginal testing.

With the inspections, Pap smear, and STD cultures complete, the speculum is removed and the manual part of the exam begins. Your doctor will insert two gloved fingers inside your vagina, gently pushing upward on your cervix (which moves the uterus) while pressing down on your lower abdomen with her other hand. This manual examination allows your doctor to actually feel the uterus and ovaries, checking for any abnormalities, enlargements, or unusual masses in the area of your ovaries and fallopian tubes. She'll check for any pain, as well. You will feel mild pressure during this part of the exam, but if you keep your abdominal and vaginal muscles relaxed, it really shouldn't hurt. If you do feel actual pain, tell your doctor.

Last, your doctor will insert her middle finger into the rectum while her index finger remains in the vagina. This is called a recto-vaginal (R-V) exam, which enables your doctor to check (1) the strength of the back wall of your vagina from the side closest to the rectum; (2) for masses deep in the pelvis; (3) the texture of your stool, if any is present; and (4) for blood in the stool.

Pap Smears

You've just read how a Pap smear is performed, but do you know why it is so important? It screens for cervical cancer, a disease that hits black women hard. Sisters are three times as likely as white women to get the disease, and twice as likely to die from it, according to the American Cancer Society. The good news is that cervical cancer is curable if caught early enough. That's why it's crucial that we be tested regularly.

Cervical cancer stems from abnormal changes in cervical cells. However, it takes time for cells to progress from normal to abnormal to cancerous—years, in fact. This gradual process, the precancerous stage, is called *dysplasia*. The hope is that by performing Pap smears regularly, doctors can detect changes in the cells early, resulting in less invasive treatment.

The standard recommendation is for women to have annual Pap smears. At times, depending on your condition, it may be recommended that you have them more frequently.

In recent years, various health organizations have come out

with other guidelines, some suggesting once every three years as sufficient, especially for women who have had hysterectomies. On one level, that suggestion does make sense for some women. The problem, however, is that most women equate getting a Pap smear done with getting their annual pelvic examination. I fear that if most women resort to the once-every-three-years schedule, they will neglect the rest of the pelvic exam, which should be done every year. And it could turn out to be a deadly decision, because a cancer may be brewing in or on the vagina, the vulva, the ovaries, or the fallopian tubes.

Also, if a woman has had surgery for cervical cancer, she still needs to have the cells of the vaginal vault examined regularly to help detect any recurrence of the disease.

For these reasons, I encourage women to have a pelvic examination and a Pap smear every year, like clockwork. It's sad to say, but sometimes the unimaginable happens. And this one little test (the Pap smear) may pick up on a minor cell change that would otherwise go undetected, ultimately saving your life.

Breast Exams

Forty years ago, a woman's risk of developing breast cancer was 1 in 13, according to the National Cancer Institute (NCI). Today, it's one in eight. For African-American women, the numbers tell an especially chilling story. Sisters are ten times more likely to die from breast cancer than white women. Studies by the National Cancer Institute show that black women have the highest mortality rates for the disease. Late detection is the primary reason. Typically, by the time we are diagnosed with breast cancer, it has already spread.

It doesn't have to be that way, not if sisters take three very important steps:

1. Perform a breast self-examination once a month

2. Have an annual breast exam by your doctor or other health professional

3. Have regular mammograms

These three steps, as well as overall breast care, are so important that I have devoted an entire chapter to the subject. Turn to Chapter 9, "Caring for Your Breasts," for complete and comprehensive information on how to keep your breasts healthy.

Prenatal Care

Early and consistent prenatal care is the key to having healthy babies. Patients who receive prenatal care, for the most part, have a decreased risk of miscarriage, prematurity, underweight babies, and severe medical complications.

Before pregnancy, both partners need to "think healthy." That means to eat healthy foods, drink plenty of water, avoid alcoholic beverages, quit smoking (if applicable), and avoid stress. Be sure to review all your social habits and current medications with your doctor.

See Chapter 10, "The ABC's of Pregnancy," for more information.

Vaccination Updates

If you think vaccinations are just a part of childhood, think again. For an adult, it is equally important to review your vaccination status with your doctor and make sure everything is up to date. For instance, did you know that you should get a booster for tetanus every ten years? Your physician can tell you what other vaccines you may need, depending on your medical history.

If you are thinking of having a baby, make sure you have been vaccinated for rubella and mumps before conceiving. It's best to take care of this well before attempting pregnancy, not just before conceiving, and certainly not during your pregnancy.

Bone Density Test

As a woman ages, the thickness of her bones decreases, and they become more brittle. This is due, in large part, to the drop of estrogen levels as she ages and becomes menopausal. In order to best evaluate bone thickness, a bone density test is now available. This test checks for bone conditions such as osteoporosis, a condition that can be very debilitating and accounts for a large number of hip fractures in menopausal women.

Occult Stool Test

The older you get, the more important it is to be screened for blood in the stool, as it is a sign of colon cancer. Make sure your physician performs a rectal exam during your annual physical, especially if you are over age 35.

Electrocardiogram (EKG)

This noninvasive, painless test produces a tracing, or "image," of your heart's beating pattern through the use of small electrodes attached to your skin at various points (chest, arms, legs). The tracing lets your doctor know if your heart is under strain, if you have an irregular heartbeat, if you have heart disease, and, in some cases, if you've ever had a heart attack.

Blood Tests

By simply drawing a blood sample and sending it to the lab, your doctor is able to check for cholesterol, anemia, leukemia, thyroid problems, and much more.

Urinalysis

Tests for the presence of sugar, blood, protein, and acids in the urine provide information that helps detect diabetes, kidney disease, and bladder infections. Urine tests can also determine pregnancy.

AGE-BY-AGE TEST GUIDE

The following table maps out the various tests every sister should have at different stages of her life. Keep in mind, however,

Age 18 to 35	Age 36 to Menopause	Menopause and Beyond
• Annual physical exam (which should include breast exam, PAP smear, STD cultures, pulse check, blood pressure reading, respiration check, urinalysis) • Cholesterol check • Vaccination status review	• Same as age 18 to 35, *plus:* • Bone density tests • EKG • Mammogram • Diabetes screening • Full biochemical testing	• Same as age 36 to menopause, *plus:* • Occult stool test • Yearly bone density test • Blood tests to check not only for cholesterol and diabetes, but also for anemia and thyroid disease • Flu vaccine

that these are general recommendations. Your complete medical history should be taken into account when scheduling medical tests. Therefore, make sure to consult your doctor for more specific recommendations tailored just for you.

RX: A PRESCRIPTION FOR YOUR SOUL

Taking a health inventory puts you on the path to wellness. But that's just part of the journey, as I'm sure you know. Spiritual inventory is equally important. Asking yourself the right questions, seeking internal truth, getting to know yourself on a deeper level— these are necessary pursuits if you are to achieve total well-being. One cannot exist without the other. You may feel good. Your blood pressure may be normal. Your cholesterol may be under control. You may be on track with your checkups and screenings. But if your spiritual life is not in order, then you are lacking a key ingredient. Good health for good health's sake is a fine start. I *want* you to focus on being in the best health possible. But I also want you to realize that to truly enjoy good physical health, to take full advantage of your strong heart, powerful lungs, boundless energy, and overflowing stamina, your inner self must be just as strong, powerful, boundless, and overflowing. Without that equilibrium two things may happen:

1. You take your health for granted and don't allow yourself to revel in your physical blessings. Why? Because you are too caught up in the downward spiral that results from spiritual need. By this I mean that instead of cherishing and enjoying the good health you've worked so hard for, you keep your attention focused on what you don't have. Maybe you're facing difficulty on the job, or you've been fighting with your man, or a good friend has hurt you, or you're simply

feeling overwhelmed by life in general. Whatever it is, it's pulling you in a negative direction and you don't have the means to fight back. You don't have the tools to see beyond the surface skirmish, get to the underlying problem, fix it, and rejoice in the positive outcome. Do you know why you aren't able to do this? That's right: because your spiritual house is not in order. Which leads me to,

2. The imbalance begins to take a toll on that which you thought you had under control—your health. Stress, anxiety, worry, frustration, sadness, depression, and anger all flow from the same stream—spiritual deficiency. Research shows that illness isn't far behind when you are constantly barraged by these negative states of mind. Your immune system starts to falter, and the next thing you know, your good health has turned poor. Without a strong connection to your Higher Power, your loved ones, and yourself, you invite emotional maladies. You thrust open the door to psychological hurts. You clear a path for soul sappers.

Take heart, my sister. You *can* prevent this from happening. The secret lies in taking spiritual inventory. Doing so follows the same basic principles as taking a health inventory. You ask yourself specific questions, ponder specific relationships, and closely examine your spiritual life. As with the health inventory, I recommend that you find a quiet, peaceful spot to conduct your spiritual inventory: someplace away from distractions, away from other people. If need be, ask your husband to take the kids to the movies one Sunday afternoon. This is part of your inner work. You *must* find time for it. Block out an hour or two, or do a little bit at a time over consecutive days—whatever works best for you.

Be sure to make your quiet place conducive to serious inner

work. I love the idea of lighting aromatherapy candles. The fragrance and the flame have a calming, soul-opening effect. And that's exactly what you want.

Have pen and paper on hand, as well. You may even want to use this inventory process to begin a spirituality journal. Journaling is a wonderful way to get in touch with yourself. It allows you to expose your innermost feelings in a safe and loving way. Only you will read your spirituality journal, so dig deep, bare your soul, be brutally honest. This is difficult work—good inner work always is. But the result is so worth it. Use this inventory exercise to start your spirituality journal, then continue writing in it every day. Let the writing process purge you of your pain, anxiety, sadness, or stress, and replace those spirit- and soul-depleting feelings with blessings. Write out your blessings daily, and soon you will feel them overtake the painful emotions, not just on the journal page but in your heart as well. Try journaling. Your spirit will thank you.

Cleansing the Soul—A Spiritual Inventory

Begin by examining a few key relationships. Really think about each of the following questions before writing down your answers. Be totally honest.

Your relationship with God

1. Is God a part of your life? In what way?

2. Do you pray? How often? For what reasons?

3. How active are you in church?

4. Do you dialogue with God every day?

5. Has God ever spoken to you? What did He say?

6. How would you define God?

7. Do you believe God lives within you? If yes, how so? If no, why not?

8. Do you believe God loves you? Why or why not?

9. When was the last time you spoke to God? What did you say?

10. In what ways are you blessed? Be as specific as possible.

*Your relationship with
your spouse or lover*

(If you are unmarried or unattached, skip to the next section.)

1. Do you love him? Do you tell him you love him? How do you show him your love?

2. Does he love you? Does he tell you he loves you? How does he show you his love?

3. How has he blessed your life? If you could start your life over, would you marry him (or become involved in a relationship with him) again? Why or why not?

4. When was your last argument? What was it about? How was it resolved? What do you regret about it?

5. How is your sex life? How would you describe it? Who usually initiates lovemaking? When did the two of you last make love?

6. How often do the two of you spend "quality" time together (just the two of you)? What sorts of things do you tend to do together? What would you like to do with him if you had more time together?

7. How well do the two of you communicate? Does he know your lifelong dreams and desires? Do you know his? When did the two of you last have a long, in-depth conversation that did not have to do with the kids, work, bills, household chores, or extended family? What did you talk about?

8. Is he your friend? If yes, describe how. If no, why not?

9. Have the two of you been faithful to each other? If yes, why do you think your fidelity has remained intact? If no, why did one of you stray? If you don't know for sure whether he has been faithful, what is causing your uncertainty?

10. What are the weaknesses in your relationship? What are the strengths? How do you feel when you think about him? Do you trust him? Why or why not?

Your relationships with your children

(If you don't have kids, skip to the next section.)

1. How have your children blessed your life?

2. What makes you a good mother? Describe your relationship with your kids. In what ways could you be a better mother?

3. What do you hope for your children's future?

4. Are you lenient or strict? Describe your disciplinary style. How do your kids view your style?

5. Have you ever felt extremely angry or impatient with any of your children? If yes, why? How did you resolve the situation? How often do you feel this way?

6. What do you regret when it comes to your children and your role as their mother?

7. How do you have fun with your kids? How often do you have dinner together as a family? Do you think you spend enough time with them? How do you feel when you are with your children?

8. How well do you communicate with your children? Do you have conversations with them that don't revolve around school, chores, or bad behavior? What do you talk about?

9. Do you tell your children you love them? How often? Do they tell you they love you? Do you praise and compliment your children regularly? Do you attend their school plays, concerts, basketball games, and similar functions regularly?

10. How are your children similar to you? How are they different from you?

Your relationships with friends

1. Do you have close friends? Why or why not? If you do, what about these particular people makes them so special? Have you met any of your friends through your house of worship?

2. How often do you see your friends? What do you do together? What do you talk about?

3. Has a friend ever helped you when you were at a low point or having a hard time in your life? How did she or he help? How did it make you feel? Have you ever done the same for a friend? What did you do and how did it make you feel?

4. Specifically, what do good friends bring to your life?

5. Have you ever had a falling-out with a friend? What happened? How did it make you feel?

6. Do you have any fair-weather friends who only want to be with you when you are upbeat, but not when you're having problems? If yes, how do you feel about that?

7. Have you ever felt used by a friend? If yes, what happened? What did you do about it?

8. Define "friend."

9. What type of friend are you?

10. Who is your "best" friend, the one person you feel closest to (other than your husband or lover)? Why is this person your best friend?

Your relationship with yourself

1. Describe yourself.

2. Do you ever spend time alone by choice? If yes, why do you think it's important? What do you do while you are alone? If you don't spend time by yourself, why not?

3. How do you think other people see you? How do you think others feel about you?

4. Do you think you have high or low self-esteem? Why?

5. What is your best trait? Your worst?

6. How often do you feel stressed out? What do you do to relieve stress?

7. When was the last time you felt sad? Depressed? Angry? Frustrated? Worried? Why did you feel this way? What do you do when you experience these types of negative emotions? How do you handle them?

8. Do you meditate? Why or why not?

9. If you had two hours of total and absolute free time, what would you do and why?

10. What are your strengths? Your weaknesses? What would you change about yourself if you could? What would you never change about yourself? Do you love you?

Use Your Answers to Change Your Life

Now look back over your answers. There is no right or wrong, only your own personal spiritual truth. The point of this exercise is not to tally up a score and figure out what it means, but to help you get in touch with yourself. When you take time to let your feelings flow through the tip of a pen, you're putting much more than words on the page. You're putting down the core of your soul, your innermost essence. That's *you* on the page, my sister, in brilliant black and white, for your eyes only. Truly see what you have written. Truly see who you are. It's right there in front of you. Read your answers with an open heart and mind. Read deeply. Let the message and the meaning of what you have written seep inside. The patterns will become clear. The information you need to bring more spirituality into your life will reveal itself—if you are open to receiving it.

Read your answers. Truly see the message and the meaning. I know it may be painful. Often when we reveal our feelings, the truth hurts. When you don't have that strong spiritual base, it hurts even more. But therein lies the revelation. The pain we all feel inside at times can be lessened if we walk with God. When our divinity is powerful, so too are we.

So ponder your answers. Which of your relationships are lacking? Where do you need to effect change? Are you not as close to God as you believed? Do your answers tell you so? Have you lost a loving connection with your husband? Do your answers reveal it? What else do your answers show? Are you spending too little time with your children? Do your friends have your back? Are you in tune with yourself? Wherever your answers lead you, have courage to make that change. Doing so will bring more balance, peace, and joy into your life.

Only you can correct the spiritual deficiencies your answers reveal. And be assured, they *are* spiritual deficiencies, whether you recognize them as such or not. That's because spirituality rests not only in your relationship with God, but in your life as a whole. And that includes all of your relationships. It may start with Him, but that's not where it ends. Your divinity influences every facet of your life, from your marriage to your role as mother to your friendships, and of course, to your relationship with yourself.

Let your answers guide you in your quest for heightened spirituality and total wellness. I can't do it for you. But what I can offer are twenty guiding principles that will help you on your wellness journey. These life-affirming truths will restore your equilibrium, thus strengthening your spirit and safeguarding your health. Do what you must in order to salve the areas of your life that are hurting. Trust me, if you follow the path your spiritual inventory answers have set forth, you will find your way to those tender, needy areas. Don't be afraid of what you've written. You have stripped yourself bare on paper and that's a good thing. Use it to change your life for the better. Then rely on these guiding principles to maintain the improvement.

Twenty Guiding Principles of Life

1. Learn to forgive yourself and others. Letting go of blame frees you to discover the true blessings of your life.

2. Make reparations, if necessary. Creating a fresh start with the people who matter most enables you to heal wounds.

3. Let go of toxic people. Sometimes you will have to walk away from folks who jeopardize your well-being. These people have to make changes within themselves, just as you do. If they insist upon bringing negativity into your life, you need to have the strength and sense of self-love to move on. In the end, one true friend is greater than hundreds of false friends.

4. Recognize God's drumbeat for *your* life. Listen to what He is saying to you; don't worry about what He is saying to others. Remember this truth from Kent Nerburn's book *Native American Wisdom:* "When you lose the rhythm of the drumbeat of God, you are lost from the peace and rhythm of life."

5. With inner peace comes inner strength, so always make time to do spiritual work and to nurture your relationship with God. Begin each day by praising His name.

6. Love yourself. Create change within your heart and soul in order to be the best person you can be.

7. The Bible says: *Whatever state I am, therewith to be content.* You are blessed. Recognize and acknowledge that fact and be happy with what you have.

8. Be at one with nature. Appreciate the beauty and grandeur of flowering buds, rich soil, flowing water.

9. Relish your solitude and quiet time. Don't feel guilty about it—revel in it. Your mind, body, and spirit crave it.

10. Be of a giving nature—but don't be self-sacrificing. Helping others nurtures the soul; giving of yourself until you are spent does not.

11. Keep it simple: do unto others as you'd have them do unto you.

12. Don't strive for perfection; it's not possible. Instead, strive for excellence. All you can do is your best. That's all He asks of you.

13. Be real with yourself and with others. There's no room for pretentiousness, pettiness, dishonesty, and superiority in a well-kept house of the soul.

14. Bring down the curtain on drama. Simplify your life by vowing to stop turning minor upsets into major blow-ups.

15. Realize that you can't always choose the external circumstances, but you can choose how you respond to them. With grace, spirit, and character you can handle anything.

16. When faced with hardship, seek the lesson. Ask yourself, *What am I to learn from this?*

17. Remember: No God, no peace. Know God, know peace.

18. Taking care of yourself does not make you self-centered. It makes you centered.

19. *A merry heart doeth good like a medicine* . . . (Proverbs 17:22). So bring more laughter into your life each day. Doing so boosts your immune system.

20. Trigger personal growth by stepping outside your comfort zone. In our comfort zones, we feel secure because we're used to the usual routine. But always playing it safe can cause you to become stuck, even depressed, and leave you feeling unfulfilled. Even Susan L. Taylor, publication director of *Essence* magazine and one of the most admired sisters in the country, felt this way. In a recent column she wrote: "While I'm loving my work, I'm not loving my life. I've been living in sweet discomfort. So *I'm* taking the reins, composing a life that also includes time to reflect, create, and grow. To be with God and myself, with family and friends. I wish for you, beloved sisters and brothers, what I wish for myself: that we always have the courage to follow our hearts, to give ourselves our deepest love, so that our joy and our gifts to our people will be full." I couldn't agree more.

4

The Doctor's Office

· · · · · · · · · ·

There is something very special, something truly extraordinary, about doctoring, about being the healer, about having the skill, the knowledge, the capacity to reach out, to help others through the highs and lows of life in the uniquely powerful role of physician.

—Dr. Robert Witzburg, past president,
Alumni Association, Boston University School
of Medicine

NEWS YOU CAN USE

· The better your relationship with your doctor, the better your level of care. You should feel a sense of comfort and trust with your doctor.

· When looking for a doctor, make sure to select one with a good reputation, excellent credentials, and hospital affiliation.

· Always ask questions during your doctor visits. If you don't understand something your physician tells you, speak up. Ask her to clarify.

*I*F YOU'RE the type of person who puts off going to the doctor, you're not alone. Many sisters don't see a physician on a regular basis, and by not doing so they are putting their health at risk. It's not unusual to get nervous at the thought of going to the doctor. In fact, it's quite common. Many of us fear doctor visits because we worry about what the doctor might find, especially if we are experiencing the same symptoms as a friend or family member who turned out to have a serious illness. Even when we're just going in for a routine checkup, some of us start to imagine the worst. *What if the doctor finds this? What if the tests results show that?* We tend to let our imaginations get the best of us.

Fear isn't the only reason many sisters avoid the doctor. Some are simply squeamish and can't stand to get shots or have blood drawn. Others are shy about getting undressed in front of anyone other than their man. They feel exposed and vulnerable. I've found this to be especially true among overweight patients. (And since more than 60 percent of African-American women are overweight according to *Health, United States, 2001,* that's a lot of self-conscious sisters.)

For some black women, time is the culprit. They just don't have any, or so they think. With their busy schedules, the thinking goes, they simply don't have time to sit around waiting in a doctor's office. Cost and lack of insurance are yet two more reasons sisters often cite when explaining why they don't go to the doctor. The list could go on and on. But, the truth is, all of these "reasons" are nothing more than excuses. Let's be blunt. When you really want to do something, you find a way, don't you? My sisters, it's time to let the excuses go. Good health has to be a priority. You can't allow anything to stand in the way of it.

Once you resolve to overcome your self-inflicted roadblock—be it fear, lack of time, whatever—and put your health first, then you can go about the business of finding the best doctor for you. Having a trusting, comfortable, one-on-one relationship with a good doctor can make all the difference in your overall, long-term health. The key words here are *trusting, comfortable,* and *good.* You have to trust and be comfortable with your doctor, and make sure that doctor is good. It all comes down to finding the "right" physician. A doctor who's right for your next-door neighbor may be all wrong for you. As important as referrals from friends and family are, you are a unique, individual sister with unique and individual needs. There are many factors to consider when looking for a doctor. You and your physician need to be in sync in order for you to get the best care possible.

In my opinion, trust is one of the most important elements. Your health care involves you, so it should go without saying that your input is important to any decision being made about your body. There should be a sharing of information and discussion about the possible diagnoses, treatment options, and potential risks.

Your doctor is obligated to give you the best medical care possible and to provide you with pertinent information so you can make informed decisions about your health. For this reason, it is important that you pick a doctor you can trust to make sound medical decisions. Trust is paramount because, many times, very difficult decisions have to be made, and the doctor has the expertise to anticipate things that you, as a layperson, haven't even thought about, and to recommend necessary procedures that you otherwise may not want. For instance, if your obstetrician tells you that you need a C-section, your initial reaction may be negative. This is where trust comes in. You must be able to trust your doctor's knowledge and recommendation. You have to feel confident that your doctor is making the best determination for your health.

In return, your doctor must be able to trust you, too. How, you ask? For one, your physician needs to feel certain that you are being totally honest, not only about your symptoms but also about your lifestyle—how much alcohol you normally consume, if you are taking any medications, whether you smoke, if you currently use (or have ever used) illegal drugs, and so on. When asking you questions of this nature, your doctor needs to be able to trust your answers. This is so important, because any ultimate treatment will be impacted by your life choices. Let me give you an example.

As a surgeon, I love being in the operating room. I know that may sound a bit macabre to some folks, but I find being in the OR a fascinating, pleasant, and rewarding experience, especially when all is going well. Knowing that a patient will be leaving the OR in much better shape than when she entered is a wonderful blessing. But when something goes wrong for reasons you can't identify, it can be the most concerning experience in a doctor's life.

I remember one patient vividly: a young woman who was having fibroid tumors removed. Other than the tumors, this young woman was a normal, healthy patient—one who had given no history of any adverse social activities when I'd questioned her about her lifestyle. Given that, the OR staff (anesthesiologist, anesthetist, nurses, and myself) was expecting a routine, uncomplicated, uneventful, successful surgery.

To our grim surprise, even before the incision was made, the patient began to experience severe erratic fluctuations in her blood pressure, among other problems, shortly after the anesthetic drugs were administered. Everyone was shocked by this turn of events, because the problems this patient experienced during surgery are consistent with what happens when anesthetic drugs are given to people who are actively using cocaine. The unforeseen problems were so severe that everyone in the OR had to work extremely hard to bring this young woman back from a critical, near-fatal state. Fortunately, we got her vitals under control. I performed the surgery; she went to the recovery room in stable condition and had an uneventful night's rest.

The next morning, I fully informed the patient about what had happened and asked her point-blank if she'd used cocaine recently. She looked shocked at the question but admitted that she had used cocaine "more than she should have." I quickly informed her that she should not be using the drug at all and the fact that she had—and hadn't been up-front with me about it—almost killed her on the operating table. She was at death's door for two reasons:

(1) using the substance, and (2) not telling me, especially before an operation, despite being asked about it during her exam in my office.

I gently, but firmly, talked to her about what she was doing, what happened during the surgery—including the fact that she almost died—and what she could do from that point on to turn her life around. I also talked to her about allowing God into her life and turning to Him for guidance. I'm happy to report that a few weeks later, this young, beautiful black sister told me how she had found the Lord, turned over a new leaf, and was no longer doing drugs. In fact, she has become active in her church, much to the disbelief—and joy—of her family. She is truly blessed.

It's unfortunate that this sister had to learn such a valuable lesson in such a frightening and life-threatening way. But I hope that sharing this true experience with you will help you to understand and appreciate that trust and communication with your doctor is a two-way street.

In addition to being on the level about your lifestyle, you also need to be honest about your medical history, including your sexual partners, sexual habits, and sexual history. Have you had any abortions or pregnancies that no one knows about but you? Have you ever had any sexually transmitted diseases? Are you in a monogamous relationship, or do you have several sexual partners? Should these issues come up when you talk to your doctor, please don't be afraid or ashamed to tell the truth. And if your doctor doesn't bring it up, you should. Grit your teeth and fill her in, because your physician needs to know this information. Let me share another true-life anecdote with you that underscores how important your honesty is on this issue.

A young professional sister who was thrilled and excited about the baby she was carrying was not 100 percent honest with her physician about the total number of abortions she'd had over the years. Sadly, she ended up miscarrying the baby she wanted to have. If she had been honest about the number of previous abortions, her doctor would have had a discussion with her early in her pregnancy about the need to place a stitch in her cervix in order to keep it closed. You see, repeated manipulations or procedures (in this case, abortions) through the cervix can weaken it and cause late miscarriages. This patient was ashamed of her history and, though she felt comfortable talking to her doctor, just couldn't move past her shame and bring herself to talk about this topic openly and honestly. Unfortunately, her silence resulted in a devastating loss.

The reciprocal trust we've been talking about goes beyond being honest with your doctor, however. He or she also needs to be able to trust that you will be responsible. By that I mean you follow directions, take prescribed medications as instructed, care for surgical wounds as advised, limit or increase activity according to recommendations, etc. And finally, your doctor needs to trust that you will ask questions if you do not understand something. Don't be afraid to speak up and inquire.

ARE ALL DOCTORS ALIKE?

The answer is no. Different doctors do different things. So before we move on to how to find the right doctor, I'd like to spend a few moments discussing the various types of physicians available to you. As a woman, you likely realize the importance of having a gynecologist. But what about an internist? Do you need one of those, too? Can a gynecologist be your primary physician? Is having just one doctor enough? Well, you can't answer these sorts of questions until you know exactly what different general care doctors do.

Internist—also called a general practitioner (GP), this doctor sees men and women and treats most general conditions. He or she does not perform operations. If an internist discovers a particular problem during your exam, you will be referred to a specialist who can treat the problem more specifically.

Family Practitioner (FP)—this doctor treats men, women, and children. Family practitioners in rural areas may even deliver babies, since he or she is often the only doctor in town.

Obstetrician/Gynecologist (Ob/Gyn)—though trained in general medicine, this doctor specializes in the female body, structure, and function. He or she provides general health maintenance and pelvic care, delivers babies, and performs surgery.

Midlevel Practitioner—these professionals have more training than a nurse but not as much as a full physician. Most midlevel practitioners have attended college, plus have at least two additional years in a medical training program at a university or medical school instead of four years of medical school. They also do a rotation in a hospital or medical office setting, with patients. After special testing, most become certified.

Nurse Practitioner (NP)—though not a doctor, a nurse practitioner performs many of the tasks of a physician. He or she is a licensed registered nurse who has received advanced medical training. Nurse practitioners are trained to provide health services such as preventive care, monitoring of chronic conditions, physical examinations, and health counseling under the supervision of a physician. They can make diagnoses, prescribe medication, and offer treatment.

In the past, men and women simply went to an internist and received all of their care from that one doctor—whatever the diagnosis. While there are benefits to having only one doctor, there are also great benefits to utilizing the expertise of physicians who specialize in a particular area.

Once a woman becomes sexually active or turns age 18, she should definitely have an ob/gyn. Yes, the internist can do your Pap smear, but do you call a roofer when your television is broken? Of course not. The same thinking should apply when it comes to your reproductive system. The internal workings of the female body are so special and intricate that it's best to have a doctor with expertise in the field.

Most women use their ob/gyn as their primary doctor, thereby forgoing the need for an internist or family practitioner. For the most part, and for the large majority of women, this is fine. Your ob/gyn has been trained in general medical diseases and treatments, so he or she can readily evaluate, diagnose, and treat general complaints such as mild headaches, colds, flu, earaches, mild hypertension, and so on.

However, your ob/gyn will usually refer you to an internist if your medical problem is more involved. Take high blood pressure, for instance. If your pressure is borderline, your ob/gyn will most likely perform certain blood tests and make recommendations on how to bring your blood pressure down. In this scenario, the typical treatment is to increase exercise, decrease salt consumption, and eat a healthy, balanced diet. You may be prescribed medication for mild hypertension if you don't respond to these initial measures.

But if your blood pressure is very, very high or is unresponsive to medication, you will likely be referred to either an internist or directly to a cardiologist, depending on the severity of your hypertension.

On the other side of the coin are those sisters who turn to their internist for procedures generally performed by an ob/gyn, such as

Pap smears. I strongly recommend that every woman have her Pap done by an ob/gyn. This is a very special and delicate area of the body, and the ob/gyn's eye is trained to identify any abnormalities during the pelvic exam. Also, an ob/gyn is more likely than other types of doctors to know what new advances have been made in female reproductive procedures. It stands to reason, since ob/gyns mostly attend obstetrical and gynecological medical conferences, cardiologists mostly attend cardiology conferences, and so on, to stay current in their respective fields.

To sum up, if you are a young, healthy woman and you want your ob/gyn to be your primary physician, that's fine. Women with more advanced medical problems (diabetes, hypertension, lung or heart disease, intestinal problems, etc.) should have, at the minimum, an internist, and better still, a doctor who specializes in that particular field. Here's a quick run-down of some common specialists and descriptions of what they do:

Cardiologist: diagnoses and treats problems related to the heart

Endocrinologist: specializes in diseases and disorders of the endocrine system, which consists of a collection of hormone-producing glands

Gastroenterologist: diagnoses and treats disorders of the digestive system, including the stomach, esophagus, and intestines

Hematologist: specializes in diseases of the blood, like leukemia and sickle-cell anemia

Immunologist: investigates and treats problems related to the immune system, including allergies, autoimmune disorders, and immunodeficiency disorders such as AIDS

Oncologist: specializes in the diagnosis and treatment of cancer. Many oncologists specialize in a particular type of cancer.

Nephrologist: specializes in the diagnosis and treatment of kidney disease

Neurologist: diagnoses and treats diseases and disorders of the nervous system

Reproductive Endocrinologist: specializes in problems related to reproduction and infertility

Rheumatologist: diagnoses and treats arthritis, rheumatism, and other problems of the joints, muscles, or connective tissues

Urologist: diagnoses and treats disorders of the urinary system

FINDING THE RIGHT DOCTOR

It's not always easy to find the right doctor, especially in this era of HMOs and managed care. In an ideal world, you would be free to select the doctor of your choice and feel confident that your insurance would cover the bill, whatever the cost. Unfortunately, cost keeps many sisters from enjoying that level of freedom. Yes, there are private insurance carriers that allow you to select your own doctor, and leave test and hospitalization recommendations up to the physician's discretion, but the premiums are usually quite high. If you are part of a managed care plan, such as HMOs and PPOs (preferred-provider organizations), you have to pick a doctor who is also a part of that plan. And picking from a list can be limiting. The same holds true for referrals. Say your doctor wants to refer you to a specialist for care. Well, that specialist had better be on that managed care list, too. Here's how it works:

Every doctor has a network of colleagues he or she refers patients to in order to meet the total needs of the patient. But not every doctor is on every HMO plan. There are thousands of such plans, each with its own rules and methods of referral. If you are on a particular plan and need to be referred to another physician, your doctor will likely want to refer you to someone she or he knows and trusts. But if the referral is not in your HMO plan, and your doctor doesn't know any of the physicians listed, you might end up getting a blind referral. This should not happen, but it does because of the limitations managed care places on the health care system. Some insurance plans make allowances for these situations, allowing you to go "out-of-plan." But with that usually comes additional expense.

Fortunately, many insurance plans allow an ob/gyn to be a woman's primary care physician because they have finally realized that women will typically turn to their ob/gyn first for their basic health care needs. Though this seems basic and simple to most, it has taken years of fighting with insurance companies to get them to allow this.

I strongly believe that these "provider" lists limit a patient's access to many doctors. Again, there are thousands of "plans" your doctor could apply to. But even doing that takes time; the applications are lengthy. Also, each plan has its own set of rules and its own payment allowance. Having to deal with all of these plans takes away precious time from the patient.

In times past, a patient could see the doctor of her absolute choice—not just the doctor of her choice *from that list!* I firmly believe that patients should stress to their insurance companies that they want open access to their doctor of choice. Do away with these lists. Besides, if you want to see a particular doctor, you should be able to do so. It's that simple.

Whether you're part of an HMO or a plan that allows more freedom of choice, there are some key things to keep in mind when looking for a good doctor. As I've mentioned before, trust and comfort level are very important. A few other important factors:

Reputation: This is crucial. You want a doctor who has an excellent reputation, superb bedside manner, the respect of peers, a clean malpractice and disciplinary record, and who is timely in answering pages and emergency calls. Many patients learn of physicians through ads, but a better way to find a doctor is through word of mouth. A happy and satisfied patient is the best advertisement for a doctor. Be sure to get as much input from others as possible.

When one patient refers her friends, family, and coworkers to a doctor, it's safe to assume that that patient feels comfortable with that doctor and is confident in his or her skills.

In today's medical world, however, many patients are given a "provider handbook" from which they must pick a doctor, often blindly. I strongly suggest you try to check out any doctors you are considering. Ask your family, friends, coworkers, and neighbors if they've ever used the doctors you're thinking about seeing. Call the hospitals they are affiliated with. Do a little background check. And don't be shy about setting up a consultation visit with the doctors you are considering before scheduling an actual examination visit. No, your insurance company may not pay for the previsit, but this is your health we're talking about—you can't let just anyone care for it. By going in and meeting the doctor, you get to assess a few things. First, how does the doctor's staff function? Is the office clean and well-kept? Do they run on schedule? If not, how long do patients normally have to wait? During your visit take note of how many people are in the waiting room. Does the office seem to be overly busy? A too-bustling practice may indicate that the doctor is not able to spend quality time with each patient. Talk to a few of the folks in the waiting room. Do they have to cool their heels for an hour or more each time they come? While lots of patients and long waits could indicate the doctor's popularity, it could also be a sign that he or she is trying to see as many patients as possible to help compensate for the lost income caused by HMO rules. Bear in mind, too, that some doctors overextend themselves purely for their own egos. If you approach your consultation as a way of "checking out" prospective doctors, you'll be able to see behind a fake persona and a sugarcoated manner.

Credentials: The first absolute requirement is that the doctor be licensed to practice medicine in your state. You want to make sure she or he has completed medical school and post–medical school training (internship and residency from an accredited residency program). There are several sources you can use to find out this information—your state licensing board, the American College of Obstetricians and Gynecologists Physician's Directory, your local hospital referral service, and the Secretary of State's office (to check liability claims against a doctor). Many medical web sites also allow you to access this sort of information.

You can readily check a doctor's status and standing at local hospitals and with the state's medical board. In our society, it is preferable to have a physician who is board certified. This means the doctor has taken and passed the board exam (similar to a standardized test), has knowledge consistent with the standard of care, and is well trained in her or his field.

Hospital Affiliation: If possible, it's beneficial to have a doctor who is affiliated and on staff at a teaching hospital, mainly because teaching hospitals are often on the leading edge of medical advances.

GETTING THE MOST FROM DOCTOR VISITS

After talking to everyone you know, checking with various sources, and paying a consultation visit, you have finally found a doctor you trust and feel comfortable with, one who has excellent credentials, a great reputation, and is on staff at a good hospital. You've done the legwork and it has paid off. Now what? Well, my sister, the ball is in your court. As much as your doctor is responsible for the level of care you receive, so too are you. Remember what I said before about this being a two-way street? You have to do your part to ensure that you get the best health care possible. *How?* you ask. *What can I do?* Plenty. And it all starts with your doctor visits. Here's how to make the most of them:

Don't wait until the last minute to schedule appointments. Unless, of course, it is a medical emergency. Otherwise, check your work calendar and any other schedules carefully before calling the doctor's office for an appointment. This way you are less likely to have to reschedule later. Make your doctor's appointment a priority, just as you would a business meeting. Remember, your health comes first.

If you must reschedule, give as much notice as possible. If you reserve a spot on your doctor's schedule and then are a no-show, you've wasted your physician's time as well as kept another patient from making use of that long-awaited slot. Notify the doctor's office as soon as you can if you will not be keeping your appointment. A minimum twenty-four-hour notice is expected in most non-emergency situations, but the sooner you can notify the staff the better.

Some offices charge a fee for missed appointments. Check with the office regarding your doctor's cancellation policy.

Give the reason for your visit when calling for an appointment. A simple *It's time for my annual checkup,* or *I only need a Pap smear,* or *I will be a new patient* is all it takes. Let the receptionist know specifically why you are coming in. The staff will be better able to gauge the time needed to see you and can work you into the doctor's schedule more efficiently.

Think ahead. Have you ever been scheduled to have an examination plus some sort of test or procedure (usually performed by a nurse) on the same day? There may be no need for you to sit in the waiting room waiting for both. For example, let's say you are pregnant and in addition to your regular prenatal visit you are also scheduled to have an ultrasound or fetal monitoring done. Remind the receptionist of the procedure when you sign in and ask if you may start with the procedure while waiting your turn to see the doctor. No one else may be having an ultrasound or fetal monitoring done at the moment, thus leaving the room and equipment free for you. Not only will it save you from having to wait to have the procedure done *after* your exam, it also enables the doctor to have the results in hand *before* examining you. It can't hurt to ask.

Make use of office amenities. Most doctors today provide various in-office educational tools for their patients. Take advantage of them, especially while you are waiting to be seen. It's a good way to pass the time and also learn more about your body and your health. Find out if your doctor offers:

- *Patient education rooms*—These provide excellent opportunities to learn more about how your body works and the various diseases that can affect you. Many patient education rooms have numerous brochures you can take with you and short medical videos you can view while waiting. Often these rooms are easily accessible from the waiting room. If not, ask the receptionist if you can go in while you wait.

- *Breast models*—These tabletop models are usually available in the ob/gyn's office and help teach women what breast lumps may feel like. The bust models contain lumps in the breast, and you can test yourself to see if you can find the lumps. Doing this will give you a better idea how breast lumps feel and how deeply you must sometimes press in order to find them. Practicing on the models can help you improve your breast self-exam techniques (which you should be performing regularly at home).

- *Satellite TV stations*—Some offices may have special hookups to patient education television. These TVs are usually located in the waiting room.

Be prepared for your office visit. If it is your first visit, review and be knowledgeable about your past medical history, as well as your family's medical history. Think about it before you get to the office. Write the information down and bring it with you. Also know the names of any medications you are currently taking (bring the prescription bottles with you, if it's easier), and know the full names of any other doctors you are seeing and the reasons you are seeing them. Try to think of any other information your doctor will need to know. Preparing ahead of time will greatly decrease the time it takes you to complete the new patient information forms.

If you are a returning patient, be prepared to update your doctor on any new developments since your last visit. Did another doctor prescribe medication? Have you had foot surgery, say, or any other procedure? Again, try to think of anything and everything that has happened to you medically since your last visit.

Be specific about any symptoms you are experiencing and about how you are feeling in general. It is important for your doctor to know how much something has been troubling you and for how long. Think *how long, how much, where,* and *in what way.* Describe any ailments as thoroughly as you can. And make sure to give specific, measurable answers such as "for the past two months." Answers such as "for a long time" won't help your doctor make a diagnosis.

Have your questions ready and written down. So often patients freeze up and walk out of the doctor's office having forgotten questions they'd wanted to ask. They are already in their car or back at home when they suddenly remember. Write down any and all questions *before* your visit so that all of your concerns may be addressed. And don't forget to bring the list with you.

While you are with your doctor, don't be afraid to ask for an explanation of anything you don't understand. Most doctors will go over it again because they realize how important it is for you to comprehend your diagnosis and the treatment being recommended. Often your doctor will have pictures, drawings, brochures, or body models available to help explain things more clearly and thoroughly. Ask if any of these items are available.

If you are diagnosed with a certain illness, it's particularly important to speak up and ask specific questions, such as:

- What is the exact name of the illness? (Have your doctor spell it or write it out, if necessary.)

- How did I get this illness? What causes it?

- Can you go over the treatment with me step by step? What are the side effects of the treatment?

- If I need medication, will it be oral or will I have to have shots?

- Does this illness run in families?

- Will I need surgery?

- (If you have an infection:) Is this transmittable to my husband or partner?

- What precautions should I take while being treated?

- What about follow-up? Will I need to come back in to see you? If so, how soon?

Request prescription refills in a timely manner. Before calling your doctor's office for a refill, check your previous bottle or pill pack to see if refills are already indicated on the label. If they are, you don't need to call your doctor's office. Just call the pharmacy and they can have a new bottle ready for you by the time you get home from work.

If your prescription bottle or pill pack says "No refills" or "Refills 0," it could mean one of two things: (1) the doctor did not think you would need more of the medicine beyond the time frame of the original prescription, or (2) it's time for you to go in for a checkup.

Occasionally, your doctor may honestly forget to write intended refills on your original prescription, thereby making it necessary for you to call the office and request that they call the pharmacy. When calling your doctor's office for a refill, be sure to have the complete name of the drug and the dosage you are taking (usually written as milligrams or mg on the bottle) handy. Also, have your pharmacy's phone number at the ready. Keep in mind too that it's best not to call in for refills on Mondays and Fridays, as those are typically a doctor's busiest days. You should also try to avoid calling in for refills on weekends, unless it's an absolute emergency.

Be aware that different doctors' offices have different ways of calling in refills. Some may call them in as soon as you make the request. Others may call them in at scheduled times, such as midday and just before the end of business. Find out your doctor's procedure ahead of time.

UNDERSTANDING INSURANCE

As important as it is to do all that you can to find the right doctor and make the most of your doctor visits by asking questions and thoroughly understanding what your doctor tells you, there is another element of your health care that is just as important: insurance. There are so many variables involved, so many rules and procedures, so much to comprehend, that it can make any sister's head swim. But you need to be in the know. Too often we simply meet with our benefits manager at work, make our insurance selections, sign the forms, see the Benjamins deducted on our paycheck stubs, and leave it at that. On the surface, we feel pretty comfortable in our understanding of our health insurance. But do we really understand everything we should? Do we know exactly what's covered and what's not? Do we know the amount of our deductibles? Do we know what rules apply to what medical procedures? If we are totally honest with ourselves, we have to admit that we probably don't know or understand everything when it comes to our health insurance.

Unquestionably, today's health care industry is in a terribly confused and disruptive state. In the old days, medical care and medical decision making was a very personal and direct interaction between doctor and patient, and it was a long-term relationship. Patients commonly had the same doctor for ten, twenty, thirty years or more. Now, in this era of managed care, decisions about you and your health involve total strangers.

As a patient, you may have heard the term "precertification," or "precert" for short. This term basically refers to your doctor's office having to get approval in order for you to receive a particular procedure, test, or surgery that your doctor recommends. The concept stems from insurance companies having a cookbook-style method of determining what you need done, and they approve or deny your physician's recommendation without even seeing you. As a result of these protocols and procedures, doctors and their staffs are battling insurance companies every day while trying to meet the demand of providing patients with timely visits and quality care. Often, you, the patient, are not even aware of all that your physician and his or her staff have to go through to take care of you.

Additionally, in today's society, there is more *you* must do concerning your health care decisions. Certainly time has changed things. Years ago, whatever the doctor advised was done with little, if any, significant input from the patient. It is a good thing that the "me doctor, you patient" mentality has all but vanished. For sure, that type of doctor-patient relationship is not the ideal. The bottom line is that this new millenium brings with it more responsibility for the patient—you. You have to take a more active role in your health care. Educate yourself, ask questions, be fully informed. Nowhere is this more important than with health insurance, because as times have changed and as the medical industry has altered the way it does business, it has increasingly become in your best interest to understand your insurance do's and don'ts as completely as possible.

Know the Requirements

It is impossible for your doctor and her staff to keep up with the rules and regulations of every HMO, PPO, and other insurance policy, though they try. For this reason, the more you know about what your insurance company requires of you, the easier it will be for everyone.

The doctor's office may carry thousands of patients, each with a different plan. You only have to know about *your* plan. Study your policy book and compare its rules with your health care schedule. Do you need a referral before you can be seen by your ob/gyn? Have you had more visits than your insurance company is willing to pay for? Does your plan cover a particular procedure that your doctor has recommended? Can you see a doctor who is not listed in your provider book? If so, is there an additional charge? What about going to the emergency room? Do you need to call your insurance company first? Do you have a limit on the number of visits you can have in a year? What happens if you go over that limit?

As you can see, there are myriad questions that can come up. My best advice? Go over your policy book very carefully and, if necessary, schedule an informal meeting with your benefits manager at work. Have her go over the rules and procedures with you. Many companies often arrange periodic informational sessions for their employees with representatives from their health insurer. Take advantage of these sessions. Attend, take notes, and ask questions. If your company does not offer them, speak with your benefits manager about doing so.

RX: A PRESCRIPTION FOR YOUR SOUL

Behind the reputation, credentials, and busy schedule of every doctor lies the person he or she truly is deep down inside. We tend to put physicians on pedestals because of their ability to save lives, but at the end of the day, when they've taken off the white coat and put away the stethoscope, they are regular people, just plain folk. And as such, they connect with their patients on a human level—on a personal level. Some doctors are much better at making this connection than others. Those are the physicians you want. Why? Because at the root of human connection exists the essence of spirituality. It is that indescribable, seemingly unknown entity that endows each of us with the ability to touch another through kindness, compassion, caring, and love. It's not so hard to understand, really. When you are in tune with your own spirituality, you can be in tune with others'. It is God's grace flowing through you, directing your actions, empowering you to reach out with a loving heart. Why should doctors be any different? They are human beings too, possessed of the same inherent spirituality as all of us. Whether or not they have tapped into that inner divinity is another story. But if you can find a doctor who has—not only in word but also in deed—then you will be in much better hands.

Understand, though, that how a physician expresses his or her spirituality may not be obvious. Doctors may simply extend their divinity by their day-to-day actions, by the way they live their lives, by the manner in which they care for their patients. A quiet, unheralded wellspring of spirituality is truly a joyous thing. When we stumble upon it in others it uplifts us. It gives us renewed hope and faith in humanity. It reminds us that God lives within each of us in vastly different ways. The point of all this is for you to learn to look for those divine signs in your doctor. Go a step further and actively assess whether or not your physician possesses spiritual qualities, even if they are different from your own.

It goes back to the notion of comfort and trust. Spirituality is simply another component of that. A link exists between your personal spirituality and your relationship with your doctor. That's because when you feel as though you are in sync with someone in a spiritual sense, no matter how their divinity may be manifested, you are going to be more comfortable with them and more trusting. You will feel more at ease. That's exactly what you want between patient and doctor. You know how you get a certain "feeling" about someone—about his or her innate goodness, caring, and concern? Well, it's perfectly okay if you heed that "feeling" in regard to your doctor. Listening to your heart, soul, and spirit always leads you on the right path in other areas of your life, right? So it shall be with your health.

The Bible speaks of not being "unequally yoked" with certain people. That can apply to your spouse, to friends, and certainly to your doctor. No one is saying that your physician has to be of your exact faith or denomination; you need your doctor to be in tune with your best medical interests, to understand you and the importance you place in your faith, and to have a spirit that is open to hear your concerns.

Think of a troubled marriage. I'm sure you know a couple who are still together although they probably shouldn't be. Unfortunately, everyone tends to know at least one couple like this. On every issue this husband and wife seem to be on completely different pages. Sometimes, certain people just don't belong together. But many couples try to stick it out, because that's what others expect them to do, even though they are not equally yoked. When it comes to your health you can't afford to make the same mistake. You and your doctor have to be on the same page spiritually. Does that mean a Protestant doctor can't take care of a Catholic patient? Or that a Muslim doctor can't care for a Baptist? Of course not. Surely the majority of doctors are wholly committed to the Hippocratic oath and will do the best they can for their patients, whatever their faiths. However, it is important to be with a doctor who not only recognizes his or her role in the doctor/patient relationship, but also recognizes and respects your role—and your spiritual needs. How can you tell if your doctor is right for you spiritually? Here are a few things to consider:

- Does your physician speak about God? When something is a part of you, it's a part of your conversation. So if your doctor is truly invested in her own spiritual growth, you will likely notice divine references now and then, though they may be extremely subtle. You don't necessarily want her to preach to you, just to openly acknowledge a Higher Power in some fashion.

- Does your doctor conduct himself in ways consistent with a person of spiritual practice? What sense do you get of how he lives his life?

- Does your doctor's bedside manner mesh with your emotional needs? Does she have a warm, patient, caring spirit, or does she treat you and others quickly and coldly?

- Does your doctor listen attentively and treat everyone, including you, with the utmost respect?

- Does your doctor exude a calming presence at all times? Does she consistently appear to be reflective, thoughtful, and somehow meditative?

Try to perceive your doctor's spirit. Often a child of God can tell a child of God. Your spirits will recognize each other.

5

Common Illnesses, Simple Cures

· · · · · · · · · · ·

*There's more of us to give to others if we give a little bit
to ourselves first.*

—Yanick Rice Lamb, former editor in chief of *Heart
& Soul* magazine

News You Can Use

· Symptoms of trichomoniasis include inflammation and itching of
the vagina and vulva, and yellow/green discharge.

· Symptoms of candidiasis include white/yellow cottage cheeselike
discharge, and itching and burning of the vagina and vulva.

· Symptoms of bacterial vaginosis include grayish/white frothy, fishy-
smelling discharge, and itching and burning of the vagina.

WHEN IT comes to the female body, certain illnesses are far more
common than others, specifically vaginitis and bladder infections.
Both are forms of reproductive-tract infections, which start in the
external genitals, vagina, and cervix—and they affect millions of
women each year. Most women who contract one of these infections
can usually take care of it quickly and easily, as long as it is detected
early and they get proper treatment in a timely fashion. Left untreated, however, these infections may lead to a host of problems,
including pelvic inflammatory disease, infertility, and cervical cancer. That's why it's important to understand these illnesses, recognize their symptoms, and know how to treat and prevent them in an
early stage. Let's take a look at some of the most common ones.

VAGINITIS

We tend to think of bacteria as a bad thing, but that's not always the case. A normal, healthy vagina does harbor bacteria; however, it's a mixture of particular bacteria with a pH, or acidic, level of 3.8 to 4.4 (the average is 4.0). When the vagina is at its proper pH level, it helps to ward off "bad" bacteria. The hormone estrogen and a sugar substance called glycogen are also very important in maintaining a healthy vaginal environment.

This normal, healthy environment can be disrupted by a variety of things, however, including douching, allergic reactions, medications such as antibiotics and birth control pills, estrogen deficiency associated with menopause, forgotten tampons, or restrictive clothing (pantyhose, tight pants, etc.) that do not allow the vagina to "breathe." All of these things can throw off the proper balance of the vagina's normal bacteria, causing the unwanted bacteria to grow and giving you an infection that can irritate the cells of the vagina and cervix.

If you develop a case of vaginitis, you may not be able to put an exact name to it, but you'll know that something's not right. Symptoms may include itching, irritation, burning, abnormal vaginal discharge, odor, and painful intercourse. The more in tune you are with your body, the more easily you'll be able to detect anything that seems out of sync.

Even though vaginal infections are very common, it's not impossible to prevent them from occurring. Heed this advice to cut your risk of infection:

• After using the toilet, always wipe from front to back. If you wipe from back to front, you can bring bacteria from the rectal area toward the more delicate vaginal area, causing infection.

- Drink plenty of water, at least eight glasses a day.

- Dry off well after a shower or bath. Pat the genital area dry with a clean towel. Don't use other folks' towels.

- Since some women have an increased sensitivity to scented or perfumed toiletries, including tampons, vaginal sprays, bubble bath, soap, bath oils/salts/crystals, and douches, you may want to avoid these types of products.

- Speaking of douches, the American College of Obstetricians and Gynecologists recommends that women not use them. You don't need them to clean your vagina. The vagina has its own natural cleansing process. And if you do your part by washing your genital area regularly with a mild, gentle cleanser, there really is no need to douche. However, if you nevertheless decide to do so, it's best to simply use clear water.

- Change tampons frequently.

- If you use sex toys, use them hygienically. If one has been inserted into the rectum, do not place it into the vagina without first cleaning it thoroughly. Otherwise you risk transferring bacteria from the rectum to the vagina.

If you are being treated for vaginitis, make sure to complete the prescribed treatment regimen. Don't stop taking the medication just because the symptoms disappear or you no longer have abnormal discharge. If you stop treatment too soon, you don't allow the medication to do its job. You may think you're cured, but in all likelihood the infection is still present and will reappear. Also, during treatment, it's best to avoid intercourse and other sex acts that involve the penis, fingers, or sexual aids; otherwise you risk introducing new bacteria before the medication has had a chance to work.

There are many specific types of vaginitis, from yeast infections to bacterial vaginitis to parasitic infections. Here, a quick rundown of a few of the most prevalent.

Trichomoniasis

Also known as "trich" (pronounced "trick"), this parasitic infection is extremely common, affecting millions of men and women each year. One in five women harbor the infection. Trich is caused not by bacteria but by a protozoan called *Trichomonas vaginalis*. Although this infection is usually transmitted during sexual intercourse, it can also be contracted from shared washcloths and towels. Typically there are no symptoms; however, if any do occur they usually include somewhat painful inflammation and itching of the vagina and vulva, a profuse, frothy, yellow/green discharge, and in some women, a vague pelvic pain.

During the physical exam, your doctor will notice a reddened labia and reddened vaginal walls. You will have a "strawberry" cervix—so named not only because of the redness but also because the infection causes little "pimples." Trich causes the pH of the vagina to reach 5.1 to 5.4, which is higher than normal and less acidic.

Trichomoniasis is diagnosed by examining a sample of vaginal discharge under a microscope, a procedure called a "wet mount" or "wet prep." The standard treatment is to prescribe an antibiotic drug called Metronidazole (trade name Flagyl), which may be given as a one-dose treatment or a seven-day regimen. It is important not to drink any alcoholic beverages while being treated with Flagyl because the combination will cause intense nausea and vomiting. Possible side effects of the drug include headache, nausea, and diarrhea. If you are diagnosed with trich, make sure your sexual partner is also diagnosed and treated. If he isn't treated and the two of you have sex again, you can become reinfected.

Candidiasis

This is a type of yeast infection that occurs when a fungus called *Candida albicans* multiplies and overgrows. Like trich, candidiasis is also an extremely common infection. Symptoms include a thick, white/yellow discharge that resembles cottage cheese, and itching (pruritis) and burning of the vagina and vulva. Women with diabetes, who are pregnant, or who are taking antibiotics or oral contraceptives have an increased risk of contracting candidiasis because all of these conditions encourage growth of fungus that causes the infection.

Diabetic women in particular need to be concerned, because yeast loves sugar. We all have a slight amount of yeast in our vaginal tract. Usually it's of no significance because the acidic nature of the vagina helps to keep it under control. But in diabetic women, the existing yeast can feed on the high sugar content, multiply, and grow, giving the women a florid infection.

Candidiasis is diagnosed by examining a sample of the discharge under a microscope. The infection is treated with an antifungal cream, usually prescribed in the form of a vaginal cream or suppository. Occasionally an oral treatment is prescribed, though it may not be as effective.

Bacterial Vaginosis (BV)

This particular infection used to be known as nonspecific vaginitis or was sometimes called *Gardnerella vaginitis* or *Hemo-*

philus vaginitis (names that refer to specific types of bacteria). As the name implies, bacterial vaginosis develops when normal bacteria in the vagina have grown out of control. Although an exact cause is not known, it may be due to a staph or strep infection, or *E. coli.* Symptoms of BV include a grayish/white, frothy discharge that gives off a foul, fishy odor. Woman with bacterial vaginosis may also experience itching and burning of the vagina. BV is diagnosed by examining vaginal secretions under a microscope and is treated with an antibiotic such as metronidazole.

Atrophic Vaginitis

See Chapter 11, Managing Menopause.

BLADDER INFECTIONS

Another common ailment facing women is the bladder infection, also called cystitis or urinary tract infection (UTI). A bladder infection is basically inflammation of the inner lining of the bladder caused by bacteria. Fifty percent of all women get bladder infections at some point in their life. We get them more often than men do because women have a much shorter urethra (the narrow tube through which urine exits the body), making it easier for bacteria to travel to the bladder. The bacteria may be introduced to the urethra and bladder when a woman wipes herself from back to front after having a bowel movement. Or sexual intercourse may be the culprit, since the thrusting motion can push bacteria into the bladder. Cystitis can also stem from a bladder that is not emptied completely. Anytime your bladder is not fully emptied it encourages infection, because stagnant urine in the bladder or urethra provides a good breeding ground for bacteria.

Symptoms of a bladder infection include pain, burning, or

stinging during urination. You will also feel the urge to urinate frequently, though when you do, oftentimes not much urine will come out. You may experience difficulty getting your urine stream to flow. The urine will have a strong or foul odor, and occasionally blood will be present. Painful intercourse is yet another symptom of a bladder infection.

A urinalysis coupled with an assessment of symptoms and a thorough discussion of your medical history is usually enough for your doctor to make a presumptive diagnosis and begin treatment. A urine culture should also be taken to identify the actual type of bacteria causing the infection.

Once the diagnosis is made, your physician will prescribe antibiotics that work against the majority of bacteria that cause UTIs to fight the infection. It is very important that you follow your doctor's instructions and take all of the medication prescribed. If treatment is not completed, a bladder infection can lead to a persistent infection that will ascend from the bladder toward the kidneys (via narrow tubes called the *ureters* that course along the deep, inner sides of the body). A kidney infection is much more serious than a simple bladder infection, so it's best to treat cystitis immediately and fully.

To reduce the chances of recurrence, drink plenty of fluids, especially cranberry juice, which encourages acidity of the urine. Empty your bladder fully each time you use the toilet, and never try to "hold it." If you have to go, go. Try to urinate after sexual intercourse to flush bacteria out of the bladder. And always wipe from front to back after using the toilet.

OTHER MINOR CONDITIONS

Vaginitis and bladder infections may be two of the most common ailments women face, but there are a whole host of other conditions we have to deal with as well. Some may be less prevalent, others less serious. Either way, if you want to have good all-around health, it's important that you know what they are, what they can do, and how to treat them.

Folliculitis

You know how the fellas get "hair bumps"? Well, guess what, ladies; we get them, too. In our case, however, these little bumps usually occur in the mons pubis and are a result of bacterial growth at the base of the pubic hair follicles. The bumps may be small and self-contained, but they can get very large and painful. An abscess may form and the pus may eventually burst out of it.

The key to preventing folliculitis is good hygiene. When you shower or bathe, make sure to clean your pubic hair thoroughly. Think in terms of "shampooing" your pubic hair. Regular soap will do fine; just be certain to lather the area well and rinse it meticulously. Drying off well is equally important. If you leave any water or moisture in the pubic area, then cover it up with underwear or pantyhose, you create a breeding ground for bacteria to grow—a dark, warm, and moist area. Bacteria love that kind of environment, so make sure you do all that you can to prevent it.

For mild folliculitis, good hygiene is usually all that's needed to clear things up. However, if the infection is severe, antibiotics may be necessary. Occasionally an "I&D," or incision and drainage, will be required to lance an abscess.

Bartholin's Cyst

A pair of oval, pea-sized glands called Bartholin's glands are located on either side of the entrance to the vagina. The glands' ducts open into the vulva, and during sexual arousal these glands secrete lubricating fluids. Infection of Bartholin's glands causes bartholinitis, in which an intensely painful red swelling forms at the opening of the ducts. This infection can develop into a Bartholin's cyst, a swelling in one of the lips of the vagina that is filled with either clear liquid or, more likely, pus, causing an abscess. These cysts or abscesses can be extremely large, and if filled with bacteria and pus, extremely painful.

Treatment entails cutting open the mass and draining the fluid. Afterward, the abscess cavity is irrigated well with a saline and peroxide solution, then packed with gauze, or more commonly, a drain is placed inside until the cavity closes up, expelling the drain. Treatment will also include antibiotics, analgesics (painkillers), and warm sitz baths (only the hips and buttocks are immersed in water). You should definitely abstain from sex during recovery to allow the area to heal completely.

Occasionally, women have chronic bartholinitis, in which the Bartholin's gland becomes infected repeatedly. If this is the case, surgery may be necessary to remove the affected gland. It is an outpatient procedure and you would be able to go home the same day. The remaining gland, and others, can still provide vaginal lubrication.

Sebaceous Cysts

These firm, raised bumps appear in the vulva area as a result of blockage in the gland openings in the skin of the vulva. The bumps are filled with a cheesy, greasy material. Although harmless, sebaceous cysts may grow very large and sometimes become infected by bacteria, in which case they are very painful.

Good pelvic hygiene helps diminish the occurrence of these usually benign masses. Sitz baths and hot, moist compresses can also help. However, if the cyst is large or is infected, a doctor can remove it using a local anesthetic. The physician makes a small incision in the skin and removes the cyst.

Cervical Polyps

These are usually small, fleshy growths that protrude from the opening of the cervix. They typically are found on a pedicle (stalk) that extends upward into the cervical canal. The polyps are painless and predominately noncancerous. A woman won't be able to tell if she has cervical polyps; however, her doctor will be able to detect them when she goes in for her routine pelvic exam because they will be visible. Sometimes, bleeding after sexual intercourse is an indication of cervical polyps. The friction of the penis against the polyps is what causes the bleeding.

The polyps are easily removed by simply clipping the pedicle at its highest point, then using a small cauterizing stick to prevent bleeding at the site of removal. You won't be able to have sex for a few days while the tissue heals. Malignancy is rare but recurrence is fairly common.

As you can see, the glory of being a woman is not without its minor problems. However, if we know what common feminine ailments might affect us and how best to take care of ourselves, we may not have to suffer through too many of them at all.

RX: A PRESCRIPTION FOR YOUR SOUL

Mark Twain once said, "I am an old man and have known a great many troubles, but most of them have never happened." How many of us can say the same thing? How many times have we worried ourselves over events that had yet to occur—and rarely, if ever, did? Too often people allow themselves to become over-anxious about absolutely nothing.

That's not to say that we shouldn't be concerned about certain matters, especially when it comes to our health. But we need to keep things in their proper perspective and not make mountains out of molehills. When we allow anxiety to override common sense, it diminishes our ability to take care of business. It's so easy for undue concern to escalate. The next thing you know, you're frozen in fear, unable to take action. Worrying never solved or resolved anything.

I once heard a preacher say that worrying is like being in a rocking chair; once you get through, you're still in the same place. He has a point, doesn't he? Just think about how much energy you burn with needless, toxic worrying. What is toxic worrying? Worrying that causes you to go off on a tangent, magnifying even the smallest, most insignificant things. You start jumping to conclusions that, many times, aren't reasonable. Too often we get caught up in the "oh my gosh, what if it's this," or "what if it's that" mentality. What we need to do is first, acknowledge the problem. Next, pray to God for courage, direction, and wisdom. And finally, take action. How does this advice impact your health? Well, think of it this way: If you're not feeling well, or you notice something out of the ordinary, rather than sit and worry (which is simply inaction in action), find out what's wrong (if anything) and then have it taken care of. All it takes is a visit to your health care professional for an accurate diagnosis. You'll set your mind at ease. You won't waste precious time fretting over something that may be nothing. And, most important of all, you'll be able to get your health back on course with proper treatment, if in fact you are ill.

Keep in mind too that chronic worrying itself can have an adverse affect on your health. Now wouldn't that be an ironic turn of events? Here you are worrying that you might be sick and all of that worrying may, in fact, make you sick. Not convinced? Then consider this: Constant worrying raises your pulse rate, can increase your blood pressure, heightens your stress level, and can cause you to lose your appetite (or, conversely, to eat more). The possible problems don't end there, though. Being in a constant state of anxiety can also wreak havoc with your state of mind. Worrying occupies your mind with needless, useless, and unproductive thoughts, causing you to lose track of what's truly important in your life. It can be paralyzing, preventing you from fully engaging in your normal, everyday activities. When you worry it's as if you are not trusting God to look after you. It's as though you've removed Him from the process.

The Bible says "Be anxious for nothing, but in everything, by prayer and supplication with thanksgiving, let your requests be known to God. And the peace of God, which passeth all understanding, shall keep your hearts and minds . . ." (Philippians 4:6–7) The message is clear. The time you spend worrying could best be spent praying to God to comfort you, calm you, and encourage you to act toward resolving your problem.

So trust in Him. Yes, pay attention to what your body tells you and heed its messages. See your doctor if you notice anything out of sync or unusual. Take action rather than sitting and worrying. But let God guide you as well. Don't fret in solitude. Turn your fears and worries over to Him. The relief you feel will free you to do what has to be done. It will empower you to get the answers you need from a health professional you trust. How do you spell relief? K-n-o-w-i-n-g. Knowing what your actual diagnosis is brings great relief, as compared to not knowing and freaking out at home about the wrong thing. Chances are the problem is far more common and less serious than your worry-fueled imagination leads you to believe.

Let me also reiterate the importance of getting regular check-ups. Doing so keeps you in tune with your body and its normal functions. As I've said before, the more in touch you are with your body, the better you'll be at keeping your worries in check. For instance, women who see their doctors regularly and who've had, say, a yeast infection (or any other minor concern) before will have some knowledge about the signs of the condition. They'll have a better idea of what the symptoms indicate and therefore won't be consumed by worry and anxiety. They'll have a degree of comfort in knowing that it's a relatively minor ailment—one that can be treated simply and easily.

Calmness, rationality, and reliance upon a Higher Power to help us keep all things in proper perspective go a long way toward enabling us to lead stress-free, worry-free, healthy lives. And it's not just about physical health. We fret about a wide variety of issues, some great and some small. It's the small ones—the little things in life—that can really do a number on you if you let them career out of control. Keep minor worries reined in and you'll do both your health and your state of mind a huge favor. So how can you stay calm during times of uncertainty, whether health-related or regarding life in general? Try these methods:

- Acknowledge that there is a problem, but don't blow it out of proportion. You can't and won't be able to seek help until you first admit something's going on. Just try to keep everything in perspective until you know for sure what you're dealing with. It may turn out to be quite minor.

- Remember, you are a child of God. His eye is on the sparrow, so you know He's still watching over you. There's no need to feel that the worst will happen.

- Pray to God with thanksgiving, especially in the midst of worry. Pray for His comforting spirit to guide you as you proceed with what you have to do.

• Take the appropriate action. If you are concerned about a health matter, call your doctor. Make an appointment, then go in for the checkup. Go in armed with the facts—your symptoms, how you are feeling, etc.—not what your worried state of mind may have conjured. Don't allow your fear to cause you to embellish or self-diagnose. Be specific about the facts and let your doctor do his or her job.

• Trust that God has led you to the right person and is over-seeing your doctor's care of you and guiding his decision-making.

• Give glory to God for all that He has done and continues to do concerning every aspect of your life.

• Do the right thing. If you are prescribed medication, take all of it as directed, not just until you feel better. Follow all of your physician's instructions.

• Rejoice when you are healed!

6

A Woman's Body—
Dealing with Serious Illness

· · · · · · · · · · ·

We are now faced with a situation where African Americans are suffering from diseases that are totally preventable, and dying from conditions that are the result of chronic diseases that can be prevented.

—Dr. Stephen Thomas, director for the Center for Minority Health at the University of Pittsburgh

NEWS YOU CAN USE

· African-American women are three to four times more likely to develop fibroid tumors than are other women.

· Up to an astounding 71 percent of women with chronic pelvic pain suffer from endometriosis.

· Blacks are nearly 1½ times more apt to contract a sexually transmitted disease than are Caucasians.

· Research shows that AIDS is the number one killer of African-American men and women ages 25 to 44.

· Sisters have the highest endometrial cancer mortality rate among all races of women.

· While more whites are diagnosed with breast cancer, blacks are more likely to die from it.

ALL OF us wish to live our lives as vitally and healthfully as possible. And if we take care of ourselves—eat right, exercise regularly, get routine checkups, heed our body's messages—odds are we won't have to deal with anything more serious than the common illnesses discussed in Chapter 5.

However, ensuring long-lasting good health encompasses more than doctor visits, proper diet, and the like. You also have to be armed with the facts about serious illness. You can't afford to stick your head in the sand when it comes to your health, for there may come a time when you're faced with a medical crisis, and knowing the facts can help you get through it. Remember, African-American women are more at risk for a multitude of diseases, including hypertension, diabetes, stroke, heart disease, and certain cancers, to name a few. You've heard the phrase "forewarned is forearmed." Well, nowhere is that sentiment more true than when it comes to your well-being.

As much as you have to face up to the health risks inherent in being a black woman, it doesn't mean a serious illness is definitely in your future. The diseases that affect us most aren't inevitable. While it's true that race and heredity may place you at higher risk, you still have the power to take control. In her book *Dream the Boldest Dreams,* Dr. Johnnetta B. Cole states, "An African-American proverb correctly asserts that you can't know where you're going if you don't know where you've been. But let history and past experiences instruct rather than determine your destination." Yes, race and heredity may play a major role in our health, but we can take the lessons we learn from that and alter the direction for our own health. Leading as healthy a lifestyle as possible will add years to your life.

Part of being able to lead that healthy lifestyle is understanding the serious illnesses that can affect you and knowing what you can do to try to keep them at bay. With that goal in mind, I have put together a sort of primer of the serious female-specific illnesses African-American women face. Here you'll learn what each illness is, its symptoms and warning signs, its causes and effects, and how it is treated.

FIBROIDS

Fibroid tumors are extremely common among black women. In fact, sisters are three to four times more likely to develop them than any other group of people. While 20 to 30 percent of all women over age 30 have fibroids, an estimated 50 to 75 percent of African-American women do. Chances are someone in your family has had them—perhaps even you.

When a sister learns she has fibroids, a myriad of questions come to her mind: *What are they? Where do they come from? Can I still get pregnant? Will I have to have a hysterectomy?* While black women appear to be more susceptible to fibroids, the reason why remains a mystery. Is it dietary? Genetic? No one knows for sure. But just hearing the words "fibroid tumor" can evoke a sense of fear. That's understandable, considering that many people automatically associate the word "tumor" with cancer. However, *tumor* simply means an abnormal overgrowth of cells. Fortunately, most fibroids are completely benign (noncancerous). Less than 1 percent of them turn out to be malignant.

Exactly what are fibroids?

Fibroids are well circumscribed but non-encapsulated "balls" of smooth, musclelike tissue that can grow in a woman's uterus. They are firm growths, often called masses. The correct medical name for them is *myomas,* though the word "fibroids" is most commonly used. They have also been called *leiomyoma, fibromyoma, leiomyofibroma, leiomyomata,* and *fibroma.*

Fibroids can range in size, with some as small as a pea and others growing as large as a ten-pound baby or more. In fact, the medical textbook *Danforth's Obstetrics and Gynecology* cited a myoma that reached a weight of 147 pounds!

What causes them?

Although the definite cause is yet to be confirmed beyond all doubt, it is now widely believed among health care researchers and clinicians that these tumors form and grow in response to the hormone estrogen. Estrogen is one of the hormones naturally produced by the ovaries, and it plays a vital role in maintaining various body functions, including heat regulation, vaginal moisture, emotions, heart and bone strength, and ovulation.

The actual way in which estrogen contributes to the growth of fibroids is still unknown, however. It is believed that the hormone serves as a nutrient to the tumors, reaching them via the blood as it flows normally through the uterine vessels. What *is* known, though, after years of observation, is that when estrogen levels are low or depleted (typically because of menopause or antiestrogen medication), fibroids usually shrink. Women who have had their ovaries removed but their uterus left in place for possible embryo implantation, also have low or no estrogen and do not produce fibroids. All of these findings suggest that estrogen can be linked to the growth of fibroid tumors. So as long as a woman has functioning ovaries that are still producing estrogen, she is at some risk of developing the tumors.

Since estrogen is the likely culprit, anything that increases levels of the hormone may be considered a contributing factor to the development of fibroids. Birth control pills used to be one of those factors. During its early years, the Pill often contained very large doses of estrogen. As a result, many women who were on the Pill and also had fibroids experienced an increase in the size of the tumors. This is not as much of a problem now because many of today's oral contraceptives have extremely low levels of estrogen. The amount of hormones in the pills was reduced to help decrease side effects and potential complications.

Another contributing factor that is still very much a problem is obesity. Body fat can produce a form of estrogen; therefore, women who are overweight may run a slightly greater risk of developing fibroids. This is of special concern to sisters because statistics show that more than 66 percent of African-American women are overweight. Although a definitive correlation between weight and race has not been proven to be the reason why sisters get more fibroids than other women, it's still important to know that being overweight may increase your risk.

What are the symptoms?

Many fibroids are totally asymptomatic and are usually not noticed until a routine gynecological exam is performed. For many women, fibroid tumors cause no problems at all, especially early in life and/or when the tumors are small. Usually, though, as time progresses, many women do begin to experience some problems, including heavier menstrual flow, prolonged periods, bleeding in between periods, pelvic pain, painful intercourse, bladder pressure, increased pelvic girth, urinary urgency, or constipation. Some women may also have difficulties with pregnancy, having trouble either conceiving or carrying the baby to term. Fortunately, most women are able to successfully complete their pregnancies despite the presence of fibroid tumors.

In general, the location of the tumors in or on the uterus often dictates the type of symptoms a woman experiences.

Where can fibroids be located?

As depicted in the diagram on page 116, there are four different types of fibroid tumor, each characterized primarily by its location:

- *Subserous myomas* cause a distortion of the basic shape of the uterus, giving a "knobby" feeling; project from the exter-

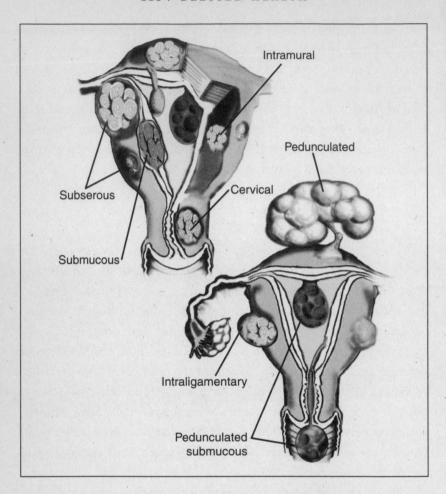

nal surface of the uterus; may continue growth resulting in fibroids on a stalk (called *pedunculated myomas*). These may
attach to other organs in the pelvis or abdomen, latching on
to that organ's blood flow. When this happens it's called a
parasitic myoma.

• *Intramural myomas* are the most common; situated in the
muscle wall of the uterus, they distort the cavity and the gen-

eral shape of the uterus; may significantly block the endome-trial cavity, which is a concern in terms of pregnancy.

• *Submucous myomas* are present just beneath the lining of the womb (the endometrium); because of their proximity to the womb's lining these tumors are the ones most prone to caus-ing bleeding problems in women; can become pedunculated and fall downward into the cervical canal. These tumors may cause additional irregular spotting or bleeding due to infec-tion, the use of tampons, or intercourse (the irritation of fric-tion is the culprit).

• *Cervical myomas* are tumors that grow in the actual muscle walls of the cervix; because this area is extremely vascular (full of blood vessels), removing the tumors may cause a great deal of blood loss.

How are fibroids diagnosed?

There are two major components to diagnosing fibroid tumors: a pelvic exam and an ultrasound. If you have fibroids, they will usually be detected during a pelvic exam by your gynecologist, his or her physician's assistant, or a nurse practitioner. A trained exam-iner who does pelvic exams daily is well trained to feel the "lumps and bumps" these tumors cause in or on the uterus, or to recognize one protruding from the cervix.

If the tumors are very large, they may be readily apparent even to you, because they can distort the abdominal wall, often giving the appearance of a pregnancy.

A pelvic ultrasound or sonogram is often in order, as well. This test, which employs sound waves and emits no radiation, takes a picture of the growths, though very tiny tumors (smaller than a green pea) may not be detected. The objective picture of the ultrasound allows your doctor to check the relative size, location, and number of tumors present. All of these factors can be very important when deciding the best course of treatment and whether a woman needs surgery.

How are fibroids treated?

The treatment you receive for fibroids is largely determined by your symptoms, physical findings on exam and ultrasound, and your plans for future childbearing. Options can include observation and periodic monitoring, hormone therapy, or surgery.

If the tumors are small and are not causing any symptoms, your doctor may simply have you come in for exams periodically so that he can monitor the fibroids. He will check them to make sure they haven't grown and ask whether you have experienced any fibroid-related problems.

If the tumors are large, your doctor may utilize a treatment known as hormonal manipulation. With this treatment, specific drugs, such as Lupron, Synarel, and others, are prescribed in an attempt to shrink the tumors in preparation for surgery, or to relieve the symptoms (though temporarily) if the patient is not a surgical candidate because of medical reasons.

Here's how hormonal manipulation works: Because it is widely believed that the hormone estrogen plays a key role in the development and growth of fibroid tumors, doctors now prescribe medications that counteract estrogen's effects. These medications, which—as a group—your doctor classifies as *gonadotrophin-releasing hormone (GnRH) agents,* act to decrease and ultimately eliminate estrogen production for the time period in which the drug is used. Without estrogen, the fibroids lose their source of nutrition, so to speak, and end up diminishing in size. Such a reduction is often desired when the woman has tumors large enough to cause problems, but wishes to maintain her childbearing capabilities.

The medication is usually given in the form of an injection once a month for three to six months (typically three). Once the tumors shrink, surgery is performed to remove them.

Some may ask, why not just continue taking the medication and avoid surgery altogether? GnRH agents are powerful drugs whose primary action is to stop estrogen production. As a result, women using the drugs experience the same symptoms as women going through menopause: hot flashes, decreased sex drive, occasional mood swings, and the possible onset of osteoporosis (loss of bone density, which leaves bones brittle and easily fractured). What's more, drug treatment is not a panacea. Once the medication is stopped, the tumors will grow back. Because of these factors, the standard recommendation is to administer the drugs for three months, reevaluate the fibroids, and, in all likelihood, proceed with the *myomectomy* (a surgical procedure that removes the tumors and leaves the uterus in place).

If certain drugs can shrink fibroids, why can't they get rid of them for good? you may wonder. Why do they grow back? Think about what happens when you go on a diet. You diligently cut back or eliminate the foods that go right to your hips. Three months without them, and the pounds have melted off. What would happen if you suddenly began constantly eating all of those foods again? That's right—you'd regain the weight. The same thing happens with fibroids. When the drug treatment stops, your body begins producing estrogen again, thus feeding the shrunken tumors and causing them to grow. With a diet, you are able to exercise self-control, but your hormones occur naturally and spontaneously. That makes it tough for you to control their effects.

Another form of hormonal manipulation is the administration

of progestin-only birth control pills or injections, such as *norin-thindrone, medrogesteone,* and *medroxyprogesterone acetate.* (No, I don't expect you to remember these words, but should your doctor mention them, you can at least have a point of reference). These drugs also seem to inhibit prehormone secretion from the brain. However, as with the GnRH agents, these progestational agents are not a permanent treatment. They will temporarily decrease the size of the tumors, not eradicate them. Once the medication is stopped, the tumors will grow back.

What are the surgical options for fibroids?

Just because you are diagnosed with fibroid tumors doesn't mean you'll have to have surgery. Remember, these tumors cause no problem at all for many women. Your doctor may simply advise you to get regular checkups (something you should do anyway) so that she can monitor the fibroids and make sure they haven't grown or are causing you any problems.

If bleeding is a symptom you experience, your doctor will likely check for other possible causes of bleeding abnormalities before subjecting you to a specific operation for the tumors.

If, however, it is determined that you do need surgery for the tumors because of pain or other symptoms, you do have options, depending on the severity of the tumors (including their size and the symptoms you experience) and your plans for future childbearing. Prior to making a decision on a surgical procedure, you should carefully and thoroughly consider your plans, since the childbearing organ (the uterus) is directly involved.

If you require surgery for the fibroids, there are various treatment options available that your doctor should review with you, depending on the size of the tumors, the symptoms you are experiencing, and your future childbearing plans.

If you wish to keep your womb (i.e., *not* have a hysterectomy), then depending on your examination, symptoms, and ultrasound findings, a *myomectomy* may be recommended. This simply means removal of the myomas, or fibroids. (Note: anything ending in "-ectomy" means "removal of." *Tonsillectomy*: removal of the tonsils; *appendectomy*: removal of the appendix, etc.). Women choosing this procedure are able to keep their fertility options open, of course. This procedure is more fully discussed in the next chapter, as are other surgical procedures.

As difficult as these decisions can be, the good news is that thanks to technological advances and scientific research, women have more options than ever before. One of these new options is *uterine artery embolization*. This procedure cuts off the fibroids' blood supply and may decrease the symptoms. It is performed by an interventional radiologist—a specially trained x-ray doctor. Pellets are inserted into the uterine artery via suppositories and act to block blood flow—and thus, estrogen—to the fibroids. Without estrogen, fibroids' source of nutrients, the tumors aren't able to grow. The procedure has mostly been used overseas, but more and more U.S. hospitals are performing it with good results. Uterine artery embolization is not currently recommended for women who want to have children. However, instances of pregnancy have been reported in some women who have undergone minimal embolization. Uterine embolization is relatively new in this country, so statistics are still coming in—though reports are favorable concerning treating the fibroids.

ENDOMETRIOSIS

This is a condition in which fragments of the endometrium (the lining of the uterus) are found in other parts of, or organs within, the pelvic cavity. Normally, when the endometrial lining is shed each month during menstruation, it flows down and out through the cervix into the vagina. But with endometriosis, some of the blood and endometrial tissue flows upward, into the uterus, through the fallopian tubes, and into the pelvic cavity. Basically, the endometrial cells flow in reverse, a condition also described as "reverse menstruation."

The cause for this reversal is uncertain. But the wayward cells can adhere to and grow in or on the fallopian tubes, ovaries, cervix, bladder, intestines, pelvic ligaments, and other locations within the pelvic area. The displaced cells continue to act as if they were still in the uterus, and every month, often respond to the menstrual cycle by bleeding.

Under normal conditions, this blood would be expelled in the menstrual flow, but because these endometrial cells are not where they are supposed to be, the blood has nowhere to go. It is trapped in the pelvis, where it causes the formation of slowly growing cysts. The growth and swelling of the cysts are responsible for much of the pain associated with endometriosis—pain that is often severe and, at times, debilitating for many women. In fact, endometriosis has caused many days, weeks, and years of pelvic pain in a large number of women, resulting in lost wages and decreased production in the workforce. Endometriosis also causes inflammation, scar tissue, and even infertility.

Another possible factor in this disease process involves the body's immune system. Our immune systems, which usually help clear up and clean out abnormal cell processes, don't completely respond to the implantation of cells, and, thus, the cells can keep growing. Perhaps, since the endometrial cells are actually our own, the immune system doesn't kick in, failing to recognize their presence as abnormal.

Incidence of Endometriosis

Some reports put the incidence of endometriosis at 10 percent of American women. Whether this is an accurate figure or not, an accurate determination of its occurrence in black American women is even more difficult to ascertain, because this disease usually presents as pelvic pain. For many years, black women's "pelvic pain" that had no identifiable cause was often called pelvic inflammatory disease (PID), not endometriosis. The latter was considered a disease of more educated, higher-income women, while PID was and is due to pelvic infection, often acquired from sexual activity.

Was this just another attempt to disparage black women? Perhaps. But now, most clinicians see that endometriosis is an equal opportunity affliction that affects women of all races. And, since many black women have delayed childbearing in deference to their careers, the incidence of endometriosis in this population has increased significantly.

Studies show that anywhere from 15 to 71 percent of female patients—including black women—with chronic pelvic pain do, in fact, suffer from endometriosis.

What are the symptoms?

The signs of endometriosis can vary widely depending on where the displaced cells have adhered. As I've mentioned, pelvic pain, especially before and during menstruation, is a common symptom. Others include painful intercourse (known as *dyspareunia*), painful bowel movements, rectal bleeding, constipation, heavy menstrual bleeding, and irregular spotting between periods.

Making the Diagnosis

Based on these symptoms and a physical exam, a presumptive diagnosis of endometriosis may be made, but a laparoscopy or other surgical procedure that actually lets your doctor view the affected area is needed to confirm the diagnosis. During this procedure, a viewing instrument inserted through an incision at the navel is used to examine the abdominal cavity.

How is the disease treated?

Endometriosis may be treated with surgery or drug therapy, depending on the severity of the disease as well as other factors, including a woman's age, overall health, and her desire to have children.

During laparoscopy, the cell implants can be burned away, or vaporized, with a laser or a cautery instrument. However, the disease can recur because a woman will continue to have periods. A hysterectomy may be considered if a woman is not planning to have any more children or is near menopause. This option eliminates periods once and for all, so the disease will not recur. Many times, though, the ovaries may also need to be removed if they contain *endometriomas* (large cysts filled with aged menstrual blood).

If hormone drug therapy is advised, a woman may be prescribed GnRH agents to stop menstruation. These drugs will also help shrink the endometrial implants, which in turn will reduce pelvic pain. Some women may need to receive the drug for longer than the usual three-month regimen. Because of this, many doctors now provide a secondary medical regimen called *"add-back" therapy* in which small doses of estrogen are prescribed to help prevent the side effects of prolonged GnRH therapy. Remember, GnRH agents act to stop estrogen production, leading to menopausal side effects such as hot flashes, decreased sex drive, mood swings, and the possible onset of osteoporosis. However, the add-back estrogen dosage is not high enough to override the GnRH therapy's desired effect, according to recent research, including a study at Brigham and Women's Hospital of Harvard Medical School.

Other antiestrogen drugs that may be used to treat endometriosis include Depo-Provera and Danazol.

Depo-Provera, an injection often prescribed for birth control, makes the body think it's pregnant and stops the menstrual cycle, causing the endometrial implants to regress and disappear for as long as the drug is used.

Danazol also prevents menstruation, but this particular drug has a more masculinizing effect, similar to that caused by the male hormone testosterone. As a result, women taking Danazol may experience hair growth in unwanted places.

Low-dose oral contraceptives are yet another drug treatment choice, although they are usually prescribed to women who have received some form of surgical treatment and don't want more radical surgery, because they want to maintain their childbearing ability. In this circumstance, a woman may take low-dose oral contraceptives until she wishes to attempt conception.

In severe cases, or when the woman has tried other less invasive treatments, a hysterectomy may be recommended to permanently resolve this oft-debilitating condition. Simply removing the uterus can help, but since endometriosis can affect the tubes and ovaries, it is not uncommon to have the uterus, tubes, and ovaries removed together in order to completely eradicate the condition.

ADENOMYOSIS

Also called *internal* or *uterine endometriosis,* this is a condition characterized by the presence of endometrial glands and tissues *in* the uterine wall (the myometrium). Like endometriosis, adenomyosis also begins with a reverse menstrual flow: instead of leaving the body, the menstrual fluid flows to areas it shouldn't. With adenomyosis, however, the endometrial cells actually implant themselves in the walls of the uterus and get trapped between the muscle fibers. Why this happens is not certain, but some research suggests that it may be due to a disturbance of the closely knit uterine muscle fibers caused by a prior pregnancy or a previous surgical procedure such as a dilatation and curettage (D&C).

What are the symptoms?

Pelvic pain is the most common one. The implantation of misplaced endometrial cells in the uterine walls causes the uterus to become very tender, especially when touched, as with an examination, or when manipulated or moved, as during intercourse.

Women suffering from adenomyosis will also experience irregular and heavier periods. Patients often describe the bleeding as periodic and crampy.

When a doctor physically examines a woman with this condition, he will usually feel a boggy, soft, mildly enlarged uterus. Because pregnancy can also cause irregular bleeding, pelvic discomfort, and a soft uterus, it's important to have a pregnancy test done to make sure a woman with these symptoms isn't with child.

How is adenomyosis diagnosed?

The condition can be hard to diagnose judging solely by a woman's symptoms. That's because a definitive diagnosis can only be reached by examining the uterus microscopically after it has been removed via hysterectomy (usually to end chronic pelvic pain).

Because diagnosis is difficult, it is also difficult to determine how many women suffer from adenomyosis. According to recent research, about 15 to 25 percent of chronic pelvic pain cases that result in hysterectomy are determined to have been caused by adenomyosis. Of course, no one wants to have a hysterectomy in order to find out if this condition is the underlying cause of abdominal pain and irregular heavy periods. Fortunately, doctors have had some success in using *magnetic resonance imaging* (MRI) to detect the condition. MRI is a diagnostic technique that provides high-quality images of organs and structures in the body without using X rays or other radiation. CT scans, however, are not reported to be as accurate. Laparoscopy is not usually helpful in detecting adenomyosis either, since the endometrial cells are within the uterine walls, and a laparoscope allows only the surface of the uterus to be seen.

How is adenomyosis treated?

Since the majority of cases are diagnosed after the uterus is removed, this, by definition, solves the problem for good. For women with a milder form of the disease, or those wishing to preserve their childbearing ability, other treatment options are available, including GnRH therapy, progesterone IUDs, endometrial ablation in which the doctor cauterizes the endometrium, or the surgical removal of a wedge of the uterine wall following an MRI.

PELVIC CONGESTION SYNDROME

Most people know what varicose veins are, and what they look like. Pelvic congestion syndrome is similar to varicose veins, only instead of affecting blood vessels in your legs, it affects the blood vessels supplying your pelvic structures, specifically those alongside the uterus and those supplying blood to the fallopian tubes and ovaries. When pelvic congestion syndrome occurs, these particular blood vessels become so engorged with blood that they appear ready to burst.

No one knows for sure why this condition occurs, but it can cause intense pelvic pain, especially during menstruation, sexual intercourse, and exercise.

How is it diagnosed?

The condition is usually diagnosed during a laparoscopy—the most common procedure performed to evaluate a woman's complaint of chronic pelvic pain. Occasionally a CT scan or MRI will uncover the problem.

How is it treated?

Nonsteroidal anti-inflammatory drugs (NSAIDs), such as aspirin or ibuprofen, may be used to relieve pain if the swellings are small. But in most patients they only provide temporary relief, and surgery is required to remove the veins. Unfortunately, this may involve removal of the ovary or fallopian tube on the most affected side.

ADNEXAL MASS

This term may sound very specific, but *adnexal mass* is actually a vague, often-used, "catch-all" phrase that means the doctor feels something abnormal in the lower right (right lower quadrant or RLQ) or left side (left lower quadrant or LLQ) of the pelvis, medically referred to as the adnexa, the area next to the uterus. This is the area where the ovaries are located.

An adnexal mass can result from many things. Usually it stems from an enlargement of the ovaries or fallopian tubes, or from a tumor with a stalklike base hanging off the uterus into the adnexal area, or some other abnormal growth from other internal structures such as the intestines.

What are the symptoms?

Pain or discomfort in the affected area is a common sign. If the mass is large, there may also be increased abdominal girth and a feeling of fullness in the area. If the mass is an ovarian cyst or an endometrial growth, irregular vaginal bleeding may occur as well.

How is it diagnosed?

The mainstay of diagnosis is the pelvic exam and an ultrasound. Since your physician knows what normal ovaries feel like, he will classify anything over that size as an adnexal mass. An adnexal mass can usually be felt by your doctor during a pelvic exam. He will feel fullness in the lower left or right side of the pelvis. In most cases, a pregnancy test should be performed to make sure the mass is not an *ectopic pregnancy* (a pregnancy that develops outside the uterus, most commonly in the fallopian tube). Once pregnancy is ruled out, an ultrasound may be done to determine if the enlargement is a simple clear cyst on the ovary, if it contains blood, or if it has solid components.

There are also other pelvic abnormalities such as cancers, or benign processes that can create this type of mass. Some of these are very strange growths. One in particular, called a *teratoma,* is an ovarian tumor that can actually contain all the components that your body is made of. These ovarian cystic teratomas can enclose hair, teeth, bone, cartilage, and fat (really!). Interestingly, these tumors are very common in black American women.

Other radiologic studies can be done (CT scan or MRI), but

these are much more expensive, and the ultrasound usually gives enough information about the mass to consider cause and treatment plans.

If a cancer is suspected of causing adnexal masses to form, further procedures will be required to confirm this.

How is it treated?

Treatment will vary depending on the size and characteristics of the mass. Repeated observation may be in order for simple ovarian cysts that are small and not causing severe pain. In this scenario, patients are given nonsteroidal anti-inflammatory drugs for pain relief and advised to apply heating pads and take warm baths for two to three weeks. After that time, they are re-examined to see if the mass has diminished.

If it is still present, a laparoscopy will be performed. If you recall, this is the procedure in which an internal viewing instrument is used to view the abdominal cavity. This procedure is used when a mass persists past the observation period. A laparoscopy is also done when the diagnosis is unclear and cancer must be ruled out, when pain is severe, when the mass appears to be growing, or when unusual characteristics were seen on the ultrasound. Most adnexal masses can be removed during the laparoscopy. In some cases, this means having to remove the structure containing the mass (such as the ovary), but in other instances, the mass can be excised while leaving the organ in place.

If the mass is too large to be handled through a laparoscope, a laparotomy may be performed. Unlike a laparoscopy, in which a viewing instrument is inserted through a small abdominal incision, a laparotomy calls for the abdominal cavity to be opened. The doctor may opt for this operation if widespread cancer is of concern, because he will be able to explore the entire abdomen. However, with the advanced laparoscopic techniques available today, most adnexal masses are treated through the smaller, less invasive laparoscopy procedure.

CHRONIC PELVIC PAIN (CPP)

Ask any obstetrician/gynecologist, and they'll tell you that the four most common problems women seek services for are pregnancy, vaginal discharge, bleeding problems, and pelvic pain. Chronic pelvic pain (CPP) means that you have been experiencing pelvic pain continuously over time, usually for at least six months. The problem with this term is that it's somewhat vague, covering a wide array of possible problems. The trick is to get to the underlying cause of the pain, then something can be done to alleviate it.

What causes CPP?

The culprit may be one of many things and therefore, we're going to take a little extra time discussing the possibilities for CPP, to try to help you distinguish between normal discomfort and a potential medical problem. So many times, we may hastily assume that a twinge we feel is a sign of a problem when really it's a normal process. Contrarily, we are just as likely to ignore certain twinges and pains that we need to pay attention to. Additionally, not every discomfort we feel is necessarily of gynecologic origin—or "female-related."

So how do you determine what's normal discomfort as opposed to abnormal discomfort? *Normal discomforts* can include pains or cramps associated with ovulation and/or the menstrual cycle. Many women experience periodic cramping just before the onset and mostly during the monthly period. These menstrual cramps are due to the release of certain body chemicals called *prostaglandins* that act on the uterus, causing contractionlike activity.

Menstrual cramps should not be debilitating, however. If they are, a pelvic examination may help reveal problems like fibroids, cysts, or other conditions.

Some women get pain midway between their cycles. This is usually due to ovulation, when the egg "pops out" from the ovary. The official name for this midcycle pain is *mittelschmerz*. This pain usually stops after two to three days or may last until the onset of the cycle.

Abnormal discomforts may be related to one's female organs or be caused by other organs like the bowels or bladder.

Gynecological problems that can cause pain include fibroid tumors, tubal pregnancies, or pelvic infections such as gonorrhea, chlamydia, trichomonas, and other bacterial inflammations of the pelvic structures. Endometriosis is another common cause of gynecological pelvic pain.

There are, however, other causes of pain that involve other pelvic structures. Let's review some of these other body parts and the most common conditions that may cause pelvic pain. (Be sure to review the box on page 135, listing many causes for CPP.)

Bladder—Bladder infections are a common cause of pelvic pain. These infections usually cause frequent and painful urination, difficulty urinating, or blood in the urine.

Other urinary tract conditions include *stones* (hardened clusters of a body chemical), which may come from the kidney. As the stone leaves the kidney and passes through the narrow tube that connects the kidney to the bladder (called the *ureter*), severe, excruciating pain may be experienced.

Bladder *spasms* (a crampy tightening or contraction) are also uncomfortable.

Intestines—Intestinal diseases include *ulcerative colitis* and *Crohn's disease,* which are major bowel diseases that often need medical and even surgical intervention. Depending on which one is present, the patient may see blood or mucus in the stools; have loose, watery stools; or abdominal cramping or distention.

Constipation can also cause discomfort, especially if your bowels are very dry and hard to move. Eating a high-fiber diet and drinking at least eight glasses of water each day helps to keep your bowels moving freely.

Intestinal obstruction can also cause severe pelvic and abdominal pain. This is usually associated, however, with nausea and vomiting.

Also, don't forget *appendicitis* as a cause of pain. The appendix is on your lower right side.

Muscles, Bones, and Ligaments—Patients may have pain from musculoskeletal problems. Have you pulled some muscles? Strained some ligaments? Twisted the wrong way or too hard? Have you fallen or bumped into furniture or some other hard object?

Adhesions—*Adhesions* are a common cause of pelvic pain. These are scar tissues that essentially cause internal structures to stick together, resulting in mild or severe pain. Internal infections such as gonorrhea, previous surgery, or conditions like endometriosis can cause the formation of adhesions.

Unfortunately, the best way to remove adhesions is to have surgery, which can cause the possibility of forming new adhesions at a later time. However, there are some products on the market that doctors can use to help prevent adhesion formation at the time of an operation.

As you evaluate your pelvic pain, run through the following checklist to help determine the possible source:

- When was your last period?

- Was it normal?

- Are you in midcycle?

- Is the pain brought on by certain foods?

- When did you last move your bowels? Was the stool normal?

- Have you had any nausea and vomiting?

- Are there changes in your urine?

Remember, an occasional twinge here or there may just be a normal process. Persistent or worsening pain should always be evaluated by your health care professional and appropriate X rays or other diagnostic studies performed.

The box opposite will give you a clearer idea of just how many conditions can be at the root of chronic pelvic pain.

Incidence of CPP

The impact of CPP is significant. According to *Women's Health Reports,* chronic pelvic pain accounts for 20 percent of all laparoscopies and 12 percent of the hysterectomies done, and can cause loss of wages and productivity exceeding $1 billion annually. Additionally, CPP is often a source of frustration, anger, marital discord, and depression for patients, while doctors and their staff can also experience similar frustration when a patient seems not to show signs of improvement with her symptoms or complaint of CPP.

Primary Causes of Chronic Pelvic Pain

Gynecological diseases

endometriosis
ovarian cysts or tumors
adenomyosis
pelvic adhesion
fibroid tumors
genital tract obstruction
pelvic congestion syndrome

Urological disorders

urinary tract infection (UTI)
urinary stones (kidney, bladder, ureteral)
interstitial cystitis
pelvic relaxation

Infectious disorders

pelvic inflammatory disease
(resulting from a sexually transmitted disease)

Gastrointestinal disorders

inflammatory bowel disease (Crohn's disease, colitis)
irritable bowel syndrome
peptic ulcer
cancer

Musculoskeletal disorders

muscle strain or pain
gait disorders
osteoporosis and other bone disorders

Psychological disorders

depression
anxiety
post-traumatic stress disorder

Surgical disorders

hernia
poor healing of wound

What are the symptoms of CPP?

The first indication that chronic pelvic pain is not simply due to your menstrual cycle appears when the pain persists throughout the month, not just right before or during your period. The pain is, for the most part, constant and not usually relieved by over-the-counter medications. Once these two things occur, you need to make an appointment with your doctor to determine the cause of the pain.

Diagnosis

In addition to taking your complete medical history and giving you a physical exam, your doctor will likely order tests such as an ultrasound, CT scan, MRI, or other procedures to find the source of your pain. If the tests reveal a mass or growth, your doctor will prescribe the necessary course of action to treat the mass. But if the ultrasound or other tests don't reveal a growth, and a conservative treatment approach (prescription medication, for instance) fails to ease the pain, many patients then undergo an exploratory surgical procedure—usually a laparoscopy—in order for a concrete diagnosis to be made.

Laparoscopy is usually the surgery of first choice: the incisions are small, it's done as an outpatient procedure, many growths can be not only diagnosed but also removed through the scope, and the recovery time is short. Laparoscopy also allows the doctor to take a picture (or even a video) of findings at surgery. This is very helpful with CPP patients, for actually seeing what was causing the problem—and knowing that it is no longer present—provides additional emotional relief after a long episode with a particular problem.

On the other hand, for those patients in whom no physical

cause was first identified, but the complaint of pain persisted—meaning their CPP is likely psychological in nature—sometimes the laparoscopic pictures may give the patient assurance there is nothing there. For some, the pictures help; for others, it only makes them want to look further, and their physical complaints persist. Again, most times, a definite cause for the pain is found, but when it is not, frustration can mount for all involved.

Unfortunately, some women who complain of CPP do so not because of true pelvic problems but because of a psychological need or cause. These patients have been known to seemingly live in their doctor's office, never finding any relief despite a thorough workup, diagnostic studies, and even surgery to search for a cause. They can run up tens of thousands of dollars in medical bills or insurance claims searching for an answer. These situations cause a great deal of frustration for the patient, her family, the doctor, and his/her staff. As a result of frustration, some patients jump from doctor to doctor, especially if their physician makes the suggestion to the patient that her condition is, or seems to be, psychological in origin.

Fortunately, most patients with CPP have an actual disease that can be diagnosed with laparoscopy and treated, with mostly good results.

Treatment for CPP

As mentioned, initial treatment plans are based on the diagnostic findings. If a mass is found, observation, then medication and/or surgery is in order. If there's no mass or other definite finding, a continued search for a cause must take place. A laparoscopy may be performed to look inside for anything that may not be showing up on the studies. Adhesions, for example, rarely—if ever—are visible on X rays and ultrasounds but are readily apparent at laparoscopy, and can be removed or broken down. Other treatments are used as indicated, including emotional support and a nurturing spirit on the part of the doctor and staff as well as the patient, her family, and her friends. Last, for complicated cases, a multidisciplinary approach may be indicated, utilizing specialists in intestinal, urological, musculoskeletal, and other diseases. Psychiatric assistance may also become necessary.

PELVIC RELAXATION

Over time the musculature of the pelvic organs weakens through the normal occurrences of life—pregnancy; sexual intercourse; long-term increases in intra-abdominal pressure caused by laughing, coughing, and weight gain; increased age; decreased estrogen; and, of course, gravity. Vaginal walls become weak and flaccid. They are no longer firmly in place. As the vaginal walls lose their tone, the structures behind them—the bladder and/or rectum, for instance—can "slip down." This dropping down of the pelvic structures, and the possible problems that can arise as a result, are called *pelvic relaxation*—or more precisely, pelvic organ prolapse. Simply put, part or all of a pelvic organ is displaced from its normal position, and patients often say their "parts are hanging out."

Incidence

While this condition is more common in white women than black women, it does affect us, especially if we have had numerous children, tend to carry excess abdominal weight, smoke and/or have respiratory diseases, and work at jobs that require a lot of standing (such as cashiers, salesclerks, and waitresses).

Nearly half of women (40 percent) who suffer from pelvic relaxation are over age 60, and 22 percent are age 70 or older. With women living longer than ever, the numbers are bound to increase.

What are the symptoms?

A feeling of pressure in the vagina is the primary complaint of women with pelvic relaxation. Painful sexual intercourse is also common. Other symptoms include vaginal dryness, urinary problems (incontinence, a sense of urgency, frequent urination), and intestinal problems (incomplete bowel movements, frequent bowel movements, straining during a bowel movement).

How is it diagnosed?

Diagnosing this condition is fairly easy because in many patients some protrusion of their pelvic structure is readily visible during the examination. For an accurate and definitive diagnosis, however, your doctor will begin by taking a thorough medical history. You will be asked a series of specific and pertinent questions, such as:

• your age

• the number of pregnancies you have had and how much each child weighed at birth (especially vaginal births)

• your current weight and whether or not you have gained weight

• if you have any chronic medical conditions, like respiratory problems that may cause you to have frequent periods of intra-abdominal pressure. You'll also be asked about illnesses and habits associated with chronic coughing, such as asthma, emphysema, bronchitis, chronic obstructive pulmonary disease, cigarette smoking, and others.

- if you have had any pelvic surgical procedures (they may have affected the tissue strength in the vagina)

- your hormone status—whether you are menopausal or taking any hormone/estrogen treatment

- if you are experiencing any of the symptoms associated with pelvic relaxation

After taking your medical history, your doctor will move on to the physical exam. This will be an overall assessment, with special attention given to your abdomen and pelvic region. (You will probably be given a lung exam, too, to check for diseases that cause you to cough a lot or otherwise cause pressure in the pelvic area.) You can expect the following to occur during your exam:

- While lying on the exam table with your feet in stirrups, you will be asked to "bear down" as if you are trying to move your stool. If you have extensive pelvic relaxation the inner tissues will push down and out without the doctor's even having to separate the vaginal lips. Many times when this is the case, the tissue gives the appearance of an uncircumcised penis.

- If the pelvic relaxation is not severe, the doctor will gently separate the vaginal lips, have you bear down again, and then make an observation. (The "grade"—or degree—of pelvic relaxation is determined by how far down the tissues protrude.)

- Next, your doctor will have you stand, bend over, and bear down once more so that she can assess the pelvic relaxation from a different angle.

- An internal vaginal exam and a digital rectal exam will also be performed to further aid in the diagnosis.

Depending on which pelvic structure is relaxed, you will get a diagnosis of either:

- Cystocele—weakness in the front (or upper) vaginal wall, causing the bladder to hang down

- Rectocele—weakness in the back (or lower) vaginal wall, causing the rectum to protrude in toward the vagina

- Enterocele—an internal condition in which the intestinal sacs become situated between the folds of the vagina and the rectum inside your body

*Can any of the symptoms ever
be a sign of something else?*

Yes, especially incontinence. Patients with urinary problems associated with pelvic relaxation will often experience incontinence. Because the vaginal walls have weakened, giving less support to the bladder, the opening of the bladder (the urethra) will not be in its normal position. This shift in position leaves the bladder susceptible to simple daily functions like laughing or coughing. Any increase in intra-abdominal pressure (from, say, a laugh or a cough) is likely to cause urine to leak.

To assess the incontinence, diabetes must be ruled out, as well as any other diseases that affect the nervous system's control over the bladder. You will probably have a test called cystometrics, also known as urodynamics. This procedure actually tests the flow and control of your urine. Small pressure-gauge tubes are placed in the vagina, the urethra, and/or the rectum. As you urinate, measurements of your bladder are taken. This test is important because if your incontinence is due purely to a structural abnormality such as pelvic relaxation, surgery will likely help. But if the incontinence is the result of a nerve condition, surgery won't do any good. Medicine may be prescribed instead. Urodynamics will help your doctor determine your best course of treatment.

How is pelvic relaxation treated?

As you've just learned, treatment depends on whether or not your symptoms stem from a neurogenic problem or a structural one (actually due to the weakness in tissue strength).

If your medical history, physical exam, and test results indicate that you have some type of nerve condition—diabetes, for instance, which can affect the nerve supply to the pelvic organs causing similar symptoms—then you will be treated for that primary disease. However, if your problems are truly due to pelvic relaxation, surgery is usually the treatment of choice.

For patients who may not be good surgical candidates (or who opt not to have surgery), a prosthetic device, called a pessary, may be placed in the vagina to help alleviate the symptoms, but it does not correct the condition.

Your doctor will discuss the various surgical options with you. As with any operation, there are risks; and with surgical procedures for pelvic relaxation, in particular, recurrence is a very likely possibility, especially if the conditions causing it remain unchanged. For instance, if you are older and have a cystocele that can be linked to decreased estrogen and overweight, even if you have surgery, you may experience pelvic relaxation again if those factors stay the same.

Can the condition be prevented?

While you can't do anything about certain contributing factors, like age, previous pregnancies, and the laws of gravity, you can fight back on other fronts:

- Maintain a normal weight and pay special attention to your midsection. Having a trim, toned, strong abdomen helps stave off pelvic relaxation. If you are currently overweight, begin a sensible exercise and nutrition plan to shed those excess pounds.

- If you smoke, quit. And if you take asthma medication, make sure to take it regularly as prescribed by your doctor. Be diligent about getting treatment for any respiratory ailments, like asthma, bronchitis, and so on.

- If you suffer from diabetes, follow your doctor's recommendations to keep it under control. Better still, try to rid yourself of it altogether by dropping excess pounds if you are overweight and limiting your intake of sweets. Talk to your doctor about other ways to battle diabetes.

- Do Kegel exercises. They are easy to do. Simply tighten then relax your vaginal muscles several times during the day. You can do them while sitting, lying down, driving—anytime, anywhere. And no one will even know you're doing them.

These movements help maintain muscle tone in the vagina. Kegel exercises are often advised for women with minimal pelvic relaxation to help strengthen the vaginal walls.

- Avoid constipation by making sure to have enough fiber (whole grains, fresh fruit, vegetables) in your diet and by drinking plenty of fluids each day.

- Don't hold your urine. Whenever you feel the urge to go, go.

- If you notice any of the symptoms associated with pelvic re-laxation, see your doctor. Don't put off having a physical exam. The sooner the condition is caught, the easier it will be to treat.

MENSTRUAL DISORDERS

For many of us, our "time of the month" is often accompanied by cramps, bloating, and moodiness. Some sisters must also con-tend with irregular periods, while others of us see our cycles arrive like clockwork, the same time every month. Mild physical discom-fort and possible irregularity are common aspects of menstrua-tion—things we learn to cope with as women. Other occurrences, however, aren't so normal and may be caused by several factors. Let's take a look at a few of these menstrual disorders.

Amenorrhea: This terms refers to the absence of menstruation. While it's not that unusual for some women to miss a period on oc-casion, repeatedly missing your cycle could signal an underlying problem. The most common reason for a missed period in women of reproductive age is pregnancy. If you are older, it may indicate the onset of menopause. Other causes of amenorrhea:

- Certain contraceptives can affect your menstrual cycle, such as Depo-Provera and birth control pills. Talk to your doctor to see if your method of contraception is interfering with your menstrual cycle and if you need to alter your birth control.

- Uterine abnormalities, like structural deformities either from birth or as a result of a medical condition, can also contribute to the cessation of menses.

- Stress can upset the stability of your hormones, resulting in missed periods.

- Fluctuations in weight can also be the culprit, especially in women who suffer from *anorexia nervosa,* an eating disorder in which a person has a distorted body image and diets to such a degree that she becomes emaciated.

- Strenuous exercise can play a role as well. It's not uncommon for high-level athletes, such as marathon runners, Olympic competitors, and other athletes of that class who train heavily, to stop menstruating. The amenorrhea can last for months, even years. In most of these cases, stopped periods are due to a deficiency of body fat, a vital part of estrogen production, which is necessary for normal menstruation to occur.

- Certain illnesses, such as diabetes, thyroid disease, ovarian cysts, and anemia, can also impede menstrual flow.

- Aside from contraceptives, other medications may be at the root of amenorrhea. Chemotherapy agents, hormone medication, steroids, and other drug therapies can stop or alter menses.

Hypomenorrhea: This means lighter and/or shorter periods. Birth control pills are the most common reason for hypomenorrhea. The hormones in the pills affect the endometrium, causing it not to thicken as much as it normally would. Therefore, once it's shed, the menstrual flow seems much lighter. Weight fluctuations can cause lighter periods as well because of the disruption that weight gain or loss causes in your hormone levels. Another culprit could be early pregnancy. During the first one to two months of pregnancy, some women experience spotting instead of a normal full flow when their period is due. Finally, hypomenorrhea can also be caused by stress or by certain medications.

Hypermenorrhea: This condition of heavier and/or longer periods may be the result of fibroid tumors or other growths in the womb, such as polyps. It may even be a sign of endometrial cancer, though fibroids are the more common culprit, especially in black women. At one time, IUDs were a very common cause of hypermenorrhea because the device irritated the lining of the womb. But today, the newer IUDs make this less of a problem, though it may still occur in some women. Another less common cause of heavy, long periods is bleeding abnormalities, such as sickle-cell disease and hemophilia.

Oligomenorrhea: This term refers to infrequent periods—more than thirty-five days apart. Unusually long stretches between cycles are often due to either obesity or being underweight, both of which upset your body's hormonal balance, specifically estrogen production. With obesity comes an excess of estrogen. Being underweight diminishes estrogen production. Having few periods may seem like a blessing—after all, what sister actually enjoys this time of the month?—but it may not be. You must see your doctor to determine the underlying cause, especially if you are sexually active. Pregnancy, ectopic pregnancy, and other conditions must be ruled out. Your physician may try to stimulate your period. This helps her determine if your basic hormonal makeup is sound.

Intermenstrual Bleeding: This condition means bleeding between periods. Spotting between cycles can be caused by any number of things. Sometimes it's simply ovulatory bleeding—as the egg is released from the ovary, a small amount of blood may be released as well. This type of spotting usually appears for just a few months, then stops. Other times, bleeding between periods can also be caused by stress, certain medications, IUDs, or sexually transmitted disease. Abnormal growths such as fibroids, cysts, or cancerous tumors can also cause intermenstrual bleeding, as can bleeding abnormalities, including sickle-cell disease. If you notice spotting after sexual intercourse it may indicate an infection, polyps, or inflammation of the cervix or vagina.

What are the signs and symptoms?

The good news about menstrual disorders is that recognizing a problem may exist is easy. You get your period every month. You know it's coming and you know what your normal side effects are, be it a little bloating, cramps, or minor irritability. The point is, after all of these years you know what to expect. So when something unexpected occurs—you miss your period, it's heavier or lighter than usual, you've been spotting in between cycles—you know immediately that something is up. If you notice a change in or anything unusual about your period, see your doctor to find out what's causing it. To best do this, it is always important for you to know the first day of each cycle and how long it lasts.

Diagnosis

In addition to thoroughly discussing your symptoms with you, your doctor will give you a physical, take a blood count, and perform a pregnancy test to rule out pregnancy or miscarriage. From there, you will likely have an endometrial biopsy in which a sample of womb tissue is checked for chronic inflammation, hormonal disorders, and other problems. You may also be scheduled for an ultrasound to check for fibroids, cysts, or other growths.

Treatment

Treatment is determined after a full diagnostic workup is accomplished. Depending on the cause of your menstrual abnormality, medication or surgery may be recommended. Commonly, patients will be given medication to stimulate a period if it's been absent (after pregnancy has been ruled out, of course).

If there's been excessive bleeding, either pills or injections may be prescribed; or, if the bleeding is very excessive—or the patient is unresponsive to previously prescribed medications—she may undergo a hysteroscopy or a *dilation and curettage* (D&C).

As mentioned earlier, hysteroscopy involves looking into the uterine cavity with a long, narrow scope. This allows your doctor to actually view the lining of the womb and any excessive tissue growths, polyps, tumors, etc., that may be present. Also, a sampling of the tissue can be obtained under direct visualization. Small fibroids may be removed through the scope if the tumors are on the innermost wall of the uterus.

A D&C is the actual scraping of the entire uterine lining (endometrium) from the inner wall of the uterus. This procedure not only allows the tissue to be tested for cancer, infections, and hormonal problems but also causes the lining to be renewed. Usually a more normal, less heavy flow returns.

Endometrial ablation is a procedure wherein, after a hysteroscopy, the lining of the womb is touched by a very hot rolling ball. This can actually cauterize the bleeding points causing the problems. This procedure is not recommended for women who desire to have more children, as the long-term effects of cauterizing the lining of the womb on future pregnancy potential are still undetermined. Many women report improvement with this procedure, though the excessive bleeding may recur in others.

More definitive surgical procedures may be employed when all other, lesser modalities have failed to rectify the problem. These more involved procedures include myomectomy (if fibroids are present) or hysterectomy, when necessary.

Can you prevent menstrual disorders?

Yes, there are things you can do to cut your risk of developing problems with your period. Maintain a healthy weight. Try to avoid stress. Keep track of your menstrual cycles on a calendar, noting the start and end dates and the nature of the flow. Get regular checkups and pelvic exams. If you take birth control pills, make sure to take them as directed. It's best to take them at the same time every day. Be certain that any medication you are taking has not expired; if it has, its effectiveness may be compromised. Finally, if you do notice a change or abnormality in your period, see your doctor about it right away. Don't assume it will pass. Your body is trying to tell you something. Listen.

UTERINE ANOMALIES

What are anomalies? An anomaly is a deviation from the normal way something is supposed to be. So a *uterine anomaly* refers to the instances in which the uterus was not formed properly, giving it an abnormal structure, which can affect reproductive function later in life. Also, as we grow older, things like fibroids can give an anomalous shape to the uterus.

Fortunately, true genetic uterine anomalies are not extremely common, but they do occur with enough frequency to merit mention. Should you be diagnosed with a genetic uterine anomaly, be sure your doctor thoroughly discusses all the possibilities for treatment with you, and that you have a clear understanding of what is discussed in order to achieve the best outcome for your reproductive future.

SEXUALLY TRANSMITTED DISEASES (STDS)

Today, in the new millennium, we are much more educated about the risks of unsafe sex. There's no denying that the AIDS epidemic has opened many eyes. We hear about sexually transmitted diseases on the news. We read about them in newspapers and magazines. We are informed through public service announcements. Yet, despite our increased knowledge the sad fact is that the rate of sexually transmitted diseases is on the rise. And the effects are far-reaching. STDs can wreak havoc on your health since many of them have chronic, long-lasting, even life-threatening effects. And they can harm you psychologically as well. That's why it's so important to not only know the facts but also heed their message.

What are sexually transmitted diseases?

An STD—now also called STI for *sexually transmitted infection*—is an infection that is contracted through sexual activity, which includes vaginal and oral intercourse, and oral sex. There are various types of STDs, and we'll be taking a closer look at some of the most common ones. One thing you need to realize right off the bat, though, is that sexually transmitted diseases are serious business and need to be treated as soon as possible. Otherwise they can lead to a host of problems, including pelvic inflammatory disease, infertility, and more.

According to the United States Department of Health and Human Services Office on Women's Health, more than 12 million cases of sexually transmitted diseases are reported in this country every year. Unfortunately, African Americans are 1.3 times more likely to contract one than are Caucasians, according to a 1999 University of Chicago study. What this means for sisters is that we are at heightened risk. Right now the incidence of syphilis, herpes, chlamydia, and venereal warts (warts caused by human papillomavirus, HPV) is increasing at an alarming rate. In the early 1990s, gonorrhea was the only STD to see a decrease in occurrence. But *Health, United States, 2001* reports an increase in the condition since 1999, with 133 cases per 100,000 population, with the highest incidence in African Americans.

There is reason for hope, though. STDs are preventable. The key is safer sex. Whenever you engage in sexual activity, whether oral, anal, or vaginal intercourse, use condoms or dental dams to avoid contracting an STD. Barrier contraceptives, such as diaphragms, can also protect against STDs when used with a spermicide. Bear in mind, though, that the only way to guard against HIV, other than abstinence, is by using condoms. Barrier contraceptives alone won't protect you against that. As you can see, there is much

SEXUALLY TRANSMITTED INFECTIONS

ORGANISMS	DISEASES

Bacteria

Neisseria gonorrhoeae	Gonorrhea
Chlamydia trachomatis	Chlamydial infection
Treponema pallidum	Syphilis
Haemophilus ducreyi	Chancroid
Calymmatobacterium granulomatis	Granuloma inguinale
Gardnerella vaginalis, anaerobes	Bacterial vaginosis
Group B β-hemolytic streptococcus	Group B strep infection

Mycoplasmas

Mycoplasma hominis	Mycoplasma infection
Ureaplasma urealyticum	Mycoplasma infection

Viruses

Herpesvirus hominis	Genital herpes
Cytomegalovirus (CMV)	CMV infection
Hepatitis B virus	Hepatitis B
Human papillomavirus (HPV)	Genital warts
Molluscum contagiosum virus	Molluscum contagiosum
Human immunodeficiency virus	HIV/AIDS

Protozoa

Trichomonas vaginalis	Trichomoniasis
Entamoeba histolytica	Inflammation of rectum

Fungi

Candida albicans	Candidiasis (yeast infection)

Parasites

Sarcoptes scabiei	Scabies
Phthirus pubis	Crab lice infestation

Source: from Danforth's *Obstetrics and Gynecology*

to know when it comes to sexually transmitted diseases. You can also see in the table opposite that there are numerous STDs out there, some you probably haven't even heard of!

For the sake of this writing, we'll focus on the primary culprits. So let's take a more in-depth look at a few of the most common STDs.

Chlamydia: Spread through vaginal and anal intercourse, chlamydia is the most common STD, with 4 million cases reported each year. Chlamydia can be a "silent" infection, existing undetected for months because it sometimes presents no symptoms. All the while, however, the infection is causing damage to a woman's inner reproductive organs. If symptoms are present, they typically include pelvic pain, abnormal vaginal discharge, painful or burning urination, and painful intercourse. A cell culture performed by your doctor can detect the disease, which can be treated with oral antibiotics such as doxycycline or metronidazole.

Sexual partners should be tested and treated (if necessary) for the disease to prevent reinfection. If left untreated, chlamydia can cause inflammation or scarring of the fallopian tubes, leading to infertility and inflammation of the cervix. A pregnant woman infected with the STD can pass it on to her baby, who may develop eye infections or pneumonia as a result.

Gonorrhea: This STD is spread through vaginal and anal intercourse, as well as through oral sex. If fellatio is performed on an infected partner, the woman can get gonococcal pharyngitis— gonorrhea of the throat—which is characterized by the appearance of yellow-white curdlike patches on the throat and soreness in the throat. Though gonorrhea is most prevalent among teenage girls between the ages of 15 and 19, black women are disproportionately affected as well. According to the Department of Health and Human Services, the incidence of gonorrhea in African-American women ages 34 to 39 is more than 20 times that of white women.

As with chlamydia, gonorrhea is a major cause of pelvic inflammatory disease (PID), which can severely affect the internal reproductive organs, possibly rendering them scarred or blocked and causing infertility. Gonorrhea is also similar to chlamydia in that often women exhibit no symptoms. The bacteria has a short incubation period of just a few days. It only takes about two days after infection for the bacteria to grow in your system. If symptoms do appear, they will start a few days after the incubation period. When symptoms are present they may include a thick, yellowish-white puslike discharge, burning or pain when urinating, urinary frequency, spotting, painful intercourse, swelling around the vulva, and possible fever.

Your doctor can test for gonorrhea by obtaining a cervical culture. The lab results should take about two days. Gonorrhea is treated with antibiotics. Oral antibiotics may be prescribed in conjunction with antibiotic injections. Because gonorrhea and chlamydia are often present at the same time, the antibiotics prescribed will effectively treat both STDs. "Pelvic rest" is also recommended. You will be advised to abstain from sex and strenuous activity during treatment. Make sure sexual partners are tested and treated, too.

If left untreated, gonorrhea can lead to many other serious problems in addition to pelvic inflammatory disease and possible sterility, including arthritis, disorders of the central nervous system, heart problems, and eye infections in newborns.

Hepatitis: Hepatitis is an inflammation of the liver that can lead to liver damage, liver disease, and even death. Hepatitis may be either acute (of limited duration) or chronic (continuing). Acute hepatitis is typically brought on by a viral infection, although it can also be caused by heavy alcohol consumption. There are three primary types of viral hepatitis: hepatitis A, B, and C.

Hepatitis A (formerly called infectious hepatitis) is spread primarily by an infected person's feces contaminating food or water. Ingesting contaminated food or water isn't the only way to contract the virus, however. Someone with hepatitis A can spread the virus to others who live in the same household (especially if he or she is not diligent about hand washing after using the bathroom), or to a sexual partner through anal sex. So good personal hygiene and a sanitary environment are extremely important.

Symptoms of hepatitis A may include dark urine, whites of the eyes that take on a yellow tint (jaundice), tiredness, loss of appetite, possible nausea, vomiting, fever, or stomachache.

Someone with hepatitis A can spread the virus 1 to 2 weeks before and up to a week after symptoms appear. It is possible to have hepatitis A and not exhibit any symptoms. But just because you don't show any signs of having the virus, it doesn't mean you can't infect others. You can. If you have symptoms, see your doctor for a diagnosis. The good news is that, unlike hepatitis B and C, hepatitis A does not cause long-term liver damage and usually doesn't cause death. The virus will not lead to chronic hepatitis. Once you have had the disease, your body becomes immune to future hepatitis A infection.

To protect yourself against contracting hepatitis A in the first place, heed these tips:

- Make good hygiene your number one priority. Always wash your hands thoroughly after using the bathroom, after changing a diaper, before eating, and before and after preparing food. Use the soap liberally and scrub every nook and cranny of your hands.

- If you will be traveling in developing countries for long periods of time, get vaccinated. Ask your doctor for specifics.

- For temporary protection against hepatitis A, you can get an injection of immunoglobin (a preparation of antibodies). Not only is this shot available for short-term protection against hepatitis A, it is also recommended for people who have already been exposed to the disease. However, immunoglobin must be given within two weeks of exposure for maximum protection.

- If you have anal or oral sex, use a condom or dental dam, and wash your hands after disposing of the used contraceptive.

Hepatitis B (formerly known as serum hepatitis) is a sexually transmitted disease that is spread through the exchange of bodily fluids during oral, vaginal, and anal intercourse. It can even be transmitted by kissing. The disease can also be spread via contact with the blood of an infected person. Drug users who share needles are at particular risk. Health care workers who may come into contact with contaminated blood are at increased risk, too. A potential hazard also lies in unsterilized tattooing, body piercing, and acupuncture equipment. Even sharing personal toiletries such as razors and toothbrushes may put you in harm's way if the other person nicked himself or herself while shaving or has bleeding gums. Pregnant women infected with hepatitis B can pass the virus on to their unborn children. According to the Centers for Disease Control and Prevention (CDC), babies who contract hepatitis B at birth may have the virus for the rest of their lives, can spread the disease, and can get *cirrhosis* (scarring) of the liver or liver cancer. If you are pregnant, make sure that you are tested for hepatitis B early in your pregnancy.

Hepatitis B is very contagious. The most infectious period is from several weeks prior until several weeks or months after symptoms occur. Some people don't have any symptoms, even though they are highly contagious. If symptoms do occur they may include jaundice (the skin—if the patient is light-skinned—and the whites of the eyes turn yellow), extreme fatigue, nausea, vomiting, fever, stomach or joint pain, dark urine, pale bowel movements, and loss of appetite.

Hepatitis B is a serious illness that can cause lifelong infection (you can carry the virus and infect others for the rest of your life), cirrhosis of the liver, liver disease, and death. Therefore, it's important to see your doctor if you exhibit any symptoms. A blood test can determine if you do, in fact, have hepatitis B. There is no treatment for the disease. Your doctor will most likely advise you to get plenty of rest so that your body can do its best to fight the virus. Fortunately, for most people the body's own healing properties can successfully combat the virus and in a few weeks' time they will have recovered. However, a small percentage of those with hepatitis B will not fully recover: they will become chronic carriers of the disease. That's why prevention is vital. The vaccination, administered in a series of three shots, is your best protection against hepatitis B. The CDC recommends that all babies receive the vaccine at birth and that children ages 11 and 12 who have not yet been vaccinated against hepatitis B should be. The CDC also advises people of any age who are sexually active and health care workers exposed to human blood to be vaccinated as well.

Hepatitis C (formerly known as non-A–non-B hepatitis) is spread through close physical contact with the blood of an infected person. Pregnant women can pass the virus on to their unborn babies. In rare cases, it may also be passed on during sex. Anyone who had a blood transfusion or organ transplant before July 1992 may also be at risk, because prior to that date donated blood may not have been screened for hepatitis C.

Many people with hepatitis C do not have any symptoms, hence it is considered a silent epidemic, affecting almost 4 million Americans and 170 million people worldwide. In fact, a person with hepatitis C may not feel sick at all. For some, the most common symptom that may occur is extreme tiredness. The only way to tell if you have been infected with hepatitis C is to have a hepatitis C blood test.

Unfortunately, most people who contract hepatitis C carry the disease for the rest of their lives and will likely develop chronic liver disease. Therefore, anyone who tests positive for hepatitis C should also be tested for liver disease. Some people with liver damage brought on by hepatitis C may develop cirrhosis of the liver and liver failure, which might take years to appear. The good news is that there are antiviral medications that may get rid of the virus and reduce liver disease. If you have hepatitis C, your doctor can determine whether or not this treatment can help you. He will also advise you on how to protect your liver from further harm. These protective steps will probably include seeing your physician regularly, not drinking alcohol, checking with your doctor before starting any new medications including over-the-counter and herbal remedies, and getting vaccinated against hepatitis A if you have liver damage.

In 2002, the new therapeutic agent called *pegylated interferon alpha* was approved by the Food and Drug Administration for treatment of this disease. This treatment required less frequent dosing than its predecessors, and many patients who participated in its clinical trials reported fewer side effects.

If you have hepatitis C, it's also important to take precautions to avoid spreading it to others:

• Don't donate blood, body organs, or other tissue.

• Don't share personal toiletries such as toothbrushes or razors.

- Cover any cuts or sores well with a bandage.

- If you have multiple sexual partners, use a condom or dental dam whenever you have sex. If you are in a monogamous relationship, talk to your doctor about how to best protect your partner and whether or not he should also be tested.

There is currently no vaccine available to protect against contracting hepatitis C. Your best bet is to avoid coming into contact with another person's blood and, if you are concerned about risk factors such as blood transfusions and organ transplants prior to July 1992, to see your doctor about getting tested for hepatitis C.

Herpes: There are two types of herpes—*herpes simplex virus type I,* which causes cold sores around the mouth or the lips, and *herpes simplex virus type II,* which causes ulcerated lesions on the genitals, buttocks, and thighs. One fourth of this country's population has type II herpes, many of them African-American women. The Office on Women's Health reports that black American women are six times more likely to be affected with type II herpes than any other group of people.

Both types of herpes are incurable and highly contagious. Within two to seven days of exposure, an outbreak of sores will appear at the point of contact. At first you'll notice itching or tingling around the affected area. Then red bumps will appear. These will turn into blisters and finally open sores. This occurrence is called the primary outbreak and is usually the most severe. The sores may also be accompanied—or preceded—by flulike symptoms such as fever, headache, and fatigue. Urination will also be painful if the lesions are at or near the vagina and the urethra. Other symptoms include pain at the site of the sores and a slight watery discharge. If untreated, the sores will eventually dry up and heal, but it may take a week or two.

Even after the primary outbreak subsides, the virus is still present. It lies dormant in the nerve roots of the lower spine until the next outbreak, which can be brought on by stress, illness, or any number of things. Therein lies the frustration of this virus. There is no cure, the virus stays with you forever, and you never really know when an outbreak may occur. Subsequent outbreaks, however, typically cause fewer sores, usually only one with each outbreak.

Your doctor can make a definitive diagnosis by examining the lesions and running a lab test of a sample of the cells in the base of the lesions. He may also order a blood test. Even though there is no cure for herpes, it can be treated with an antiviral medication called acyclovir (brand names Zovirax, Famvir, and Valtrex). This medication may help soothe the sores, decrease the duration of an active lesion, and speed healing. Some people take the medication even when they aren't having an outbreak in order to suppress future recurrences. Although this preventive measure is not foolproof (outbreaks may still occur), it usually does decrease the number of outbreaks a person has each year. In fact, health experts report a 75 percent reduction in recurrent outbreaks when the medication is used regularly. However, the drug can be very expensive, making a regular regimen quite costly. In any event, the drug's manufacturer recommends that herpes sufferers who take the medication regularly stop after one year of continuous use to reassess the recurrence rate. Because acyclovir is metabolized in the kidneys, users need to be careful. Some reports indicate that the drug may be safe to use for five to six years continuously without damage to the kidneys. You should discuss the most appropriate long-term treatment for you with your doctor.

Human Papillomavirus (HPV): This virus is the cause of *genital warts* (also called venereal warts), cauliflowerlike growths that occur in or around the pelvic structures, including the vagina, vulva, and anus. HPV is spread through vaginal, anal, and oral sex, and it can be extremely serious, leading to cancer of the cervix. You can be infected with the virus and not even know it. That's because when the warts appear on the genitals they aren't always readily detectable. They don't cause pain, irregular bleeding, or pus drainage. At most they may cause a slight itchiness. But if left untreated, they can multiply and grow larger. Because they can lead to cervical cancer, it is important to get treatment. This is a good reason to do a self-examination of your genital area regularly. There's no need to be embarrassed about it. By doing a self-check daily or weekly you can make sure that your genital area is healthy. If you notice unusual discharge, bumps, warts, or anything else out of the ordinary, have it checked out by your doctor. Making self-checks a regular habit, like going in for your routine pelvic exam and doing breast self-exams, is important to maintaining good health.

Your doctor will be able to detect genital warts via a pelvic exam. Some warts are flatter than others, and your doctor may need to use a special instrument called a *colposcope* (a sort of magnifying lens) to spot them. A Pap test can confirm an HPV diagnosis.

HPV cannot be cured. The goal of treatment is to get rid of the growths. However, they may return. The three-month recurrence rate is about 25 percent. There are several ways your doctor can treat genital warts. He may prescribe a topical medication called Podofilox that you apply to the warts yourself, after being instructed by your physician. Or your doctor may treat the warts by applying a chemical called podophyllin. It can be very caustic to the skin around the warts and can actually burn the tissue. You will be advised to wash the solution off after six hours. Another topical solution your doctor may use to remove warts is trichloracetic acid.

Aside from medications and solutions that are applied directly to the warts, your doctor may opt for a different course of treatment. One is *cryosurgery,* or freezing. This method isn't really surgery in the typical sense, in that there is no cutting involved. Rather, the doctor uses a special instrument to freeze off the warts. It's an outpatient procedure that doesn't usually take very long. Another alternative is removal of the warts with a laser or a hot cautery instrument. This procedure usually requires anesthesia.

If the warts are extremely large, they may need to be removed surgically. One of the newest treatments is to inject interferon (a group of proteins produced naturally in the body during viral infections that can also be given as a drug) directly into the warts or to administer it intravenously.

Syphilis: This is a potentially deadly sexually transmitted disease that affects many black women. The most recent studies from the Office on Women's Health show that in 1994, the incidence of syphilis was highest among African-American women. This STD is caused by a bacteria that is spread through vaginal, anal, or oral intercourse, as well as through kissing. Once in the body, the bacteria passes quickly through the bloodstream and lymphatic system to all parts of the body. If left untreated, syphilis can do major damage to your heart, brain, nervous system, and bones, to name a few areas. It can also lead to death.

Syphilis usually progresses in stages. During the *primary stage,* the first symptom is a painless sore called a *chancre* that appears at the site of initial infection (i.e., the genitals, mouth, etc.) about three weeks after exposure. The sores will heal in four to six weeks. This is a very contagious stage.

About six weeks later the *secondary stage* will begin. More advanced symptoms occur, including a rash, wartlike lesions, swollen lymph glands, fever, fatigue, and perhaps mild weight loss. During this stage you will still be contagious.

Next comes the *latent stage,* which can last for years. Although the bacteria is still in your body, you will show no symptoms and will usually no longer be contagious.

The last stage of syphilis is the *tertiary-stage,* which is very serious. It is not a contagious stage but it can cause severe illness, including damage to your heart, neurological system, brain, and lungs. This final stage can end in death.

A physician can diagnose primary syphilis by performing a procedure called a *darkfield examination* of scrapings from the chancres. Other stages of the disease require blood tests for a definitive diagnosis.

Depending on the stage, syphilis is treated with penicillin (or doxycycline if you are allergic to penicillin) or with tetracycline. Follow-up blood tests will be necessary to make sure the medication is working effectively. Your sexual partner should also be tested and treated. If you test positive for syphilis it is recommended that you also be tested for HIV because having syphilis (as well as certain other STDs, such as gonorrhea) puts you at greater risk of being infected with HIV. Some STDs can cause open lesions that provide the HIV virus easier entry. If the first HIV test is negative, a second should be performed in three months.

Trichomoniasis: See Chapter 5, Common Illnesses, Simple Cures.

HIV AND AIDS

While technically an STD, HIV and AIDS has had such a profound impact on all of our lives that I'm going to discuss it a bit more in depth. HIV and AIDS have had a devastating effect on the black community. According to the National Institutes of Health, AIDS is the number one killer of African-American men and women age 25 to 44. What's more, black women are currently the fastest-growing segment of the population to contract the virus and develop the disease. Research by the Centers for Disease Control and Prevention as recently as June 2000 show that 48 black women out of every 100,000 had AIDS. Yet only 13 Hispanic women out of every 100,000 had the disease. And even fewer white women—3 out of every 100,000—were affected. Clearly, sisters are more at risk. The question is, why?

A study published in the journal *AIDS Education and Prevention* entitled "Are African-American women worried about getting AIDS? A qualitative analysis" may hold some of the answers. A surprising 64 percent of black women respondents said that they were not worried about contracting the AIDS virus, compared to 36 percent who were. What's alarming is that regardless of whether the black women surveyed were worried about getting HIV or not, all of them were equally likely to report risky sexual behavior, such as not using condoms or having sex with questionable partners. Of the black females who did express concern about contracting the virus, some pointed to their uncertainty about their partners' sexual history as one of the reasons; and 10 percent of those who were not concerned about getting AIDS said that they trusted their partners' sexual history. Either way, whether the women were worried about their risk level or not, the harsh reality is that they were not protecting themselves by using condoms or being carefully selective about sexual partners.

And that's precisely the problem: They are not practicing safer sex. Other than abstinence, it is the only way to help protect yourself against sexually contracting the AIDS virus. It all begins with education. As I've said before, knowledge is power. Knowing exactly what the disease is, how it is spread, and how to prevent it can save your life.

For sure, the statistics are staggering, for black men and women.

Incidence

In a report by the CDC, of the 415,864 persons diagnosed with AIDS from 1991 to 1996 in the United States, 19 percent were Hispanic. The majority of causes for AIDS in white, black, and Hispanic men from 1985 to 1997 are:

	white men	black men	Hispanic men
homosexual acts	68.1%	27.6%	38.6%
injecting drug use	12.0%	**36.1%**	33.1%
heterosexual contact	5.0%	**15.6%**	11.2%
transfusion	1.5%	0.8%	0.3%

Source: U.S. Department of Health and Human Services. *Health, United States, 2001,* table 54

This table points to a few interesting facts:

- Most white men get their HIV/AIDS from homosexual activity, while black men primarily get this condition from IV drug use.

- It also shows that the women many black men are sleeping with are infected. For the most part, that means the men are getting HIV/AIDS from black women; but many black men may be getting infected by white women, too.

But for sure, African-American women are currently the fastest-growing segment of the population for new cases of HIV and AIDS in the United States.

FOR ALL YEARS 1985–2000	12 MONTHS ENDING 6/30/00
males:	
white: 49.2%	15.1 cases/100,000
black: 34.2%	117 cases/100,000 people
females:	
white: 22.8%	2.2 cases/100,000
black: 60.0%	48.0 cases/100,000
Hispanic: 16.2%	13.4 cases/100,000
Asian: 0.6%	1.9 cases/100,000
children (under 13):	
white: 18.3%	0.1 cases/100,000
black: 61.3%	2.0 cases/100,000
Hispanic: 19.3%	0.4 cases/100,000

Source: U.S. Department of Health and Human Services. *Health, United States, 2001*, table 53.

Again, interesting findings:

- The number of black men getting the disease has obviously picked up.

- Black women are at high risk.

- Black children are at high risk.

- Hispanics aren't faring very well either, but blacks . . . !

I find all these statistics utterly frightening and very concerning. This is a serious illness and we, as a people, must consider it so, 24/7.

What are HIV and AIDS?

HIV stands for *human immunodeficiency virus,* and it is the virus that causes AIDS. *AIDS* stands for *acquired immune deficiency syndrome,* and it is a condition that destroys your immune system, leaving you susceptible to various infections and diseases including pneumonia, a type of cancer called Kaposi's sarcoma, liver failure, kidney failure, and more. Although many people mistakenly believe that you can "catch AIDS" from all sorts of things, the virus, which is transported via blood, semen, or vaginal fluids, can only be spread in specific ways:

- through unprotected vaginal, oral, and anal sex

- by infected needles used during drug use, in a health care setting, during tattooing or body piercing

- from mother to baby during pregnancy, childbirth, or breast-feeding

- via infected blood during a blood transfusion

The HIV virus cannot be spread through casual contact such as hugging, shaking hands, or dry kissing. Nor can it be contracted by sharing utensils, sitting on toilet seats, or just being around someone who has the virus. An infected person's blood, semen, or vaginal fluids must enter your body in order for you to be infected with HIV.

Another "myth" surrounding the disease is that if a person has HIV she has AIDS. That's not true. You can be HIV-positive without having AIDS. The HIV virus leads to AIDS, which is the advanced stage of the disease. With the developments that have been made in treating the disease since it was first identified in the United States in 1981, many people are able to live for years with HIV and with AIDS. In fact, the phrase you're likely to hear people with AIDS use to describe themselves today is "*living* with AIDS."

Exactly how does HIV affect immunity?

Once the virus enters the bloodstream, it attacks the lymphatic system, a part of the immune system that helps the body fight infection and disease. White blood cells called *T cells* (or CD4 cells) present in the lymphatic system are crucial to defending the body against infection and disease. The body produces antibodies in response to the HIV infection, but the virus simply keeps reproducing itself. As it multiplies, it kills off more and more of the infection-fighting T cells, ultimately crippling the immune system.

What are the symptoms?

When a person is infected with the HIV virus, she may not show any initial signs for years. However, as the virus continues to attack the immune system, weakening the body's natural defense mechanisms, that person may begin to have chronic flulike symptoms that last for weeks, including fever, sore throat, and muscle aches. Other HIV-related symptoms that may also appear are swollen lymph nodes, skin rashes, ulcers in the mouth or on the anus, unexplained weight loss, persistent diarrhea, chronic cough, night sweats, and thrush (yeast infections of the mouth). Women may also have persistent yeast infections and sexually transmitted diseases. An HIV-positive person may exhibit these symptoms for years before developing AIDS. She will be diagnosed as having full-blown AIDS once she develops one of the many conditions defined as a feature of the disease. These include a T cell count of less than 200, cancers such as Kaposi's sarcoma, various infections, certain types of pneumonia, and others.

How is HIV diagnosed?

HIV is diagnosed through blood tests. Before you have an HIV test, a counselor will talk to you about the disease—not just the medical facts, but the psychological and social side as well. Once your blood is drawn, the sample is lab tested for the presence of antibodies to HIV. If the test comes back negative, that means that you currently don't have the virus. However, you should be retested in six months to be absolutely sure, because it usually takes about two months from the time of exposure before your body begins to produce antibodies to the virus.

If the blood test comes back positive, it will be rechecked by use of other tests for confirmation. A diagnosis of full-blown AIDS is based on positive test results for HIV antibodies and Western blot (a confirmation test), along with observation of the disease's characteristic illnesses and conditions, and various other tests such as a T cell count.

How are HIV and AIDS treated?

Although medical research on ways to treat and combat HIV and AIDS has come a long way in the last twenty years, there is still no cure for the disease. But the medical advances that have been made have helped people with HIV and AIDS live for years following their diagnosis. Therefore, the earlier an HIV-positive person begins treatment, the better. Antiviral drugs that disrupt the chemical processes necessary for the virus to grow are typically prescribed to slow down the progression of the disease. A three-drug "cocktail" that combines a variety of antiviral drugs appears to be having success in improving cell counts in HIV patients and slowing the progression to full AIDS. These "cocktails" may include nucleoside analogues such as AZT (Retrovir), DDI (Didanosine or Videx), and DDC (Dideoxycytidine); protease inhibitors like Saquinavir (Fortovase or Invirase), Indinavir (Crixivan), and Ritonavir (Norvir); and a non-nucleoside reverse transcriptase inhibitor drug such as Nevirapine (Viramune).

Recently scientists have discovered new drug therapies that may prove successful in the fight against AIDS, including Kaletra, a protease inhibitor manufactured by Abbott Laboratories. The drug, which received FDA approval in September 2000, is taken as part of a cocktail of standard AIDS drugs. Initial evidence suggests that, unlike other protease inhibitors, Kaletra allows a higher HIV-fighting level of drug to circulate in the blood system. However, Kaletra does have side effects, including diarrhea, fatigue, nausea, and a possible increase in cholesterol and triglyceride levels. A very small percentage of users suffered pancreatitis.

Side effects are not unusual. All drug therapies used to treat HIV and AIDS carry that risk. AZT, for example, arguably the most commonly used antiviral drug, can cause severe anemia. Each category of drug used in HIV and AIDS treatment acts differently to help keep the virus under control, but each also has an extensive list of possible side effects. Therefore, patients taking these drugs must be monitored carefully by their doctors and also need to pay close attention to how they are feeling.

Can AIDS be prevented?

Absolutely. The key is education. You must know the risks and how to avoid them. The only way to ensure that you don't contract the virus sexually is through abstinence. Otherwise you must practice safer sex. Make sure you really know your partner—sexual history, HIV status, any history of IV drug use, the works. Always use condoms and dental dams when having vaginal, anal, and oral sex. If you are not currently in a monogamous relationship, limit your number of sexual partners.

If you are going to get a body piercing or tattoo, go to a reputable shop and make sure the instruments are properly sterilized.

Don't do drugs, especially IV drugs. As a woman of God, I know this caution shouldn't even be of issue, but some sisters struggle with the grip of drug abuse even though faith exists in their hearts. My plea to those sisters: Please don't share needles.

HIV/AIDS is a disease each and every one of us can keep at bay. All we have to do is educate ourselves, live smart, and think before we act.

A Global Concern

As devastating an impact as HIV/AIDS has had on the black community in the United States, our brothers and sisters in the Motherland are literally being ravaged by the virus. Of the 34.3 million people worldwide infected with HIV/AIDS, a shocking 70 percent live in sub-Saharan Africa. And our African sisters are being affected most of all. Of the nearly 22.3 million adults in sub-Saharan Africa living with HIV/AIDS, 12.2 million—that's 55 percent!—are women. Because HIV is spread in Africa primarily through heterosexual intercourse, women there are more at risk for contracting the disease than men; the virus passes more easily from men to women. What's more, new research presented at the 13th International AIDS Conference in 2000 suggests that genetic differences may make African women more susceptible to HIV infection as well.

When we look at the devastating effects of HIV and AIDS on

our people from a global view, it underscores just how important it is for us to safeguard our health here at home.

CANCER

No other word or medical diagnosis, except perhaps for HIV/ AIDS, strikes as much fear in people as *cancer*. In the past, being told you had cancer was basically a death sentence. Today, with all of the technology, medical research, and advances, many cancers are not only treatable but curable—if they are detected early.

Unfortunately, African Americans are the least likely to benefit. Despite the medical advances and the increase in survival rates among cancer patients, brothers and sisters continue to die of cancer in greater numbers than nearly all other racial populations. Consider this sampling of statistics from the Institute of Medicine:

PERCENTAGE OF PEOPLE WHO SURVIVE ALL TYPES OF CANCER, BY RACE	
Whites	50%
Hispanics	47%
Blacks	38%
Native Americans	34%

Why are we dying from this disease more than others? Because we are being diagnosed later. Late diagnosis results in a poorer prognosis, less likely chance for a cure, and a decreased life expectancy. The fault is our own. We are less likely to see our doctors, get regular physicals, and have the tests and screenings that can detect cancer early. Sadly, we are not as serious about our health as we need to be. We may be complacent, or fearful, or blame it on a lack of funds. But in the end, the only ones we hurt are ourselves. We are dying from diseases that can be cured, and it has to stop. We have to change our behavior and our way of thinking, especially black women.

The fact is, after heart disease, cancer is the second most frequent cause of death in women. What more of a wake-up call do we need? If we want to live we must get our priorities straight. Early detection is the only way to give ourselves a fighting chance.

What is cancer?

Cancer refers to any of a group of diseases characterized by the uncontrolled growth of abnormal cells that cause malignant tumors to develop. The transformation of a normal cell into a malignant (cancerous) one begins when a carcinogen (a cancer-causing agent) alters the genetic structure and function of the normal cell, causing chromosomal damage. Once the normal cell has been changed into a malignant one, the alterations in its genetics are passed on to all of its offspring cells, thus establishing a small group of abnormal cells that multiply rapidly. Simply put, cancer develops when the normal behavior of cells is affected in a significant way, enough to alter the genetic structure and function of those cells, especially concerning changes in the DNA of those cells.

If caught early enough, some premalignant changes can be reversed or cured. But if left untreated, the cancer will continue to grow and spread, invading surrounding tissues. Cells from the cancer may also metastasize, spreading to other parts of the body through the bloodstream and lymphatic channels.

While cancer can affect just about any part of your body—your organs, tissues, blood and lymphatic systems, bones, muscles, or bone marrow—certain forms of the disease are particularly prevalent among African-American women.

Endometrial Cancer

Also called uterine cancer, endometrial cancer affects the upper part of the womb and the lining of the uterus. It is the fourth most common cancer among women in the United States and typically strikes later in life, after menopause. However, the disease can affect younger women. From age 30 to age 70 and beyond, African-American women have the highest endometrial cancer mortality rate among all races of women, according to the National Cancer Institute. Research from the American Cancer Society shows why: Black women are more likely to be diagnosed with the disease at later stages. As we have seen again and again, black women lag behind when it comes to early detection, and it's killing us at every turn. This has to stop. We must begin getting the tests and screenings that can save our lives.

What are the symptoms of endometrial cancer? In about 85 percent of endometrial cancer cases, the main symptom is abnormal bleeding. Prior to menopause, that may include unusually heavy menstrual periods or bleeding in between periods. After menopause, increased vaginal discharge is a common symptom. If the discharge is puslike or thick and tissuelike, both are indicators of cancer. Some women also have pelvic discomfort.

How is endometrial cancer diagnosed? In about 10 to 15 percent of cases, a Pap smear will show a change that turns out to be abnormal endometrial cells shedding from the uterus. However, Pap smears aren't considered reliable screening tools for this cancer because they are primarily a screening test used for detecting cervical disease, not endometrial, uterine, tubal, or ovarian disease. A D&C (dilation and curettage) is much more accurate since it allows testing of an actual sample of the uterine lining. With this method, the entire womb is scraped clean of the endometrial lining and the tissue is sent to the lab and checked for cell types. A less invasive procedure called an *endometrial biopsy* may be performed, but it is not as reliable as a D&C because it gets only some, not all, of the tissue. Another reason the D&C is the preferred procedure here is because the cells of the endocervical canal are obtained first, then the endometrial canal is entered and the womb is scraped. Why is it so important to do the endocervical scraping first? Because it allows the doctor to determine how far the cancer has extended—a crucial piece of information for staging the disease.

How is endometrial cancer treated? This type of cancer requires hysterectomy, with removal of the uterus, fallopian tubes, and ovaries. Following treatment, Stage I cancer has at least a 75 percent 5-year survival rate and Stage II has at least a 60 percent 5-year survival rate. In the later stages of the disease, patients will also receive radiation and/or chemotherapy in addition to a hysterectomy. The 5-year survival rate for Stage III endometrial cancer is 25 to 35 percent. For Stage IV it's 10 to 15 percent. As you can see in the table below, early detection can make a huge difference:

ENDOMETRIAL CANCER	
Surgical Stage	5-year survival
Stage I	75–95 percent
Stage II	60–75 percent
Stage III	25–35 percent
Stage IV	10–15 percent

Ovarian Cancer

This is the fifth most common type of cancer in American women. More white women get it and die from it, but black women aren't far behind. According to the National Cancer Institute (NCI), African-American women have the third highest mortality rate for ovarian cancer. It is a disease that, across the board, is usually discovered very late, so long-term survival is rare.

The cause of this disease is not clear, though some type of hormonal stimulation is believed to play a role. Family history is also a risk factor as certain gene mutations (the BRACA gene) cause a 20 to 40 percent risk of ovarian cancer.

What are the symptoms of ovarian cancer? Unfortunately, in most cases ovarian cancer causes no symptoms until it is widespread. One reason is that because the ovary is small (about the size of an almond) it has plenty of room in the pelvic cavity to grow before you might notice any pressure or other problem. The first symptom is usually vague abdominal discomfort and swelling. There may also be shortness of breath or fluid in the lungs if the cancer has spread to the lungs. Another sign is increased abdominal girth, either as a result of the size of the cancerous growth or, more commonly, from *ascites* (excess fluid in the abdominal cavity).

How is ovarian cancer diagnosed? A variety of tests will be given, including an ultrasound, CT scan or MRI, barium enema, and different blood tests, including the CA-125, which—though not 100 percent accurate or tumor-specific—can be used as a marker for possible ovarian cancer. Surgery is usually necessary in order to get a definitive tissue diagnosis.

How is ovarian cancer treated? The disease is treated with surgery to remove the cancer, which typically entails removing the ovaries, fallopian tubes, and the uterus. Early Stage I and Stage II patients may have a 70 to 90 percent 5-year survival rate. Unfortunately, since most patients aren't diagnosed until later stages, the 5-year survival rate drops to 45 to 50 percent. If the cancer is late stage and has spread, only 3 to 10 percent of patients survive for five years. Later stages of the disease will require chemotherapy as part of the treatment, commonly using the anticancer drugs CIS-Platinum and paclitaxel.

Cervical Cancer

Cancer of the cervix, the lower part of the uterus, occurs in two main forms—*squamous cell carcinoma,* the most common type, which is often associated with the human papillomavirus (HPV); and *adenocarcinoma,* which is much more rare. Cervical cancer stems from abnormal changes in the cells on the surface of the cervix. Minor conditions can affect the cell characteristics of the cervix, such as vaginitis, which causes inflammation of the cervix. Other risk factors include first having sex at an early age, your number of sexual partners, having had several children, a history of sexually transmitted disease, failure to get Pap smears, prolonged use of oral contraceptives (for some women), and smoking.

There are stages of cervical cancer. The preinvasive stage is readily detected by a Pap smear and can be treated and cured. *Carcinoma in situ* (CIS) is a development of cancer that is only on the surface of the cervix and has not extended deep into the cervical tissue. This stage is also curable. "Invasive" cancer means the cancer has been present for a while and has spread past the cervix surface into its tissue. In advanced cases, the cancer can spread to the body of the uterus and the pelvic sidewalls, and may also involve the lymph nodes.

Black women are more likely to develop cervical cancer than are white women, almost twice as likely, according to U.S. health figures. Worse still, American Cancer Society research indicates that sisters are twice as likely to die of the disease. Why are African-American women faring so poorly when the National Cancer Institute reports that, overall, the incidence and mortality rates for cervical cancer have declined about 40 percent since the early 1970s? The answer is simple: A Pap smear can detect cervical abnormalities and is commonly used to screen for cervical cancer. Yet, large numbers of black women haven't had a Pap smear in years. Over a third of sisters have not had one in the past year, according to government health statistics. It all goes back to the importance of early detection and to our being responsible regarding our health care regimen.

What are the symptoms of cervical cancer? Some women have no symptoms. Others may experience unusual vaginal discharge, spotting, bleeding after intercourse, and pain in the pelvic region. If the cancer has spread, there may also be urinary complications and bowel problems.

How is cervical cancer diagnosed? As you've learned, a Pap smear is the primary way to screen for cervical cancer. This procedure can detect precancerous and some cancerous cells. However, once a Pap smear shows precancerous cells (called dysplasia), more diagnostic procedures are indicated, particularly, a special procedure called *colposcopy and biopsy*. It is the cervical biopsy that will confirm the Pap findings and give an accurate diagnosis. For this reason, it's important that your doctor make his or her best effort to locate the focus of the abnormal cells. That's where colposcopy comes in.

What exactly is a colposcopy? Colposcopy is the main way to identify the site where a cervical biopsy should be done. After visualizing the area with a high-power microscope, the doctor can see where he wishes to make the biopsy to have the cells evaluated. This procedure:

• can be done in the doctor's office

• can cause some minor spotting afterward

• can be done during pregnancy

• doesn't hurt, but the biopsies that are usually done in conjunction with it may be painful to some

Once the tissue is reviewed by a pathologist in the lab, your doctor can best determine the next step, which may be freezing the cervix (cryosurgery), or a cone biopsy, in which a larger biopsy is done: A specimen of the cervix, shaped like an upside-down ice cream cone, is removed. By means of the cone biopsy, a more definitive diagnosis can be made regarding the extent and depth of the cervical neoplasia process. Cones not only help diagnose the problem but, in many milder cases, actually remove the dysplasia—for that point of time. Cones are not a treatment for actual cervical cancer, however.

How is cervical cancer treated? Using the diagnostic test results, the doctor may treat the cervix with an anti-inflammatory cream, then another Pap smear will be performed in a couple of months. If abnormalities persist, a colposcopy may be done. This procedure allows your doctor to look at your cervix with a microscope for any lesions, HPV warts, or other abnormalities. Next comes the biopsy, in which abnormal cells are removed and evaluated in the lab. Your doctor may then attempt to destroy the affected area by freezing the cervix (cryosurgery) or by doing a cone biopsy.

Hysterectomy is the primary treatment for this disease. If the cancer is caught early enough, the hysterectomy can be done vaginally, sparing the ovaries. More extensive cervical cancer may require more involved surgeries, including lymph node dissections. If the disease is in a highly advanced stage, it may be treated with radiation only.

What can you do to lessen the risk of cervical cancer? Make sure to have regular Pap smears. Use condoms, and avoid STDs, especially human papillomavirus, which is the leading cause of cervical cancer. Proteins found in sperm have also been implicated as causative agents for cervical cancer. Again, using condoms can help decrease your risk of not only STDs but possible cervical cancer.

RARE GYNECOLOGIC CANCERS

Vaginal and vulvar cancers are not very common and usually occur in older women. Vaginal cancer may occur secondary to previous involvement from cervical cancer. For this reason, it is important that patients who had cervical cancer continue with their pelvic exams and Pap smears even after a hysterectomy—this holds true for all women.

Symptoms include abnormal vaginal discharge, spotting, and urinary problems. Vulvar cancer patients may have actual lesions or bumps in the vulvar area that don't go away. They might be red in color, raw, and ulcerated, with drainage. Lymph node involvement is also common with this type of cancer, especially the nodes in the groin.

Fallopian tube cancer is also very rare, but still possible. Patients usually get a thin, watery, blood-streaked discharge from the vagina. The drainage comes from the tubes, through the uterus, down into the endocervical canal, and out into the vagina.

RX: A PRESCRIPTION FOR YOUR SOUL

Being a black woman offers so many wonderful and unique gifts. I, for one, would never want to be anything else. Peel back a sister's many layers and you will find an array of attributes—from our strong sense of spirituality, to our bold inquisitiveness, to our inherent strength and tenacity, to our unshakable familial bond. African-American women have it going on.

But for all of our qualities we still have one persistent cross to bear: the state of our health. It is truly under attack. You've seen the statistics. You've read the facts and figures. As women, we must deal with the reality that particular illnesses and diseases may factor into our lives. As *black* women, we must also deal with the reality that being African American increases our risk.

Our spirit and faith guide us through life's journey, and sometimes that journey will lead us down a rocky path—one strewn with hurdles and minefields in the guise of illness. You know that certain medical conditions can come with the female territory. But that doesn't mean we don't have the resources to get through them. Our guiding faith is always there. Though we cannot usually control everything that comes our way, we can control how we handle these things.

I know that it can be difficult to reconcile this with the reality of being hit by a serious illness. It is deeply frightening and can shake our faith. But should you ever have to face down a medical crisis like some of those discussed in this chapter, the very first thing you should do is thank God. That's right, thank Him, because the condition has been brought to your attention and now you can do something about it. As I've been saying all along, the earlier you discover a possible health problem, the better your chances of having it successfully treated. Odds are, it will be a condition that is not life-threatening. So thanking Him for shedding light on the problem will enable you to maintain your cool and to think about things rationally. He will help you prepare to take whatever steps are necessary to deal with the situation.

Remember, too, you have a doctor you can trust; one who will answer your questions and inform you of possible treatments. For this you can be thankful as well.

The next thing you must do is keep a level head. It's natural to become anxious and scared in this circumstance, even to the point of inaction. Fear will either put you into a spirit of flight (running away from the situation), or give you a spirit of fight, enabling you to become proactive and do what you must to take care of the matter facing you.

As a child led by God, you must not succumb to fear. It can immobilize you and that will delay your treatment. You will always have Him, so you need not be afraid.

For these reasons, it becomes increasingly more important for you to be knowledgeable about how God wants you to behave in difficult situations. You have to be sure you have God's word in your heart so you can draw upon it, even in the doctor's office. You have to be ready to speak God's promise to you as soon as possible, for you know the spirits of darkness are right there, too, waiting for the moment when they can attack you with toxic worrying, undue anxiety, and fear. And we all know that fear is not of God. Concern, yes; fear, no.

You have to know what to say when ungodly spirits try to talk to you and discourage you. You need to remind them and yourself that you are a child of God, and no weapon formed against you shall prosper. Remember, you are a part of the promise of God. And God has promised you that He is a healer of all your diseases, that there is nothing greater than Him, that He loves you and wants only the best for you. He is watching over you.

Third, seek God's direction for you during this difficult time. Pray. Petition God. Proclaim God, and praise Him for what He has done in your life—and what He's about to do.

Fourth, take action. Don't procrastinate. All the while you should be communicating with your doctor. I can't stress this strongly enough. Ask questions: Doctor, what causes this condition? What are my treatment options? Why are those my best options? Is there something I can do to prevent this from occurring again?

If you have a family member you can trust, or a prayer partner, share your concerns with that person. Let them be a part of the process. It may be your spouse, a parent, a sibling, or fellow parishioner, but make sure it's someone who is a strong member of God's family, who values you, and who won't divulge your business to the entire world.

As you seek God for direction and rely on His strength to get you through, listen for His voice and His leading. To do this, you may need to extend your devotional period. There is nothing greater than hearing the voice of God and knowing that He is truly speaking to you. I am a witness to that fact!

Then, go forth. Do what you must do to take care of the matter. Remember, God has made you a steward over your body while here on earth, so if you don't take care of it, who will? God's word says things should be done decently and in order. This applies to your health also.

If You Need Surgery

· · · · · · · · · · · · ·

Pursue what nourishes your soul first, and blessings be-
yond measure will be showered upon you. This is life's
promise.

—Susan L. Taylor, publication director of
Essence magazine

News You Can Use

· Studies show that 65 percent of African-American women who undergo hysterectomies are diagnosed with fibroid tumors.

· Before you have any type of surgery, be sure to ask your doctor very
specific questions about the diagnosis and the procedure.

· When it comes to surgery, always get a second opinion.

· Uterine embolization has helped decrease the number of hysterectomies performed.

"*Surgery.*" Say the word softly and it sounds almost soothing.
But the thought of actually having surgery is anything but. If a
physician ever says, "You need surgery," your immediate response
is likely to be "Oh my God," and rightly so. It's a scary thought. If
you've ever had an operation, or know someone who has, we're
sure you can testify. The doctors and nurses assure you that everything is going to be just fine. Loved ones rally around to offer their
love and support. But fear of the unknown is hard to shake. That's
perfectly understandable. Who among us can honestly say that
being wheeled into an operating room wouldn't faze us in the

least? No one we know. You're putting yourself in someone else's hands, literally, and trusting that he or she will tend to you well. But no matter how much confidence you have in the surgeon, a part of you is still afraid. We all feel that way, sister. We wouldn't be human if we didn't.

However, allowing fear and anxiety to overtake you will only make the experience more difficult for you emotionally and may even adversely affect the outcome. We know it's hard to let go of fear, and that's not what we're asking you to do. Fear is not an emotion that can be controlled at will, especially not in this circumstance. It's an instinctive, protective response. It's your mind's way of putting your entire being on alert. It is normal.

What we *are* suggesting is that you learn to get a handle on fear before it gets control of you. How can you put fears about surgery into perspective and calm yourself down? There are two keys: arming yourself with knowledge, and turning within.

KNOWLEDGE IS POWER

When we say arm yourself with knowledge, we mean know the facts. Find out everything you can about the surgical procedure your doctor is recommending—and be certain the information is accurate. Don't be afraid to ask your physician questions. In fact, make sure that you do. He is there to take care of you, and that means tending to both your physical and your emotional needs. If you have to ask questions in order to allay your fears, tell him so. A good doctor will make time to give you detailed, thorough answers. The more you know about the procedure, the better equipped you'll be to cope with it. It's the *not* knowing that sends many sisters into a spiral of anxiety. Having the facts won't totally erase your unease, but it can help you focus on the surgery more objectively. Get a second opinion as well, and know about possible alternatives. The bottom line is that you must be able to make an informed decision. This is especially important for African-American women, since we are more likely to suffer from poor health than are white women. If you're not sure how to go about obtaining the information you require, don't worry. We'll give you all the tools you need. More on that later. For now, let's start with the basics.

COMMON SURGERIES

Although heart disease, breast cancer, and diabetes cause many of us to have operations each year, one of the more common reasons we undergo surgery is to remove fibroids, noncancerous tumors that grow on the outside or inside wall of the uterus (womb). Even though these growths are usually benign, they can still lead to severe pain, abnormal bleeding, anemia, bowel and urinary problems, painful intercourse for some women, and even infertility. No one knows for sure what causes fibroids, which can be as small as a pea or as large as a grapefruit, eggplant, cantaloupe, or even a newborn baby. But they are believed to be linked to high estrogen levels. Fibroids are estimated to occur in 50 to 75 percent of African-American women, and are often treated with surgery, especially hysterectomies and myomectomies. Research shows that hysterectomies are more likely to be done on black women than on white women. In fact, a University of Maryland study found that 65 percent of black women who undergo this type of surgery are diagnosed with fibroids, compared to only 29 percent of white women who have hysterectomies. Depending on the size of the fibroids and other factors, a myomectomy may make more sense for some sisters. (See page 121.) Women also undergo surgery for problems with irregular bleeding, pelvic pain, pelvic infections, and more.

When faced with the prospect of surgery, knowing as much as possible about your diagnosis and the treatments available can make a world of difference. To help you get a handle on the most common surgical procedures, we've put together a mini primer designed to take you through each one step by step.

Cervical Cone Biopsy

Classification: Minor surgery; usually done as an outpatient; takes about ten minutes.

Reason: To remove a portion of the cervix to evaluate for abnormal cells that may be cancerous.

Anesthesia requirements: Usually done under mild general anesthesia or with a spinal.

Blood loss: usually minimal, but at times, there can be heavier bleeding.

Description: A cone biopsy is a procedure in which a portion of the cervix is removed—cut in the shape of an inverted ice cream cone, hence the name—to evaluate how deep into the cervical cells a precancerous or cancerous condition exists.

Ofttimes, doing the cone biopsy not only helps the doctor evaluate the cells, but the procedure can remove the entire focus of abnormal cells.

Postoperative course: Following surgery, you will be in recovery for approximately one hour, then released to go home. Many patients have this done on a Friday so they can recover over the weekend and return to work on Monday. There will be minimal bleeding/spotting for a few days, eventually clearing. A follow-up visit usually occurs in three weeks, at which time the cervix is examined and your report reviewed. It is recommended that you not engage in any sexual activity—nor put anything into the vagina such as tampons—during the recovery phase, until seen by your doctor.

Dilatation & Curettage (D&C)

Classification: Minor surgery; outpatient procedure; takes less than ten minutes.

Reason: To scrape the inner lining of the womb clean to check for cells that may cause abnormal bleeding; to look for cancerous cells in the womb.

Anesthesia requirements: Usually done under local, spinal, or mild general anesthesia.

Blood loss: Usually minimal.

Description: A D&C is a very easy procedure that gives a lot of information about the lining of the womb. Many women have this done in order to "clean out" the uterus when troubled with excessive bleeding problems. Gently scraping the womb of its lining causes cells to be removed. The specimen is sent to the lab and evaluated. Infection, precancerous cells, and cancerous cells may be detected, as well as other causes for abnormal bleeding.

Postoperative course: Similar to the cone biopsy regimen described above, though instead of a three-week return visit, you may be advised to return in two weeks.

Laparoscopy

Classification: Usually minor surgery done as an outpatient, though more extensive procedures may require an overnight stay.

Reason: To insert a scope into the abdomen to view the pelvis, check for disease, and treat any abnormalities that can safely be handled through the laparoscope. It can also be used to "tie tubes."

Anesthesia requirements: General anesthesia.

Blood loss: This is usually minimal, but it depends on exactly what is being done during the procedure.

Description: Now widely accepted and widely used, laparoscopy is a very common procedure that allows doctors to look inside your body using smaller incisions than were needed in times past. In today's world, laparoscopy is used extensively for many procedures including gynecological indications (to diagnose adhesions, endometriosis, infections, infertility, cysts, and other diseases that may be present.) It is also used for nongynecologic procedures such as to remove the appendix, to treat hernias, remove gallbladders, and more.

Postoperative course: Most patients recover in a couple of days if the laparoscopic procedure was for examination only. If more extensive procedures are done—such as a laparoscopic myomectomy, in which extensive dissection of the womb or another organ is done—a longer recovery is indicated. There will be some vaginal spotting or bleeding for a short while; sexual activity should be curtailed until cleared by your doctor, and the small incisions that are made should be kept clean.

Hysterectomy

Classification: Major surgery; an inpatient procedure; takes one or more hours.

Reason: To remove the uterus.

Anesthesia requirements: Usually done under general anesthesia, but may be done with a spinal or epidural, if the patient is not a good candidate for general anesthesia.

Blood loss: Varies.

Description: A hysterectomy is an operation to remove the uterus. The number one reason women have hysterectomies (the surgical removal of the uterus) is because of fibroid tumors. This operation has long been the most common treatment for fibroids. Fortunately, the rate is decreasing because of other advances in fibroid treatment.

NUMBER OF HYSTERECTOMIES IN THE U.S.	
Year	Number
1975	724,000
1985	670,000
1994	556,000

Source: Johns Hopkins University "Reproductive Endocrinology" course materials, 1999.

If you don't plan to have any more children and your fibroids are causing problems, a hysterectomy *may* be the option for you. With this operation, the entire womb is removed along with the tumors. As a result, it is impossible for the fibroids to grow back. This surgery also takes away the risk of developing cervical and endometrial cancer, and because you will no longer menstruate, bleeding abnormalities will also be eliminated. The downside to this procedure is that there is no chance for future childbearing. Additionally, some women report decreased sensation during intercourse after having a hysterectomy. Most women, however, enjoy better sex because they are free of the pain caused by the fibroids.

As you can see, there are both positives and negatives surrounding hysterectomy. It is a major operation that women should consider carefully. If you are faced with it as a possible way of treating fibroids, make sure to discuss the pros and cons with your doctor thoroughly, as well as all other treatment options that may work for you.

On the one hand, a hysterectomy will cure you of fibroids forever. Other treatments may be effective, but tumors can and often do grow back. You need to think about whether you are willing to deal with the symptoms and possible surgery again a few years down the road. On the other hand, if you want to have children— or want more children—you have to think about how making the decision to have a hysterectomy will affect you in the long run, beyond the immediate issue of treating your fibroids.

There are many things to consider on both sides. It can be a very tough and traumatic decision for a woman. That's why it's so important to ask your doctor questions, to understand all of your options, and to get as much information as you can. Your doctor should respect your wishes, and you in turn need to trust your doctor enough to respect her medical knowledge and advice. Together, the two of you can make the correct decision for you.

The most common type of hysterectomy is called a "simple" or "total" hysterectomy, in which the body of the uterus (the upper part and the lower part, known as the cervix) are removed. Many people assume that a "total" hysterectomy also includes removal of the fallopian tubes and ovaries, but that is false. Those involve two separate, less common procedures, known as a salpingectomy and an oophorectomy, respectively. A salpingectomy may be necessary in the event of a ruptured ectopic pregnancy (a pregnancy that develops outside the uterus), severe endometriosis (a condition in which fragments of the lining of the uterus implant on parts of the pelvic organs, forming cysts), or other conditions. An oophorectomy may be indicated for many of the same conditions as a salpingectomy. However, ovaries are usually removed because of the presence of large cysts.

Depending on the size of the uterus and other considerations, you may have an abdominal or vaginal hysterectomy. In an abdominal procedure, the uterus is removed through an incision in the lower abdomen. In a vaginal hysterectomy, the uterus is removed through an incision at the top of the vagina.

Possible complications include excessive bleeding, wound infection, anesthesia complications such as aspiration (when saliva and fluids from the mouth are inadvertently "swallowed" down into the airway, putting fluid into your lungs) or an adverse reaction to one of the anesthesia drugs, and injury to other organs; as with any surgery, there is always the possibility of death.

Postoperative course: Following surgery a drainage tube may be inserted at the site of the incision, though this is not usually required. There may be some scant vaginal bleeding and discharge for a few days, as well as considerable tenderness and pain. Full recovery usually takes six weeks.

After a hysterectomy you will no longer be able to bear children, you won't have any more periods, and you won't be at risk for cervical or endometrial cancer. Many sisters are afraid that having a hysterectomy will cause them to lose their sex drive, or to "feel different." While it is true that women who have oophorectomies, during which the ovaries are removed, may get such menopausal symptoms as hot flashes, night sweats, and vaginal dryness, these can be relieved by hormone replacement therapy. With a simple hysterectomy, however, hormone pills are usually not needed. In this case, feeling different or changed in some way is, in all likelihood, a psychological reaction to the operation. Give yourself time. I've cared for thousands of sister-patients over the years, many of whom have had hysterectomies. Today they are pain-free. Their sex lives are terrific. They are leading perfectly normal, happy lives. And you most likely will, too.

Hysteroscopy

Classification: Minor surgery. This technologically advanced procedure can sometimes be performed right in the doctor's office.

Reason: To view the inner cavity of the uterus to check for structural abnormalities, excess endometrium buildup, septums, fibroids, and other abnormalities.

Anesthesia requirements: Local anesthesia, usually, but if done in the hospital, spinal or general anesthesia is used.

Blood loss: Usually minimal.

Description: A hysteroscope, an instrument similar to a laparoscope, is used to view the endometrial cavity of the uterus. Your doctor will be able to see the actual lining of the womb, as well as any endometrial polyps or fibroids in or on the cavity. The growths are removed using the hysteroscope's cutting device. This is usually an outpatient procedure that doesn't take very long in most cases.

There is minimal blood loss and minimal postoperative pain. While it's true that some hysteroscopies are done in the doctor's office, riskier or more involved procedures are performed in an operating room.

As with any surgery, hysteroscopy carries standard operating risks, specifically the risk of excessive fluid administration, which could overload your lungs with fluid, causing pulmonary edema or heart failure. It's crucial that your doctor be well trained in this procedure and knowledgeable about its risks.

Not all fibroids can be removed with this method. Hysteroscopies are only for fibroids that are in the endometrial cavity and are simple to manipulate and remove. Some submucous myomas may also be removed with this technique, but there is a greater risk of hemorrhage due to the intricate nature of the surgery. I can't stress enough how important it is that your surgeon be highly skilled in these particular procedures.

Postoperative course: Since this is often done in the doctor's office or as an outpatient, most patients get up, go home, rest for a day, and return to their full activities the next day. Of course, it depends on exactly what was done and how extensive the procedure was.

Myomectomy

Classification: Major surgery; an inpatient procedure.

Reason: To remove fibroids from the uterus.

Anesthesia requirements: Usually done under general anesthesia, though may be done with an epidural, if necessary.

Blood loss: Varies.

Description: An alternative to some hysterectomies is a myomectomy, a surgical procedure in which only the fibroid tumors are removed and the uterus is left intact. Seventy percent of the myomectomies done in the United States are performed on African-American women. The good news is that this operation preserves a woman's fertility, an important consideration for sisters who want to have a child, or want more children. The bad news is that in 10 to 20 percent of cases, the fibroids grow back. This procedure has the same recovery period and carries the same risks as a hysterectomy.

Hormone medication, such as Lupron, may be given before surgery in an effort to shrink the fibroids by causing estrogen levels to drop. Smaller fibroids require a smaller surgical incision, which means less trauma to the uterus. However, the reduction in fibroid size may be temporary, and hormone drugs can have side effects, such as allergic skin reactions, hair loss, and in the event of long-term use, osteoporosis (loss of bone density, which leaves bones brittle and easily fractured).

Several crucial factors help determine whether a myomectomy is the best course of action. These include:

- *Tumor size.* If the fibroids have grown to such an extent that they cause significant symptoms, then surgery is indicated.

- *Fertility issues.* Fibroid tumors can adversely affect fertility, depending on where they are located, particularly if they are blocking the fallopian tubes, the cervix, or the endometrial cavity where the embryo implants and the fetus grows. If a woman is infertile or has had repeated miscarriages, a full infertility workup should be done to rule out other potential causes besides fibroids (see Chapter 10).

- *Persistent, heavy bleeding.* Other causes of abnormal bleeding need to be ruled out first.

- *Bladder obstruction, resulting in an inability to urinate.*

- *Rapid enlargement of tumors.* Fibroids are usually slow growing. If they suddenly increase in size, it may suggest a malignancy in the fibroid, though this is very rare.

The standard myomectomy procedure, an abdominal myomectomy, calls for an incision to be made on the abdomen, either horizontally (low, near your pubic hair) or vertically (extending down from the navel, or a bit above it). The horizontal incisions heal better and carry less risk of separating.

In the past fifteen years, a newer method, laparoscopic myomectomy, has been performed for the purpose of removing fibroid tumors. A laparoscopic myomectomy utilizes smaller abdominal incisions. In this procedure, a telescopic instrument called a laparoscope is inserted through a small incision, allowing the doctor to see an image of your uterus on a video screen. (For more on this procedure, see Chapter 6).

Laser myomectomies are another option that require only a small abdominal incision. In this surgery, the doctor removes the fibroids with a laser beam (vaporization), which may be used either with the traditional or laparoscopic methods for myomectomy.

With any of these types of myomectomies, after the fibroids are removed, the area is closed with sutures. There is no limit on the number of tumors that can be removed during a myomectomy. A patient may have one large tumor or forty of varying sizes. What can limit removal of all the tumors, though, is their location in the uterus and their proximity to or involvement with large blood vessels or other internal organs.

Be sure to ask your doctor whether he or she entered your endometrial cavity during the myomectomy. Why is this important? Because most doctors feel that a full-thickness cut in the walls of the uterus—or any extensive dissection of the uterine walls—can weaken the uterus, leaving it susceptible to rupture or excessive hemorrhage during childbirth. Find out your doctor's recommendation for handling delivery if you become pregnant—should you allow labor or plan for a cesarean?

Myomectomies can be bloody operations because the uterus is very rich in blood supply. For this reason, some doctors might recommend that you bank your own blood in advance of the surgery. This is called an *autologous donation*.

Because this type of surgery carries a risk of excessive bleeding, it is crucial that your doctor be well practiced in the procedure. The risk of excessive blood loss, infection, and operative complications decreases dramatically with an efficient and knowledgeable surgeon who has performed this operation many times.

Postoperative course: Recovery time is usually six weeks for most myomectomies. For the first two weeks, you will have to curtail your activities markedly. You'll be able to resume them in gradual increments as the weeks progress. Hospitalization for myomectomies used to be six or seven days. But in today's insurance climate, and with increased scientific knowledge, many patients go home two or three days after the operation.

BEFORE YOU CONSENT—SEVEN IMPORTANT QUESTIONS TO ASK YOUR DOCTOR

As we mentioned earlier, it's crucial that you ask your doctor several key questions before having any form of surgery. The only way you can become informed is by speaking up. In an ideal scenario, your physician would sit down with you and explain every facet of your diagnosis and the surgical procedure from A to Z. However, to ensure that you receive as much relevant information as possible, it's in your best interest to ask the right questions.

When surgery is first recommended, many doctors will give you a pre-operation (pre-op) patient information handout that addresses patients' most common questions. Once the actual surgery date has been established, it's a very good idea for you to have what's known as a pre-op visit with your doctor a few days before the operation. If he or she doesn't bring it up, make sure that you do. During the pre-op visit, your doctor will go over the procedure with you and will also likely review the operation consent form that you must sign before having surgery. If you haven't done so already, now is the time to ask the following important questions— and be sure to take detailed notes.

1. *What is the diagnosis requiring surgery?*

The answer to this question will let you know the exact problem or condition that will be rectified by surgery. When you have the exact, precise diagnosis, in the doctor's own words, you're better equipped to pass along the information accurately to your second-opinion consulting doctor. It's your body, after all; you need to know what's going on with it.

2. *What are the test findings from the ultrasound, blood work, etc., to support the diagnosis?*

The answers will help identify which objective tool specifically pinpointed your medical problem. In other words, you'll know that your condition was determined through an analysis of your blood, your organs, etc. Why is this so important? Because it provides evidence that your doctor's impression is correct and that the treatment recommendation is justified. Remember, too, that the objective findings of the test results give the consulting second-opinion physician unbiased information about your illness.

3. *What are the treatments available to me? Can my condition be treated with medication only, or is surgery absolutely necessary?*

You should be aware of all possible treatments. Some doctors may be quick to suggest surgery without first trying a viable medication-driven alternative. In general, most doctors will explain all of the possibilities to a patient, but why wonder? Be certain by being up-front. Ask for a run-down of all available treatments. In this era of HMOs, which may unduly influence some doctors' treatment recommendations, it pays for you to inquire about every option.

4. *What are the surgical options?*

There may be more than one way to approach your medical problem surgically. For example, fibroids may be removable through a small incision in the navel, rather than with the standard full-length abdominal incision. Hysterectomies can be done through the abdomen, which leaves a visible scar, or sometimes through the vagina, which leaves no external scar at all. What may seem like minor considerations to a doctor can have big implications for you. So ask.

5. *What specific risks and complications are associated with this procedure?*

All surgeries carry the risk of excessive bleeding, infection, potential injury to other surrounding organs, and complications from anesthesia (when used). But some operations carry risks particular to that type of surgery. These shouldn't be glossed over by your doctor. Ask for not only a broad overview of potential dangers, but also a pinpointed explanation of specific risk factors. Yes, it's scary to be told some of these things, but you'll need to know in order to weigh the risks and the benefits of having the surgery.

6. *How long does the procedure take, on average?*

Most surgeons try to finish operations as quickly as possible. It's not that they simply want to wrap things up and get home. The real deal is that they know that the less time you are under anesthesia, the lower the risk of anesthesia-related complications. And the less time the incision is open, the lower the risk of infection.

You need to understand, though, that a procedure can take longer than expected, depending on what the surgeon finds once the operation begins. The amount of bleeding, the existence of old scar tissue (your doctor will ask about all of your prior surgeries; be sure to fill him in fully), unforeseen complications—all of these factors, and any number of others, can lengthen a surgery. That's why it's best to ask for a "time frame" for the operation rather than specific start and end points, and pass the information on to your loved ones. This way your family will be a little less stressed as they wait.

7. *Is it likely that I will need a blood transfusion?*

The majority of operations performed do not require blood transfusions, which are mostly given for trauma cases or when there is excessive blood loss. Even though odds are that you won't need a transfusion, you should be aware that myomectomies can involve a good deal of blood loss. Since this type of surgery is one of the most common among African-American women, it's important for you to raise the issue of blood transfusions with your doctor beforehand. Although stored blood used for transfusions is diligently screened and tested, many sisters still have concerns about its purity. In some cases, you may be able to have your own blood stored ahead of time so that it will be available, if necessary, for the operation.

DO YOU REALLY NEED A SECOND OPINION?

In a word—*Yes*. No one should ever have any type of major surgery without one. While you may have an excellent physician whom you trust completely, your health is not something to be taken lightly. Just because your long-time, trusted doctor advises surgery as the best treatment, that doesn't mean he's automatically right. When you need to get your car or a major household appliance repaired you search out more than one opinion, don't you? Why would you do any less for your health? You have to make sure that the suggested treatment is the best course of action. Doesn't it make sense that if two top-notch doctors offer the same recommendation, you'll feel two times better about following the advice?

So how do you go about obtaining a second opinion? Ask your doctor to give you the names of other doctors who have experience with your particular diagnosis. If your physician is hesitant to make referrals, that's a red flag. Either he is afraid of losing you to the other physician, or he may not be giving you all the possible treatment options. All the more reason to seek a second opinion. You can also turn to female friends, family members, and coworkers you trust. Ask them about their personal physicians. If you know any operating room nurses (or know anyone who does), give them a call. OR nurses are an excellent source of referrals to good surgeons who perform the type of surgery you are considering and who treat their patients well. It stands to reason, doesn't it? These nurses see the surgeons in action; they know who does a good job and who doesn't.

Once you have decided upon a consulting doctor, call for an appointment and explain that you are seeking a second opinion. (Health plans generally cover second-opinion visits.) Make sure that you have any objective findings readily available for the consulting doctor to review, including ultrasound reports, blood tests, Pap smear results, most recent notes from your doctor, and the like. You can request a copy of these materials from your doctor's office staff.

CARING FOR THE INCISION

In the days following surgery, you will be in pain or, at the very least, sore and tired. The only thing you'll probably want to think about is getting rest and getting better. Part of that healing process involves taking care of your incision site. Most surgical wounds heal with minimal scarring. Unfortunately, black women have a high tendency to form keloids along the incision line. These thick, raised, hard, itchy scars are more common in African Americans than in Caucasians, and form when excess bacteria is present at the site of the healing scar. That's why it's so important for sisters to be diligent about wound care. You may be afraid to touch the incision because of discomfort or plain queasiness. But, unless instructed otherwise by your doctor, you must keep your incision site clean as it heals to prevent keloids from forming.

If you are prone to keloids and let your doctor know ahead of time, he may inject your incision line with a steroid medication, which sometimes helps prevent the thick scars from occurring.

RX: A PRESCRIPTION FOR YOUR SOUL

You can have all the solid, nuts-and-bolts information about surgery in the world, but if you ever need an operation, there is one important thing you must always keep in mind: The success of the surgery lies as much in your hands as in your surgeon's. Yes, you are tendering your precious physical body to his care, but your equally precious spiritual self is still completely within your control. It's up to you to prepare yourself spiritually for this journey, not just to help the procedure go smoothly and to speed your healing, but also to enable you to navigate the journey from a position of inner strength.

Surgery is serious and it's frightening. If you let the enormity of it overwhelm you, you won't be doing yourself any good. We know it's difficult to stand up to your fears and approach the experience with calm and peace of mind. But we believe you can do it, if you turn to the healing power within. Some people may scoff at the power of spirituality, but we know you're not one of them. The fact that you're reading this book and thinking about how to shore up your health through divinity says to us that you are ready to open up your soul to new possibilities. You are ready to accept what some may not understand. You are ready to tap your spirituality in ways that you've never previously considered.

Picture the day of your surgery. Do you want to feel as though you are turning yourself over to others and simply hoping for the best? Or do you want to feel as though you have a hand in the outcome, as though you are going to be a contributor to your own health and well-being? This is such an important lesson for sisters to learn. If we can create a personal environment in which we shepherd our destinies with faith and a deeply rooted spirituality, then we can get through any hardship, any trial, any test of strength, character, or belief. Do you see it? Do you see the picture we are trying to paint for you? An upcoming surgery is just one hurdle that spirituality can help you overcome. Life is sure to throw others in your path. Do daily inner work and you will be able to face them all head-on.

For right now, sister-friend, let's concentrate on surgical procedures. Your doctor gives you the news and you're visited by fear, apprehension, and anxiety. How can you tap your spirituality to move beyond to a more positive frame of mind? First, realize that those emotions will be a part of you. Don't try to put up a brave front if you're not really feeling it. Inner work doesn't mean denying the truth of your experience. It means finding a way to cope and move on. It means reflecting on what's causing those feelings, understanding them, accepting them, appreciating them, and pushing forward to a better place—a place of strength.

Second, take steps to get yourself to that better place. Every sister will have her own way of taking each step. When we look within, each of us hears different messages and responds to different calls. Heed your individual messages. If your heart and soul are telling you something specific, pay attention. That's why it's called inner work. No one else hears exactly what you hear. No one else feels precisely as you feel. Your divine self speaks to you and you alone. When you focus on your spirituality, you are focusing on the most private, intimate, sacred parts of your being. It is yours, and how you use it now, during this time of health crisis, will gently and lovingly guide you through your physical ordeal.

That said, there *are* spiritual techniques that all sisters can use when faced with the prospect of surgery. The wonderful part is that although these techniques are universal, the way in which your spiritual self interprets and manifests them will be unique and special for you. Keep in mind, your soul knows every facet of you. It will never steer you down the wrong path if you nurture it and give it the sustenance it needs to grow. That's what these techniques are: sustenance for your soul at a particular point in your life—the point at which you are told that you require surgery.

Spiritual Techniques to Help
See You Through Surgery

Find your center. By this we mean ground yourself. Take time to focus on your body, your energy source. Find a peaceful spot, away from any distractions. Sit still and calm. Close your eyes and place your hands on your torso, right above your navel. Breathe deeply. Concentrate on the energy and positivity flowing through you. Imagine it surging through your bloodstream. Now, as you continue to breathe deeply, shift your focus and think about the surgery. Begin to internally ask yourself questions. Why is the procedure being done? Is it to rid my body of pain or disease? Is it going to make me healthier? Is it going to make me stronger? Will the operation have positive effects beyond my improved health? Will it enable me to live a longer, fuller life and be with my loved ones for more years? Will it take away pain and allow me to enjoy my children in ways that have been diminished? Take time to ponder the answers. Contemplate them. Next, try to envision yourself weeks after the surgery: happy, well, rejuvenated, full of life, vigorous, surrounded by loved ones. Let the visual image wash over you.

The point of the questioning and visualization is to keep you focused on the positive, not the negative. As we've said, fear and anxiety will be there. They are normal emotions, given the circumstances. By using this centering technique whenever those feelings start to overwhelm you, you bring your thoughts back to the positive. You calm and soothe yourself, and at the same time, strengthen your immune system and lower your blood pressure. Rely on this technique as often as you need to. It is akin to meditating but goes deeper. It retrains your thought process and helps you visualize a positive, empowering outcome, one that will better your own life and those of your loved ones. So remember, when you feel scared, panicked, or deeply depressed by the pending surgery, stop and find your center.

Have a prayer partner. Quiet meditation and finding your center will help calm your nerves, soothe your spirit, boost your immunity, and keep your blood pressure down. But sharing spirituality with someone you love and trust will give you even greater peace of mind as the day of surgery approaches. A prayer partner is someone to lean on and open up to. This person will help you to stay focused on your blessings, put the risks of the operation in perspective, and not get mired down in worry and depression. It's difficult when you must rely on yourself over and over for strength. You don't want to sap your spiritual reserve; you'll need it to preserve yourself not only before the surgery but after. That's where your prayer partner comes in. He or she is there to take some of the emotional burden off you and let you know that you are not alone. When the two of you share spirituality it fortifies you.

Set up a regular time to meet with your prayer partner. When you get together make sure it's someplace quiet and private. You may want to join hands as you pray together to feel more connected, to feel the spirit flow between the two of you. Maybe select a favorite scripture or passage to recite together. Use the time also to share your feelings about the surgery and all its implications. Your prayer partner will mirror those fears by expressing her understanding, thereby validating your feelings and giving you permission to move beyond them to the better place you're seeking. Think of your prayer partner as an extension of yourself. Allow his or her faith to strengthen your own.

Surround yourself with positivity. When family and friends hear that you need surgery, those who've been through one themselves will want to offer special support, which can be wonderful. After all, they know better than anyone what you're going through. But some of them will turn those words of support into "war stories," and, truth be told, you really don't need to hear that. What good will hearing the downside of someone else's experience do for you? None. It will only add to your anxiety. Research shows that emotions are contagious. Spend a lot of time around a person who is sad, depressed, or pessimistic and it will rub off on you. Surround yourself with folks who are optimistic, spiritual, and full of faith and you'll feel the same.

So if loved ones start off giving support and encouragement, but end up stepping over the line, don't be afraid to say *"stop."* Let them know that you appreciate their concern, but their negative comments go against the positive spiritual foundation you are trying to build. Invite them to join you on your spiritual quest instead. Perhaps the reverse will occur: Your divine attitude will rub off on them.

They do love you and want to help. Here's a good way to get them on a more helpful, spiritual path: Ask them to pray for a successful surgery. Prayer is a powerful thing; research proves it. One study at San Francisco General Hospital, for example, found that a group of heart patients who were prayed for were three times less likely to have heart failure than the patients who weren't prayed for.

Dialogue with a holy presence. Although African Americans are a devout and highly spiritual people, not all sisters have the same God. Whatever your Higher Power, our point is simply to talk to Him privately and ask for guidance and protection as you approach the big day. He knows you need Him. He knows you are afraid. He is there for you whether you seek Him or not. You are His child and He watches over you even if you aren't aware. So reach out. Ask, talk, and listen for answers. Be one with His presence. Seek His continued blessing—now and always.

Back to Basics—Nutrition and Exercise

· · · · · · · · · · · · · ·

I can begin to change the way I think about healthful food and exercise—not as a necessary evil for getting thinner, but as a daily practice that gives me life, health, and strength.

—Oprah Winfrey

News You Can Use

· In order to shed pounds and keep them off, you have to make the connection between weight and health. Put the focus on how you feel instead of how you look.

· Exercise speeds up your metabolism, helping your body burn more calories.

· Regular exercise strengthens your heart and lungs, lowers blood pressure, and improves immunity, just to name a few of its many benefits.

· You don't have to give up soul food in order to eat healthfully. In fact, many of the down-home foods we love are actually good for us, such as collards, kale, sweet potatoes, and black-eyed peas.

· Keeping a food diary is one of the best weight-loss aids around.

· Herbs and spices, such as cumin, basil, curry, and cinnamon, and cider vinegar have been shown to increase your metabolism, as they are *thermogenic,* or heat producing.

· Darker vegetables and grains are more healthful than the lighter-colored choices. For example, spinach or romaine lettuce and whole wheat bread are more nutritious than iceberg lettuce and white processed bread.

· Obesity is measured in terms of Body Mass Index (BMI). Government guidelines state a BMI less than or equal to 18.5 indicates being underweight; 18.6–24.9 is normal; 25–29.9 is overweight, and 30 or greater is obese.

*T*OO OFTEN when sisters think about improving their health, they think about making more of an effort to get regular checkups, Pap smears, and breast exams, and that's it. Now, don't get me wrong. Doing these things is definitely a major step in the right direction. There's no question that visiting your doctor routinely will keep you ahead of the game. But it doesn't end there. Lifestyle is just as big a factor when it comes to bettering your health.

What do I mean by lifestyle? Simple—what you eat and how often you move. You have to work the basics if you really want to be in the best health possible. And that means eating right and exercising. It's a tried-and-true combination that's guaranteed to get results, but we tend not to focus on it as much as we should.

I can hear thousands of sisters right now: *I don't have time to work out, not with my schedule. I can't give up my favorite down-home foods. If I exercise I'll sweat out my hair. My family would go crazy if I started cooking that "healthy" stuff.* And on and on. You have to let those excuses go. The reality is that if you don't eat nutritious foods and work up a sweat on a regular basis, you're asking for trouble. We all know where a sedentary lifestyle filled with fried, fatty, processed foods leads—to obesity.

Being overweight puts you at risk for a whole slew of diseases, including high blood pressure, diabetes, heart disease, and certain forms of cancer. Make no mistake, obesity is a big problem for black women. More than 40 percent of us are obese, according to studies conducted by the Centers for Disease Control, and we are dying every day because of it. And don't think it's just extremely heavy sisters who are affected. Even if you are only 20 or so pounds overweight you can still suffer from weight-related health problems. Each excess pound places more pressure on your heart and lungs. Consider, too, that what may be just a few extra pounds now can turn into three times as many if you don't nip them in the bud. Think of it as "creeping weight." I know plenty of sisters can relate to that concept.

Fortunately, the solution is simple. You have to work out and eat well. The hard part is in the doing. I won't lie. Losing weight isn't easy. But it is possible. The trick is to change your mindset, change your way of thinking. Many people automatically associate weight with appearance. They resolve to shed pounds because they want to "look good" and wear "cute clothes." That way of thinking doesn't help you, sister. Trying to fit into a size 6 isn't the sort of motivation that sustains lifelong weight loss. Often it simply leads to a vicious cycle of yo-yo dieting. Your weight goes up and down and up and down as you battle to fit into that smaller size. We all know sisters (it may even be you) who have closets full of clothes of every size—they have to in order to accommodate their ever-changing weight. So what's the big deal about yo-yoing? It's no good for your health, either.

The goal is to get to a healthy, sustainable weight, preferably one with a 5- or 10-pound fluctuation cushion. (Your doctor can help you determine what that weight should be.) And, for my money, the best way to do that is to let go of appearance-driven motivation and adopt a health-oriented way of thinking. By shifting the focus away from how you look and onto how you feel you will begin to see the relationship between weight and health. Once you make that connection, you'll be better able to slim down for good. That's because successful weight loss comes when you commit to make an investment in your health. Keep your mind focused on lowering your blood pressure and cholesterol, getting rid of diabetes if you have it and keeping it at bay if you don't, protecting your heart against disease, and your joints against osteoarthritis. When you think of all the ways shaping up will improve your health, it keeps you motivated; it gives you a life-altering reason to shed those pounds. Wanting to "look cute" just doesn't cut it in the long run. But wanting to improve your health and add years to your life? Now that's reasoning we can all get behind.

WORK THAT BODY

Who has time to exercise? You do. I know your schedule is crazy—the job is hectic and the family is clamoring for your attention. But when good health is the goal, "no time" is an excuse you can't afford. We all have time to work out if we really want to. Once you make it a priority in your life, you'll do whatever you have to to fit it in. Get up 30 minutes earlier in the morning. Hit the gym during your lunch hour. Let your husband cook a few nights a week so you can work out in the evening. Take a hard look at your schedule and figure out ways to set aside time for fitness. Keep in mind, when you literally pencil in your workouts on your calendar or in your date book, you're more apt to do them because they are "appointments" (albeit ones with yourself). It's a psychological trick that works.

The fact is, if you want to drop pounds you have to move your body. There's no getting around it. Yes, you can shed a few pounds by drastically cutting calories, but eventually those pounds are going to come back—and you'll likely put on a couple of extra ones in the process. Why is this? Because drastic diets don't speed up your metabolism; they slow it down. And when that happens your body goes into starvation mode and hangs on to every single calorie you consume, making it harder and harder for you to lose weight.

Plus, in May 2002, researchers cited in the *New England Journal of Medicine* reported that when dieters lost 17 percent of their body weight, their stomachs made more of a "hungry" hormone called *ghrelin*. The researchers believe that this hormone contributes to the way your body fights weight loss, stimulating you to eat more. *Leptin,* a protein made in fat cells, is reported to give a feeling of satiety, but it does not do so in people who are overweight.

The way to boost your metabolism and make your body burn

more calories is by exercising. Don't get the wrong idea, though, and think that as long as you exercise you can pig out and still lose weight. It doesn't work that way. Both have to be in balance. The good thing about working out is that it helps you burn calories hours after you finish exercising; this is called *afterburn*. Your metabolism stays revved up even when you are at rest.

If losing weight isn't reason enough to move your body, think about this: Regular exercise boosts your overall cardiovascular health by strengthening your heart, lowering blood pressure, raising HDL (good) cholesterol levels, and lowering LDL (bad) cholesterol levels. All of this helps cut your risk of heart attack, according to the American Heart Association. Consistent workouts also improve your immune system, stave off osteoporosis (a disease that thins and weakens bones, making you more susceptible to fractures), relieve stress, increase stamina, and help you sleep more soundly. I'd say that's pretty impressive. Exercise is power-packed with all sorts of healthy benefits.

The crucial element, however, is consistency. Working out needs to be a part of your regular routine—at least 30 minutes (45 to 60 minutes is even better for weight loss) five or more days a week. That may seem like a lot, but if you sat down and mapped out every waking moment of your typical day, I bet you'd find lots of time that could be designated for exercise. I mean, just how important is that re-run of *Martin* or that nightly phone chat with your girl that always seems to stretch to an hour? Cut those calls short, turn off the tube, and work it out, sister. Remember, you're doing it for your health.

That said, the next question is "Exactly what do I do?" First, before you even start thinking about dumbbells and aerobics classes, see your doctor for a complete physical. You should always get the green light from your physician before beginning any fitness routine.

Now it's time to get started. One of the easiest ways to begin working out is by walking. We all know how to walk, it doesn't cost any more than the price of a good pair of walking sneakers, and you can do it anytime, anywhere. Best of all, it not only whittles off pounds, it also improves cardiovascular health, lowers blood pressure and cholesterol, increases bone strength, and puts you at low risk for injury.

Before you hit the street, map out your route ahead of time. Do you simply want to walk around the neighborhood? In the park? At the high school track? Pick a setting that suits you, or do a combination of settings if you prefer. That's one of the great things about fitness walking—you decide where and when. Speaking of when, it's also a good idea to figure out the best time of day to work out before you actually begin your program. Are you a morning person or do you have more energy later in the day? Can regular walks fit more easily into your schedule before work, at lunchtime, or after work? Think about the course of your days and plug in your walking sessions accordingly. Some people find that exercising first thing in the morning works well because they get it out of the way and it gives them extra energy for the day. Morning exercise is what most fitness experts recommend, saying it boosts your metabolism for the rest of the day. Other folks find exercising in the evening more beneficial because it helps them shake off the stress of the day. It's up to you. Do what works best for you.

A few more things to take care of before you lace up your sneakers: Wherever you decide to walk, make sure it's a safe, well-lit area. If you will be walking near traffic, always wear brightly colored clothing with reflective strips. Take a bottle of water on each walk to stay hydrated, as well as a fanny pack to hold your keys, some form of identification, and a little money.

WALKING THE WALK

Even though we all know how to put one foot in front of the other, fitness walking isn't quite the same as sauntering down the street. There's a technique to it that makes it more than a casual stroll. To truly reap the fitness benefits, you have to use good form:

- Keep your chest lifted and your eyes focused ahead.

- Use the proper heel-to-toe technique—each time you take a step land on your heel, roll the entire length of your foot on the ground, and push off with your toes.

- As you walk, keep your stomach slightly pulled in.

- Breathe deeply, in through the nose, out through the mouth.

- Swing your arms naturally at your sides when you start walking. As you build up speed, bend your elbows at 90-degree angles and pump your arms; this will help propel you forward.

In addition to good form, you also have to pay attention to the intensity of your walks. Go too slowly and you might as well go back in the house. You can't take a leisurely stroll and call it a workout. You have to put some pep in your step if you want to whittle off pounds. But if you go too fast, you'll simply poop out before accomplishing anything. You want to find a good middle ground—speedy enough to get your heart pumping and to work up a sweat, but moderate enough not to wear you out after five minutes. It's what fitness experts call the "zone." You can find out if you're walking in the zone by taking the talk test. If you are breathing hard but are still able to carry on a conversation (though you may not necessarily feel like it) then you are in the proper zone. If you're so out of breath that you can't talk, then you're pushing too hard.

Now that we have all of the must-do's and points to remember out of the way, let's get moving. First, the warmup. This is crucial. You need to get your muscles warmed and limber before hitting your stride, otherwise you risk injury. To warm up, walk a bit slower than exercise pace for five or ten minutes. (Likewise, after your workout, cool down by walking slowly for another five or ten minutes. Then do a few gentle stretches.) After you warm up, you can pick up the pace. Don't worry if you can't go quite as fast as you'd like in the beginning, or if it takes you 20 minutes just to walk around the block. You have to build up your speed and endurance. It takes time, especially if you've been leading a sedentary lifestyle. Start off slowly and at a comfortable pace. For right now, you just want to get your body accustomed to the physical activity and ease your way into a more rigorous workout.

Goal #1: Walk for 20 minutes. (You may want to keep a walking log or journal so that you can track your progress for each goal.) Build up to the 20 minutes if you need to, going a little longer every day until you are walking for 20 consecutive minutes at each outing. It may take you one week, it may take you four. The point is to keep at it until you reach this first goal. With each walk, try to go a little faster, too. Pick up the pace a bit from week to week, but make sure to maintain good form. Don't overdo it; just try your best.

Goal #2: Walk for 30 minutes at a faster pace. Once you consistently hit the 20-minute mark, it's time to nudge it up to half an hour. Increase your speed incrementally as you go, but stay in the zone. If you find yourself gasping for air, you're going too fast too soon. Remember, you want to be breathing hard but still able to talk.

Goal #3: Walk for 45 minutes at a 15-minute-per-mile pace. This translates to three miles for every walk. How do you know if you've hit the 15-minute-mile mark? You can either take a pedometer (an inexpensive gadget available at sporting goods stores) with you each time you walk to keep track of your distance, or when you're still in the "mapping out your walking route" stage, drive the route and use your car's odometer to figure out the distance between your house and various landmarks. Then, as you walk, you'll know you've gone one mile when you get to the video store, two miles when you reach the cleaners, and so on. Check your watch and see how long it took you to reach each marker.

You can continue with the 45-minute walks or go up to an hour if you like. As long as you maintain that brisk pace you will be fine. If you want to try to go a little faster as well, that's okay. Just make sure to progress slowly. A good way to test your speed ability is by doing intervals. Once you're into the swing of your workout, go super fast for 30 seconds to 1 minute, then slow it back down to your normal brisk pace for a few minutes, then do another super-fast interval. Keep alternating for 10 to 15 minutes. Not only will you build up stamina and boost your overall speed, you'll also prevent boredom. Anytime you can challenge yourself—by doing speed intervals, by adding hills, etc.—as long as you do it safely, it helps to keep your walks interesting.

If you decide to stick to walks for your cardio workout, that's fine. But if you want to spice things up and add other aerobic options to the mix, there's plenty to choose from. You can do aerobic videos at home; go biking; try in-line skating; jump rope; take an aerobics, step, or kickboxing class at a health club or the Y—any activity that gets you sweating and gets your heart pumping will work. Just remember to try new things slowly and gradually. This is a process. You want to work up to your activities so that you can sustain them. That's the key to exercising off pounds. If you overdo it, you'll simply end up stopping altogether—and no one ever lost weight doing that.

PUMP IT UP

Walking and any other form of aerobic exercise you do is just one part of your get-fit plan. Weight training is the other. Why weight-train? Because it helps build muscle, and the more muscle you have the more efficiently your body can burn calories. Did you know that one pound of muscle burns 35 calories a day? There's even more good news about pumping iron. It also increases your strength, helps combat osteoporosis, builds denser bones, and gives your body that lean, sculpted look.

If you're worried that lifting weights will make you big and bulky, don't be. You're not going to turn into a female Rocky. The women bodybuilders you see on television do intensive training and lift seriously heavy weights to get that muscle-bound look. What I'm talking about is weight training (also called strength training or resistance training) for weight loss and good health. To achieve these goals you can use dumbbells or even your own body weight—both allow you to work against resistance, which is the whole point. If you opt for weights, it's best to start off with 2- to 3-pound dumbbells and progress to heavier weights (5 pounds, 8 pounds, etc.) slowly and incrementally. As with aerobic exercise, it's important to warm up before beginning. Marching in place for a few minutes is sufficient.

There are all sorts of strength-training exercises to choose from: bicep curls, lateral raises, tricep kickbacks, lunges, squats—

the list goes on and on. For a well-rounded, safe program, I suggest checking out a class (or personal trainer) at your local health club or Y, or trying a weight-training video by a reputable professional. The point is to follow a routine developed and demonstrated by a certified fitness trainer. Make sure he or she has a degree in the fitness field and certification from a nationally recognized organization like the American Council on Exercise (ACE), the American College of Sports Medicine (ACSM), the National Academy of Sports Medicine (NASM), or the National Strength and Conditioning Association (NSCA).

Keep in mind, when you weight-train it's important to pay attention to your breathing (exhale on the action, inhale on the release) and your technique (execute each exercise slowly and with control; let your muscles, not momentum, do the work). This is why it's so crucial to work with an expert when first learning to weight-train. Proper form and technique is vital to success. Without it, you won't home in on the exact muscles you're trying to work, rendering the exercises ineffective. And you'll place yourself at risk for injury, too.

YOU ARE WHAT YOU EAT

It's sort of a silly saying but it makes sense. Think about it. The foods that fill us with long-lasting energy and enable us to perform at our peak are those "good-for-you" foods like vegetables, fruit, whole grains, and lean meat that too many of us just don't get enough of. And the foods that give us a temporary energy boost then make us crash, that leave us feeling bloated and sluggish, are the high-sugar, high-fat, high-sodium processed foods that too many of us crave. If we want to get a handle on our health, we have to start making better food choices.

That can be a tall order for many sisters because black folks have a special relationship with food, don't we? Whether it's traditional southern cooking, urban "soul food," Caribbean cuisine, or any other regionally inspired type of meal, we love the food of our people. For us, it's more than just food on a plate. It's about heritage.

On the positive side, many of our favorite foods are full of nutrients. Greens such as collards, spinach, and kale are loaded with vitamins and antioxidants that help fend off cancer and heart disease. Legumes like pinto beans, black-eyed peas, and lima beans are great sources of fiber, protein, iron, potassium, and folate. Sweet potatoes are high in beta-carotene. Catfish and shrimp offer cancer-fighting nutrients. And this is just the tip of the iceberg. Many of the foods we love contain a wide variety of vitamins, minerals, and nutrients. Unfortunately, there is a negative side, too. What sisters tend to do is take all of these good-for-you foods and cook them in ways that diminish their healthfulness. For instance, if you put ham hocks, fatback, or salt pork into your greens, you're turning a very nutritious side dish into one full of fat and salt. Likewise, if you tend to fry your chicken you're simply pumping up the fat content. Add to these cooking methods our overreliance on high-fat, high-sodium, high-sugar processed foods and you're looking at a diet that does more harm than good.

What's so bad about fat? you may wonder. Well, not everything. The truth is you do need to have some fat in your diet for balanced nutrition, but it should account for no more than 30 percent of your total caloric intake. Fat can actually be good for you. Dietary fat gives you extra energy, helps your body absorb the fat-soluble vitamins A, D, E, and K, cushions your organs and protects them from injury, offers insulation to help you stay warm, and satisfies hunger. But for good health, you have to make sure you're consuming the right kind of fat. The important thing to remember is that not all fats are alike.

Saturated fat, found in animal products (including whole milk, cheese, and butter), lard, tropical oils, and many packaged foods, raises blood cholesterol and increases your risk of heart disease. You should cut back on this type of fat.

Unsaturated fats (monounsaturated fat found in canola, peanut, and olive oils, and polyunsaturated fat found in safflower, soybean, and sunflower oils) are healthier alternatives. You must read food labels carefully to know exactly what you are consuming.

Then there are *trans fatty acids* (also called trans fats), which are found in margarine, vegetable shortening, baked goods, frozen dinners, potato chips, fast food, and various other products. Trans fats are created through hydrogenation, a process that changes liquid vegetable oils into a solid form. Hydrogenation extends a product's shelf life but also makes fats more saturated. That spells bad news for your heart, because trans fats raise LDL (bad) cholesterol and lower HDL (good) cholesterol. A study conducted by researchers at Harvard Medical School confirms that consuming trans fats increases the risk of heart disease. Unfortunately, you won't find the term "trans fats" on food labels; it's not yet required by the FDA. But you can look for the words "hydrogenated" or "partially hydrogenated." These are the red flags that the item contains trans fats.

Like saturated fats, salt is another potentially unhealthy ingredient that too often finds its way onto our tables. Although we need some sodium to keep our bodies running smoothly, many of us consume far more than our bodies need or can handle. Sodium intake can contribute to high blood pressure, a serious condition that can lead to congestive heart failure, stroke, or kidney damage. Reducing the amount of salt you eat can be a great benefit to your health.

While cutting back on fat and salt will get you off to a good start healthwise, you have to pay attention to calories as well.

That's the crux of the matter when it comes to losing weight. And, after all, that's what we've been talking about from the get-go. So how do you shed pounds without giving up all the foods you love? Follow these ten steps:

1. You've resolved to do this—to drop the weight and improve your health. The first thing you need to do is clear out your kitchen. You want to start with a clean slate, so purge those cabinets and the refrigerator. Get rid of the chips, the cookies, the soda—all of those empty-calorie foods that offer no nutritional value. (You know which ones I'm talking about.) Now it's time to shop anew. Make a list of what you're going to buy and stick to it. Also, resolve to read food labels carefully as you shop so you know exactly what you're buying. Once in the supermarket, your goal is to fill your cart with lots of nutritious, healthy, tasty foods. You have to eat a well-rounded diet, one that balances calories with nutrients. When you're trying to lose weight, you can't deprive yourself. That doesn't mean you have the green light to fill up on junk; it means you allow yourself a variety of good food eaten in moderation. (More on moderation later.) For now, let's stay focused on the choices you're going to make in the store. For a well-rounded diet, you need to eat from all the major food groups:

   - *Breads, cereals, rice, and pasta (3 to 4 servings daily).* Stay away from processed items such as pastries, crackers, refined breads, and the like. Select as many whole-grain foods as possible. Good sources include bread and pasta made with whole wheat flour (not just wheat flour), brown rice, barley, and oats. An added benefit: According to research published in the *American Journal of*

Public Health, a diet consistently high in whole grains may reduce a woman's risk of dying from cancer or heart disease by 15 percent.

- *Vegetables (3 to 5 servings daily).* Opt for a wide selection of veggies, including lots of dark leafy greens. Make sure to buy plenty of the deepest-colored vegetables. Keep starchy vegetables, such as corn and white potatoes, to a minimum.

- *Fruit (2 to 4 servings daily).* Fresh fruits are fat- and cholesterol-free and offer many nutrients. For instance, citrus fruits, like oranges, are high in vitamin C. Mangoes, cantaloupe, and peaches have lots of vitamin A. Bananas are full of potassium. Buy a variety.

- *Meats, poultry, fish, dry beans, eggs, and nuts (2 to 3 servings daily).* Make sure to select lean cuts of meat and to trim off excess fat before cooking. (Another fat-fighting tip: Remove poultry skin before eating.) Buy plenty of fish, too, because seafood contains omega-3 fatty acids, the good-for-your-heart fat. Salmon, tuna, and mackerel are particularly good sources of omega-3s. Also, try turkey-based products—turkey burgers, turkey bacon, turkey sausage—they're lower in fat and calories. Just be sure to buy low-sodium varieties.

- *Milk, cheese, and yogurt (2 to 3 servings daily).* Although dairy foods have lots of vitamin D and calcium, they can be high in fat and cholesterol. Opt for skim, low-fat, and one-percent versions.

- *Fats, oils, and sweets (eat sparingly).* When buying oils, select unsaturated ones such as canola, olive, and sunflower. Avoid coconut, palm, and palm kernel oils.

2. To shed pounds you'll need to change your lifestyle. That means exercising regularly and eating healthfully. It doesn't mean drastically cutting calories. You should never go below 1,200 calories a day. Yes, you have to adhere to some limits and cut back on how much you eat, but eating less than 1,200 calories a day isn't the way to go. When you take in too few calories your body rebels because you're not giving it the fuel it needs to run properly. You'll become fatigued, you won't think as clearly, and your health will suffer. Eating 1,500 to 1,800 calories a day is a safer and more realistic means of losing weight. Make an appointment with your doctor to discuss a daily caloric total that will work best for you in your efforts to trim down.

3. You've restocked your kitchen with healthy, nutritious foods. Don't blow it by preparing them the wrong way. You can keep the flavor without adding all the fat and calories by relying less on frying and more on baking, broiling, grilling, roasting, steaming, poaching, sautéing, and stir-frying. Also, when cooking beans and greens, don't add those old standbys salt pork, fatback, and ham hocks. Instead put a little smoked turkey neck or smoked skinless turkey into the pot. Or forgo the add-in meat altogether and cook beans and greens in low-fat, low-sodium chicken broth instead of water. Can't find low-fat, low-sodium broth? Then dilute regular chicken broth with equal parts water. All of these alternatives pump up the flavor without going overboard on the fat and calories.

4. You don't have to give up indulgences and favorite foods in order to lose weight. Simply select healthier alternatives. If you crave ice cream, have a little sorbet instead. It's lower in fat and calories. If you're addicted to potato chips, switch to equally tasty baked tortilla chips. Rather than making meat-balls or meatloaf with fatty ground beef, try ground turkey for a change. Always look for ways to cut the fat and calorie content of your meals by making healthy substitutions.

5. Why do we love fat so much? Because it adds flavor to food and satisfies our hunger. But you don't need fat in order to give greens, lean meats, and other healthy foods just the right "flava." As long as you have an assortment of herbs and spices, all your meals will be mouthwatering. And I don't mean salt and pepper. Try oregano, garlic, cumin, curry, paprika, rosemary, basil, dill, tarragon, bay leaf, thyme, and any others you wish. Experiment with season-ings and you'll discover all sorts of savory new tastes.

6. Probably the most important piece of nutritional advice I can give is to pay attention to portion size. You have to keep your portions in control. Making smart food choices is im-portant, but even the healthiest of foods can pack on pounds if you eat too much of them. Not sure how much to eat? One serving does the trick; don't go back for seconds. That said, be certain that your servings are truly *one* serving. A half-cup of cooked vegetables, rice, grits, macaroni, or beans equals one serving. Three to four ounces of meat equals one serving. A slice of bread equals one serving. Here are a few visual cues you can also rely on when cooking or plating food: One portion of dry spaghetti should be about the same diameter as a quarter. A cup of rice is about the size of a ten-

nis ball. Three to four ounces of meat is about the size of a deck of cards or the palm of your hand. An ounce of cheese is equivalent to a pair of dice. A half-cup of cooked veggies is roughly the size of your fist. Another trick that will help you get a handle on portions: Imagine your plate divided into three food group zones—½ vegetables and fruits, ¼ protein, and ¼ starch. Be sure to drink at least eight glasses of water a day, too. It will help keep you full and it's good for your overall health.

7. Plan two snacks into your day. No, I'm not kidding. You can have snacks when you're losing weight, as long as they are healthy ones (low in calories, high in nutrients), and you keep them in moderation. Figure them into your daily calories. Snacks can actually aid in your efforts to trim down. Noshing on a nutritious, filling snack curbs cravings in between meals and helps you stay on track. Perhaps have one midmorning and another in the late afternoon. Or one after work and another later in the evening. Think about the two times of day when you normally get those hard-to-resist hunger pangs. That's where you plug in your snacks. What makes a good snack? Forget cookies, potato chips, candy, and the like. And don't be fooled by their low-fat counterparts. Remember, low-fat cookies aren't necessarily low in calories. In order to compensate for reducing the fat—and thus reducing the flavor—many manufacturers load up their products with sugar. So you may be getting less fat, but you're also getting a ton of extra calories. Again, you have to check the labels. If you absolutely crave one of these items, look for versions with both reduced fat and reduced calories. It's far better, however, to find healthy, additive-free alternatives. That way you keep those goodies "good." A

cup of air-popped popcorn makes a great snack, as do two or three graham crackers, a frozen fruit bar, a handful of pretzels, a few baked tortilla chips with a bit of salsa, or a scoop or two of sorbet. When planning your snacks, also try to think out of the box. A snack can be a slice of toast spread with a little peanut butter (just check the label to make sure it is made without hydrogenated oil), a piece of fruit, celery sticks and baby carrots with yogurt dip, or half of a turkey or tuna sandwich made with low-fat, low-cal mayo. As long as you keep your snacks low in calories, you'll be fine.

8. Keep a food diary. Don't just write what you ate and when, jot down how you felt at the time. Often our emotions are tied to food and we have a tendency to eat for comfort when we feel stressed, upset, angry, sad, even bored. Seeing all of it in black and white can help you figure out what trigger foods may be connected to your emotional state. Be thorough when filling in your diary. Write down how each dish was prepared, the time of day you ate, and how much you had. As the weeks progress, you can flip back through the pages and track how well you are doing. You can also see backsliding patterns emerging before they become full-blown. This empowers you to recommit and regain control. Many times we aren't aware of what we're eating 24/7. We think we know but we may forget about nibbling on this and that during the course of the day. If you can resolve to write in your diary every single time you eat something, it will become a habit that serves you well in the end.

9. Don't sabotage yourself when you go out to eat. I know you're busy and sometimes you have to grab a quick meal

on the go, perhaps from McDonald's, Kentucky Fried Chicken, or some other fast-food place. There will also be times when you want to enjoy an evening out at a nice restaurant. Whatever the scenario, whether fast food or a sit-down restaurant, if you make the same smart choices you do when cooking at home, you can continue to successfully shed pounds. At fast-food joints, forgo the dressing-heavy burgers, super-sized fries, and soda. Go for lighter fare: for example, a grilled chicken sandwich (sans the mayonnaise or cheese; spread on mustard instead), a side salad, and a diet soda. At fancier restaurants, select entrees that are not fried, nor swimming in butter, oil, or heavy sauces. Ask that salad dressing be served on the side; this allows you to control the amount used. Opt for balsamic vinegar and lemon juice, or a bit of extra virgin olive oil, rather than the more fat-laden varieties. Speaking of salad, request that no cheese, nuts, bacon bits, or croutons be added. Can't resist that warm basket of bread? Go ahead and have a slice, but don't overload it with butter. Everyone's having dessert and coffee after the meal? You can too, just make sure to select a low-fat treat like fruit, sorbet, or angel food cake. As always, when dining out watch your portions. If your entrée is clearly more than one serving, eat only half, or split it with your dining companion.

10. Break the salt habit. The American Heart Association recommends that sodium intake be less than 2,400 milligrams a day, which is about 1¼ teaspoons of salt. But many of us regularly consume well over that amount. By reducing your salt intake you lessen your risk of developing high blood pressure; and if you're already hypertensive, weaning yourself from sodium can help bring your pressure down. Once you

acquire a taste for salt it can be hard to let go. But you can get just as much flavor and zing from other sodium-free products, like Mrs. Dash. It's all about substitution. Of course, you can't really do anything about the sodium that is in foods naturally, except to eat less of them. But you *can* do something about the salt you add to food yourself. Your first rule of thumb should be to always taste a dish before immediately grabbing the salt shaker. Sprinkling on salt has become such a habit for some folks that they do it automatically. Also, when cooking, reach for your trusty herbs and spices instead of salt to give food zest. Other tips to help you break the salt habit: Don't keep the shaker on the table. If it's not handy, you'll be less apt to use it. Shop selectively. Read food labels and buy items with low sodium content.

RX: A PRESCRIPTION FOR YOUR SOUL

Anyone who has tried to lose weight knows that there is no magic formula. As much as we may want an overnight miracle, the truth is it just doesn't work that way. We have to make up our minds to do it, and then get busy. It's hard work, to be sure; not so much the actual exercising and eating right, but the resolve to do them. That's why it's helpful to concentrate on your health when trying to shed pounds. That really is the secret to success here. Focus on how many years you'll add to your life and how high-quality those years will be. You won't be plagued by life-threatening, obesity-related illness. You'll have more energy and stamina. Your mind will be clear and sharp. Your whole attitude will be uplifted. You will attain true well-being. Isn't that what we all strive for?

Think about that term for a moment: well-being. It literally means *the state of being happy, healthy, or prosperous.* To me, that translates to happiness, health, and prosperity of your body, your mind, and your soul.

You see, fitness is more than simply how much you weigh and how much muscle you have. Yes, it reflects our physical selves, but that is only the beginning. Your body truly is a temple, one that should be cherished and protected. When we think about shedding excess pounds and getting in shape we understand that these actions are for the betterment of our temples. But the means to that end—namely, exercise and good nutrition—accomplish far more than giving you a trim, fit body. They also replenish and restore every aspect of your temple—your physical body, your mind, and your spirit. When you think of your body as a temple, think of all of its elements, not just the tissue, sinew, muscles, and organs. For when you do that, you empower yourself to see the multitude of gifts fitness can offer.

By eating well, you nourish yourself with high-quality foods, rather than polluting yourself with less-than-the-best foods. Make no mistake, what you eat affects you mentally and spiritually, not just physically. How often have you felt guilty after eating empty-calorie foods that offered no nutritional value? We tend to indulge first and feel bad later. And boy do we feel bad—beating ourselves up and berating ourselves until our self-esteem is shot. What do you think that type of self-assassination does to your mental and spiritual outlook? It leaves you feeling bereft. That sort of thinking doesn't uplift you; guilt trips and inner critics only drag you down.

But when you make smart, healthy food choices, when you give yourself nourishing sustenance, your body, mind, and spirit thank you. Eating well satiates you positively. There's no guilt baggage to weigh you down. You know you're tending your temple well, and that makes you feel renewed. Research also shows that good nutrition positively affects brain function, sharpening cognitive skills, memory, verbal acuity, and alertness.

Likewise, engaging in exercise also affects mentality and spirituality, not just physicality. When you work out, chemicals are released in your brain that make you feel good. You've heard of "runner's high"? Well, this is what it means. Exercise gives you a natural "high." Those feel-good brain chemicals contribute to a sense of peace and overall serenity. Physical fitness is as much a form of inner work as meditation. In fact, many types of exercise, such as yoga, tai chi, and Pilates, actively seek to engage participants' souls as well as their bodies. What's more, exercise increases oxygenation and stimulates blood flow to the brain, which results in better concentration and focus.

Conversely, leading a couch potato lifestyle disengages not only your body but your mind and your spirit as well.

It all comes down to one simple principle: Love yourself. It sounds so obvious, but too many sisters don't do it. Your body, mind, and spirit are a unified and sacred triad that needs to be nurtured. You must make nourishing sustenance and health-protecting movement a vital part of your lifestyle. If you dine on unhealthy foods and embrace sedentary living, you aren't genuinely loving yourself. You're basically opening the door for illness and disease. So resolve to get into your best shape possible—for your health, for your mental outlook, and for your soul. That's true self-love.

Caring for Your Breasts

· · · · · · · · · ·

What if you find a lump in your breast? What happens then? Lord, nothing has changed. You love me. Your eternal, perfect plans for me are continuing on schedule. I will praise You. I will worship You. I will rest in all You are continuing to do in my life.

—Anne Ortlund, contributor to *Joy for the Journey*

NEWS YOU CAN USE

· Current statistics show 1 in 8 women will develop breast cancer.

· The most common site for breast cancer to occur is in the upper, outer quadrant of the breast.

· The key to breast care is monthly breast self-exams, a breast exam done by your doctor, and regularly scheduled mammograms.

· African-American women die from breast cancer at a greater rate than white women, most likely because of late diagnosis.

· The sooner a cancer is diagnosed, the better the chance for cure.

· Family history is a key risk factor for the development of breast cancer, especially if found on the female side of the family (your mother, sisters, first cousins, etc.)

· Inherited mutations in genes are thought to cause about 10 percent of all breast cancers, mostly due to a mutation of the "BRCA" gene.

BREASTS COME in all shapes and sizes. Some are small and pert. Others, large and pendulous. Still others, medium and round. No matter how different each pair may be, they all hold the same power. On one hand, breasts are the object of sexual desire, exciting men by their mere presence. On the other, they are a source of sustenance, providing nourishment for our babies. Even the Bible makes clear the importance of the female breast, repeatedly referencing it as a source of pleasure and nourishment.

This enduring power is increasingly evident these days. We are, quite simply, a breast-obsessed society. Open any magazine, turn on any television show, go to any movie, watch any music video, and odds are a woman's cleavage will be prominently on display. "Boob job," "implants," and "silicone or saline" are terms that have all become a part of our national lexicon. Even the debate over whether nursing mothers should breast-feed in public can be linked to this hyped-up sexualization of breasts. Some find public breast-feeding offensive, and you have to wonder why. Could it be that they can only see breasts from a sexual point of view? As erotic as our breasts are—and that is a good thing, to be sure—we have to remember that they are more than just that.

I say let's celebrate this unique and wonderful part of the female physique. God created a woman's body to function in truly amazing ways. It really is a marvel. We should rejoice in our ability to nourish our children, enjoy the sexual arousal we can derive from our breasts, and delight in the stimulating pleasure they offer the men we love. Sisters, let's embrace all of our breasts' power. And in so doing, let us also protect this gift by ensuring its health.

THE ABCS OF BREASTS

What are your breasts made of? As you can see on page 233, the breast is primarily fat. Breasts contain very little muscle, so you can't change their size with exercise. It's the amount of fat in them that determines how large or how small they are. That's why when

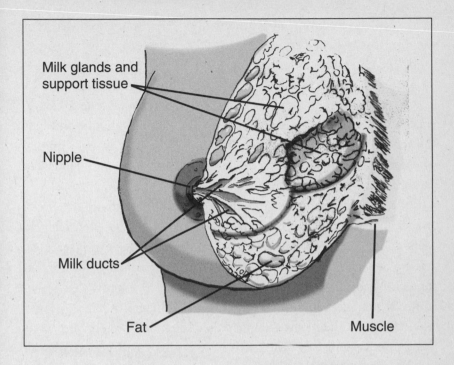

Milk glands and support tissue

Nipple

Milk ducts

Fat

Muscle

you gain or lose weight your bra size changes. In addition to fatty tissue, breasts also contain lymph glands and bands of ligaments. These ligaments and the fatty tissue support the network of milk glands (called *lobules*) and ducts in the breasts that spring into action when it's time to nurse. The milk glands and ducts merge at the nipple, which contains tiny openings through which the milk can pass.

Just as the size and shape of breasts differ from one woman to the next, so too can the nipples. Some nipples protrude while others are flat. Some are large while others are small. And some women are born with "inverted" nipples—that is, nipples that dimple inward. Inverted nipples sometimes come out when a woman is sexually aroused, and can often be manipulated out with your fingers when needed for nursing. All these types of nipples are normal. (However, if your nipple suddenly becomes inverted, see your doctor. It may be a sign of a tumor.) The nipple is highly sensitive, and when a woman is sexually aroused or cold her nipples may become erect (or more erect than they usually are).

Surrounding the nipple is a circle of darker skin called the areola, which contains sweat glands, sebaceous (oil) glands, and hair follicles. It's not uncommon to have small bumps on your areola; these are the oil glands. It's also not unusual for some women to notice a hair or two on their areola.

The areola can vary in size and color. In African-American women, it can range in color from a pinkish hue to almost black, depending on your complexion. Some women have tiny areolas, others have very large ones. And there are all manner of sizes in between. Again, these variations are quite normal. I know that sometimes we can get caught up in the idealized images of female beauty that we see in the media—images that tout the "perfect" breast as looking a certain way. The truth is, every pair is different, and all of them, no matter the shape or size, are beautiful.

FROM BUDS TO BREASTS

As a little girl you may have waited anxiously to finally sprout teeny buds. Or you may have been one of the young sisters who blossomed early and wished she could hide her shapely new form. Whatever your experience, you can be sure it's one that millions of other women have shared. From as early as the thirty-fifth day after you were conceived, your breast tissue began to take shape. As a young girl you had flat "breasts"; basically they were just nipples with a rudimentary, undeveloped system of ducts. As you reached puberty, your ovaries began to secrete estrogen, which caused your nipples to begin to protrude a bit as a result of the growth of breast tissue underneath.

The onset of menstruation brought even more changes. As you continued to grow, so too did your breasts. "Buds" began to develop as the areola swelled. At maturity (age 18) your breasts reached their full size, becoming rounded in shape, and the protruding areola flattened and took on the contour of the breast.

In our day, this period of maturation typically began at about age 10 or 11, but today puberty can start as early as 8 or 9 (and sometimes younger). Little girls are developing at shockingly early ages. That's why it's so important to talk to our daughters about the changes they can expect in their bodies while they are still relatively young. You may think five or six years old is too early, but if your daughter begins to blossom much sooner than you expect, she needs to be prepared.

A LITTLE TLC

Caring for our breasts is a hands-on experience—literally. Not only do we have to make sure to get regular mammograms when the time is right, but we have to feel and closely inspect our breasts routinely to check for lumps and abnormalities. What's more, we have to be certain that we are giving our breasts the best support possible. Take a hands-on approach, do these three things, and you'll really be giving your breasts the tender loving care they require.

Finding the Right Bra

When I talk about the best support, this is what I mean—your bra. Why do you think people in the retail industry refer to lingerie as "foundations"? Your underwear *is* your foundation; it's your support. And nowhere is this more true than with your bra.

Unfortunately, none of us can fend off gravity forever. Eventually all breasts begin to sag, even A-cup-sized ones. The ligaments in your breasts are what help to hold them up, but those ligaments can lose elasticity over time. Pregnancy, breast-feeding, and fluctuations in weight can also contribute to droop. The main culprit, however, is the clock. As we age, gravity simply takes a toll. Some women will experience more sag than others, especially if their bust is large. But wearing a good-quality, proper-fitting bra can help you combat the force of gravity. By wearing one daily you put less stress on your breasts' ligaments, prolonging their elasticity.

Most of us do wear bras every day. The problem is that we may not be wearing the right one. Too often women put on bras that just don't fit. It may be that they don't know their true bra size, or they don't know how to gauge whether a bra fits correctly, or they want to wear pretty lace numbers no matter what the size on the label, or they don't know where to go to find bras above a double D. Whatever the reason, the bottom line is you have to make sure your foundations fit. Don't worry. It is possible to find pretty, feminine, well-made bras in your size if you know where to look. They may cost more, but when it comes to support and comfort, they are worth every penny.

First and foremost, know your true size. This is where the problem starts for most sisters. They used to wear a 34C in college; ten years and two kids later, they're still buying the same size bra. Breasts change. It stands to reason that your bra size will, too. You have to measure your breasts to know for sure. Otherwise, you wind up wearing lingerie that doesn't fit properly. And we all know how annoyingly uncomfortable that can be—and worse still, bad for your breasts.

Stand in front of the mirror wearing only your bra and you'll probably notice a few obvious problems right away. For instance, if the straps dig into your shoulders, even at their loosest setting, the bra is too small. If the cups wrinkle, it's too big. If your cleavage is working overtime (and you're not wearing a push-up bra), it's not the right size. You get the idea.

So how do you get the correct measurements? While wearing a bra, use a measuring tape to measure around your diaphragm. Add five inches to the number. This is your body size. If it's an uneven number, round up. Next, measure around the fullest part of your bust. The difference between this number and your body size is your cup size. You're an A cup if your bust size is an inch larger than your body size. You're a B cup if the difference is two inches. You're a C cup if your bust size is three inches larger than your body size. A four-inch difference? You're a D cup. Five inches equals a DD, and so on.

If you're worried that your do-it-yourself measurements won't be accurate, you can ask the saleswoman at your local department store if she'd mind helping you take your measurements in the dressing room. Or you can consult a custom bra-maker at a specialty bra and lingerie store.

Once you have the correct numbers in hand, it's time to go shopping. Always try on bras before purchasing them. It's the only way to ensure a good fit. Thoroughly look yourself over in the dressing room mirror. Move around, too, to check the comfort level. Do the cups completely contain your breasts? There should be no bulges at the tops or sides. Can you comfortably slip your finger under the band? If the bra fits well you should be able to. Are the straps too tight? Adjust the length, then reassess. How about the back of the bra? Does it ride up? If it does, hook the back more snugly and/or loosen the straps. Still riding up? Then the bra may be too small. Check out the center front of the bra. If the cups separate and support the breasts properly, the center front of the bra should lie relatively flat against your breastbone. If it sticks out, you have the wrong size. And don't forget about wrinkling in the cup. That's a sign of a bra that's too big.

Don't be embarrassed to ask for the saleswoman's assistance when trying on bras. She'll most likely be happy to help. Believe me, the sales staff know that when a customer finds a comfortable, supportive bra she loves, she'll be back to buy more.

Larger-busted sisters who have trouble finding their size may want to consider specialty shops or having their bras custom-made. Check your yellow pages to find a store or bra-maker in your area.

Well, that covers everyday bras, but what about sports bras? Do you need to wear those, too? Absolutely. In fact, they may be even more important. Exercising without one can stretch the ligaments supporting your breasts, further eroding their elasticity and contributing to breast sag. Aerobic workouts, in particular, place a great deal of stress on your bust, what with all the jumping and bouncing. However, more static exercises like weight training and calisthenics can do a fair share of damage, too, because your body is still in motion, even though the movement may be less jarring overall. Either way, a body in motion equals breasts in motion, and you will need extra support.

That's where sports bras come in. They offer more stabilizing support than regular bras because of their specialized materials and construction. Sports bras compress and immobilize the breasts. As with everyday bras, make sure your sports bra is the proper size and try it on before buying. Jump around in it. Twist, bend, reach, jog in place. Assess how it responds to your actions. Your breasts should stay in place. They shouldn't bounce with your every move, nor should the bra ride up or twist as you move around. Look for wide straps and fabric that wicks sweat away. Also make sure the bra's band and straps do not dig into your skin, and avoid sports bras with underwire. The bra should feel firm and very supportive but still comfortable. It should not impede or interfere with your physical activity. If your breasts are so compressed that you feel as though you can't breathe, try another size or another style of sports bra.

Breast Self-Exams

The second part of our hands-on approach to breast care is the all-important breast self-exam. Getting to know your breasts and becoming familiar with how they normally feel is the only way you will be able to detect unusual changes. You should examine your breasts every month. Your menstrual cycle can cause changes in the texture of your breasts—in particular, increased fluid in the breasts can make them fuller and more tender, and therefore make a breast exam less accurate. Because of this, it's best to do the self-exam a few days after your period ends. It's actually a very simple process. Just follow the three steps:

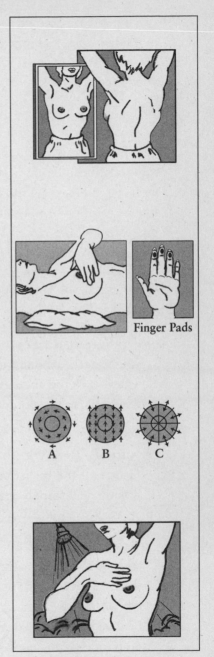

Finger Pads

1. Begin with a visual check. Stand in front of a mirror with your hands resting on your hips. Look for any changes in the size or shape

of your breasts, as well as any puckering, dimpling, nipple discharge, changes in the skin or nipples, and any other irregularities. Then raise your arms and clasp your hands behind your head and look for the same changes.

2. Now it's time to examine your breasts by touch. Lie on your back. Place a pillow under your right shoulder and put your right arm behind your head. Use your left hand to examine your right breast. With fingers flat, use the pads of your fingers to press firmly around the breast itself as well as the outer region of the breast (the underarm area, including the armpit). You can use any of three methods. Whichever method you select, use it every time you do your self-exam.

- Circular: Starting at the outer edge of the breast, move your fingers in small circles working toward the nipple. Then check the underarm area. Finish by gently squeezing the nipple to check for discharge.

- Vertical: Work your hand up and down over the entire surface of the breast and the underarm area. Afterward, squeeze your nipple gently to check for any discharge.

- Wedge: Starting at the nipple, press outward toward the edge of the breast. Then move your fingers over and do the next section of your breast, again starting at the nipple, until you have inspected the entire breast. As always, be sure to examine the underarm area and to squeeze the nipple gently to check for discharge.

Switch the pillow to the other side, position your left arm behind your head, and use your right hand to examine your left breast in the same way.

3. While taking a shower—the water helps your hand glide smoothly over your breasts—place your right hand behind your head and examine your right breast and underarm area with your left hand, using either the vertical, circular, or wedge method. Switch hands and examine your left breast.

If you feel a lump during your self-exam or notice anything else unusual, see your doctor immediately.

Mammograms

These are the final part of our hands-on approach to breast care. Far too many sisters put this important procedure off. Why? Embarrassment, lack of symptoms, fear, forgetfulness, negative attitudes about the health care system, and low income are the main reasons black women give for not having mammograms, according to a 2000 study by the Department of Community Health and Preventive Medicine at Morehouse School of Medicine's Treatment Effectiveness Center.

The sad fact is that by not having this crucial screening, black women are putting their health at risk. Breast cancer is the most common form of cancer in American women, and sisters have the highest mortality rate for the disease, according to the National Cancer Institute. This disease is killing us every day because we tend to get diagnosed too late. Breast cancer must be detected early if we are to be able to fight back, and breast self-exams and mammograms are the way to accomplish this.

Some sisters may wonder: *What about radiation? What about*

the pain? Let me assure you, the dosage of radiation used is very small, so your exposure is minimal. You won't get cancer from a mammogram. As for pain, I think that characterization is too extreme. "Slight discomfort" is a more accurate description. A mammogram does put some pressure on your breast, but just for a few seconds. You shouldn't let the thought of discomfort deter you from having the screening. Remember, we are a strong people. Besides, newest digital mammograms don't cause discomfort at all, patients say. Think of our foremothers, such as Harriet Tubman and Sojourner Truth. Would they let a little discomfort prevent them from doing what they had to do? Of course not.

Once you know exactly what to expect from a mammogram, and the benefits you stand to gain, I'm sure you'll be less apprehensive about the procedure. So let me break it down for you. A mammogram is a low-dose X ray of the breast. Both of your breasts are pressed between two plates, one breast at a time. This is what causes the discomfort you'll feel. Two X rays are taken of each breast. The entire procedure should take less than ten minutes. A mammogram can detect cancer or precancerous changes in the breast. And while they can pick up calcifications and masses that may be too small to detect during an examination, mammograms should never be your sole means for inspecting your breasts. They should be one part (albeit a very important part) of your total breast health action plan, performed in conjunction with monthly self-exams and annual breast exams by your physician.

You should be aware that, as with any medical procedure, mammograms can show false negative and false positive results. But that is no reason not to have them done. They play a vital role in detecting breast cancer early enough to save lives.

You should have your first mammogram at age 35 (earlier if you have a family history of breast cancer or other risk factors; discuss the appropriate timeline with your doctor). This initial screening will be your *baseline* mammogram. It gives your doctor a point of comparison for your future mammograms. Your risk of breast cancer increases as you age, so starting at age 40 you should have a mammogram every year.

You can find a reputable, certified mammography facility in your area by asking your physician for a recommendation, checking with your local hospital, or contacting the National Cancer Institute and the American Cancer Society. Make sure that the facility you select is approved by the Food and Drug Administration (FDA) and has certification to that effect.

BREAST BASICS

Once puberty hits, our breasts become a big part of who we are as growing adolescents and, ultimately, as fully developed women. Our breasts are one of the things that make us unique as females. By taking care of them as we should with proper bra support, self-exams, physician exams, and mammograms, we are doing our part to ensure the best breast health possible. Sometimes, however, breast conditions crop up that can range from the benign to the more serious, and some are more common than others. Knowing what these conditions are, how they affect your breasts, and what they may or may not mean for your overall health can help you handle them successfully if you need to. Let's take a closer look.

Asymmetry

When you look at your breasts in the mirror you may notice that one is slightly larger than the other. This is normal. The key word, though, is *slightly*; the difference is barely noticeable. Some women, however, have a much more pronounced asymmetry, with one breast considerably bigger than the other. This pronounced

NONCANCEROUS BREAST CONDITIONS

Congenital abnormalities:	asymmetry, nipple retraction, hypoplasia
Nipple discharge:	caused by various factors
Benign diseases:	Inflammatory—mastitis, eczema, abscess
	Solid masses—fibroadenoma, fat necrosis, sclerosing adenosis, granular cell tumors
	Cystic masses—fibrocystic disease, hematoma, galactocele

asymmetry is a genetic predisposition for many women and is not caused by anything they did or didn't do. One breast simply develops more fully than the other. Usually, the size difference does not pose a health problem unless it's a new or sudden occurrence such as with trauma, but psychologically it can be difficult for some women.

When young girls experience slight asymmetry during adolescence it can cause them a great deal of anxiety. But this, too, is normal. Their breasts may just be growing at different rates and, generally, the lagging breast will catch up eventually. But parents should be sensitive to these "growing pains" and explain to their daughter that it's just a part of her natural development. Reassure her that the vast majority of women's breasts are only slightly asymmetrical.

If you are one of those who have a very noticeable size difference and you want to make your breasts the same size, surgery is an option. You can have an implant inserted into the smaller breast, or reduce the size of the larger breast. If you are leaning in this direction, talk it over thoroughly with your doctor.

Hormone treatments aren't a good option because the effects can't be isolated to just one breast. Hormones will stimulate growth in both breasts, resulting in both getting bigger, but still differing in size.

Nipple Retraction

We've touched on this topic before, but it bears revisiting because it's a concern for some sisters. While the majority of women's nipples protrude or lie flat, some women have nipples that retract, or invert—they go into the breast rather than sticking out. Is this a major health problem? Usually not. If you were born this way, then it's perfectly normal for you. You don't need any sort of treatment or therapy to "correct" the condition. The only time you need to be concerned is if a nipple suddenly inverts when it has always been flat or protruding; that may be a sign of a tumor.

Some women with naturally inverted nipples may be concerned on a psychological level. They might worry about their appearance and about what a sexual partner will think. This may be more true for women whose inverted nipples don't become erect and "pop out" when they are sexually excited, than for those whose nipples do respond to sexual arousal.

Also of concern is how inverted nipples will affect breast-feeding. Usually the nipples can be gently coaxed out for nursing, though some women may have more difficulty than others.

Hypoplasia

This medical term literally means the failure of an organ or tissue to develop fully and reach its normal adult size. When you apply the term to breasts, it means that both breasts are under-developed. The actual breast glandular tissue is absent; it never developed or has diminished. A possible cause is a breakdown or disconnect in normal hormone circuitry.

Hormone treatment may help stimulate some growth, but its effectiveness depends on the cause of the hypoplasia. If you have this condition, consult your doctor to discuss your options.

Nipple Discharge

Most women don't usually have discharge from their nipples, except when they are lactating. Occasionally, however, some women do experience discharge from one or both breasts that has nothing to do with nursing. When this happens it can be alarming. Being aware of the various characteristics of nipple discharge can help you distinguish its significance.

Nipple discharge can be clear (like water), cloudy/milky, dark, bloody, or have a greenish hue. What do all of these color variations mean? For the most part, all but the dark or reddish-colored (bloody) discharges are usually benign. Hormonal fluctuations, stress, certain medications, and even excessive breast foreplay during sex can cause a slight discharge from your breasts. However, if you have nipple discharge plus headaches and vision problems, it could indicate a more serious problem.

A small tumor may be located in the *sella turcica,* a space near the optic nerve that supplies the eye. Tumors in this area usually induce an increase in *prolactin*—the hormone that stimulates milk production—which, in turn, causes discharge from the nipples. As this unusual tumor grows, it also causes headaches and visual changes. If the tumor gets too large and is untreated, it may compress and damage the optic nerve so severely that it leads to blindness.

Of equal concern are discharges that contain blood. There are, of course, times when an infection or a trauma may be at the root of bloody nipple discharge. But this particular symptom should always be considered a possible indicator of a cancerous growth until proven otherwise. I don't mean to scare you, but you have to take any sign of cancer seriously and have it checked out by your doctor immediately. And bloody nipple discharge is one of the signs of a possible breast tumor.

How are any of these discharges detected? The majority of women who experience nipple discharge of any type notice it themselves. You may find a stain on your bra or blouse, or you may notice it during your monthly breast self-exam. Your spouse or partner may even be the one to notice it during foreplay and bring it to your attention. Other times, you may not notice it at all; your doctor may be the one who sees it during a routine annual exam.

However you come to find out that you have nipple discharge, make sure your doctor checks it out right away. She should take a good history, perform a physical, and do a thorough breast exam while you are sitting and also when lying down. The discharge is usually easy to obtain while you are sitting upright, but it may also be obtained while you are lying down. Your doctor will gently squeeze your nipple to get a sample of the discharge, then send it to a lab for evaluation and to be checked for the presence of cancer cells.

In addition to the history taking, breast exam, and sampling of discharge, your doctor should also perform a prolactin test. If she doesn't bring it up, make sure you do. This is a blood test that measures the level of the milk-producing hormone in your system.

The treatment you receive for nipple discharge depends on the cause and the clinical findings. If the discharge is clear, white, or otherwise nonbloody, your prolactin levels are normal, your doctor doesn't feel any type of mass in your breast, and you have no other symptoms, then you'll most likely be advised to just keep a close eye on the nipple and have it rechecked in one to three months.

However, if your doctor does detect a mass during the breast exam, a biopsy is usually recommended to rule out an obscure cancer.

When the discharge is bloody, it will definitely be lab-tested to check for cancerous cells. Likewise, if a mass is also detected, a biopsy is usually advised. If no mass is felt during the exam or one is detected during a mammogram, then your doctor may order a ductogram (or galactogram) to get at the true underlying cause of the bloody discharge. This is a type of X ray that delineates the duct system in the breast, allowing possible detection of abnormalities. Although bloody discharge should raise concerns about cancer, the good news is that in most cases the cause is a noncancerous intraductal papilloma, a small benign tumor that grows in the cells lining a breast duct. In some women, it is possible for this type of benign tumor to carry a risk of eventually becoming cancerous. So it will likely be surgically removed and examined in the lab to make sure it has not, in fact, become cancerous.

Dark green or black discharge that is thick and profuse is symptomatic of a common condition called duct ectasia. Basically, a milk duct in the breast is damaged in some way and as it tries to heal itself, it forms a hard lump. What distinguishes duct ectasia from breast cancer is the fact that ectasias usually cause redness and tenderness in the affected area, while breast cancer historically does not. If duct ectasia is diagnosed, your doctor may opt for a conservative treatment to start: antibiotics and application of warm compresses. This should clear up the condition in a few days. However, if after this treatment the lump and the discharge are still present, the duct should be surgically removed. This allows it be checked for cancerous cells.

As a general rule, I'm personally very conscientious about sending discharge specimens to the lab, no matter what their particular color or consistency. I like to check, just in case. If there is even the slightest possibility of cancer, I'd rather that I and my patients know early. I'm stressing this point because some physicians may feel it's unnecessary to send a sample of discharge to the lab for testing if it's clear, because the likelihood of cancer is slim. I prefer to err on the side of excess and caution, and I'd advise you to have your doctor lab-test any type of nipple discharge you may have.

Mastitis

There are many benign breast conditions and diseases that affect women, and though they do cause concern, the majority of them are usually not life-threatening. They are perfectly treatable, and most of them do not increase a woman's risk for breast cancer. One of the most common of these conditions is *mastitis*—inflammation of the mammary gland. (Remember, "-itis" refers to inflammation.) Mastitis is common among breast-feeding mothers and occurs when bacteria (usually *Staphylococcus aureus*) enter the breast through cracked skin at the nipple. Though mastitis usually develops in nursing moms, there are cases of *nonpuerperal* (non-pregnancy/non-nursing) mastitis. Symptoms include a hot, often reddened breast, fairly moderate to severe pain, fever to about 101 degrees, and swelling of the breast. Mastitis can cause a breast abscess, which I'll discuss in a moment. Mastitis is treated with oral antibiotics that are safe to take while breast-feeding. In fact, you should continue to nurse, as emptying the breast of milk helps to relieve the symptoms.

Breast Abscess

As mentioned above, mastitis can often result in a *breast abscess*. The abscess, which is caused by a bacterial infection, is basically pus that has collected and formed a firm lump in the breast that is quite tender. This lump is actually swelling/inflammation of the tissue. An abscess is treated with intravenous antibiotics and careful observation of your vital signs. In many cases, the abscess will need to be incised and drained.

Eczema

You've probably heard of *eczema,* and if you've ever had it I'm sure you know just how bothersome this itchy skin condition can be. Eczema is a form of *dermatitis* (the medical term for inflammation of the skin). The most common type is *atopic eczema,* which is characterized by intense itching, scaling, and swelling. The disorder usually runs in families and generally occurs in people who have asthma or hay fever. Atopic eczema can be triggered by many things, including heat, wool fabrics, certain soaps, or stress. In mild cases, your doctor will probably advise you to use an over-the-counter hydrocortisone cream. If the eczema is severe, she may prescribe stronger medication. Though atopic eczema can recur, you can lessen flare-ups by avoiding irritants like wool clothing and harsh soaps and detergents, bathing and showering in lukewarm (not hot) water, keeping skin moisturized, staying cool when the weather is hot, and finding ways to relieve stress.

Fibroadenoma

A *fibroadenoma* is a solid mass in the breast that does not contain fluid. These round, firm, rubbery lumps move around when you feel them and can range in size from that of a pea to a quarter, and sometimes bigger. Fibroadenomas don't cause pain, and they are not usually accompanied by nipple discharge, inflammation, or fever. Some women develop one, others develop several. While fibroadenomas are most common in women between the ages of 20 and 30, they have been known to occur in teenagers and older women. African-American women get this type of breast lump twice as often as white women. The reason why is unclear. Fortunately, fibroadenomas are benign (noncancerous) and do not increase your risk for developing breast cancer. That said, however, I do recommend that these lumps be surgically removed (excised) and tested to make sure there is absolutely no evidence of cancer. This used to be the common way to treat fibroadenomas, but some doctors opt to leave the lumps alone and observe them over time for any changes in size, texture, and mobility. Personally, I am not in favor of allowing lumps to remain in the breast, but this is something you should discuss with your physician if you are ever diagnosed with the condition. Several factors will determine whether she advises surgery, including your age, the size of the lump, how it feels, if you have a strong family history of breast cancer, if you yourself have a history of breast cancer, and whether you exhibit any other symptoms. If you do have surgery, it will be an outpatient procedure performed using a local anesthetic. The operation is short and you can go home the same day. Unfortunately, this type of tumor can grow back.

Fat Necrosis

This condition often occurs in obese women, or in those who have had some form of breast surgery or have suffered an injury to the breast. If an area of the breast that has been damaged (by injury, a surgical wound, or some other means) affects the stromatic fatty tissue of the breast, it may scar more than normal as it heals. The resulting scar tissue feels like a mass in the breast. Fat necrosis can sometimes be mistaken for cancer masses, so a sample of the tissue should be biopsied to make sure that it is not cancer.

Sclerosing Adenosis

Similar to fat necrosis, *sclerosing adenosis* involves scarring of the glandular (adenomatous) cells of the breast. These cells become hardened (sclerosed) and feel like a thickened mass in the breast. A sample of the masslike tissue will be lab-tested for an accurate diagnosis.

Granular Cell Tumors

These tumors are more common in black women, but fortunately they are rare. Unlike fibroadenomas, which have a smooth texture, lumps in the breast caused by granular cell tumors feel grainy. Once a biopsy is performed to give a definite diagnosis, the tumor will be excised.

Fibrocystic Disease

If your breasts always tend to feel sort of lumpy, join the club. Many women have naturally lumpy or fibrous breasts. It's quite normal and doesn't mean that your breasts are not healthy. But having lumpy breasts can make it harder for you to detect a new cyst or a change in an existing one. The development of new or changing cysts is what physicians commonly refer to as *fibrocystic breast disease* (FCBD or FCD), though you'll hear many doctors call it "fibrocystic changes." For simplicity's sake, I'll just refer to the condition as fibrocystic disease.

Not only is it more difficult for women with naturally fibrous breasts to detect abnormalities, but hormonal changes that occur each month can make breasts feel even lumpier than usual. How do you tell the difference between a change in breast texture caused by hormones and changes brought on by true fibrocystic disease? If it's FCD, you will also have pain and tenderness throughout much of the breast, especially if the cyst is large.

Breast cysts are not harmful, and they are simple to treat. The cyst, which is filled with a clear or pale yellow fluid, is aspirated. Your doctor inserts a needle into the lump and withdraws the fluid. Once the fluid is drained, the lump will shrink and the pain and tenderness in your breast will subside. The procedure is usually performed in the doctor's office without anesthesia and is no more painful than having blood drawn.

While any woman can develop breast cysts, they are more common in women who have fibrous breasts. No one knows for sure why cysts develop, and even after they have been aspirated they can come back. Some women have to have periodic drainage of breast cysts.

If you have naturally lumpy breasts it's especially important for you to perform monthly breast self-exams. Become familiar with the feel of your breasts—every little bump and lump. The more thorough you are about getting in tune with your breasts, the better able you will be to detect any changes. Also, be extra conscientious about having regular mammograms and yearly breast exams. When your breasts are naturally fibrous, you have to be extra diligent.

Keep in mind, too, there are things you can do at home that may help prevent cysts and reduce the tenderness that's often associated with naturally lumpy breasts. Limit or eliminate items containing caffeine or other methylxanthines, such as coffee, soda, tea, chocolate, and cigarettes. Cut back on your salt intake to decrease water retention. Vitamin E supplements may also help. There is some debate about the degree to which these measures actually help, but they may be worth a try.

Hematomas

Hematomas are blood clots that form after a trauma to the breast causes a blood vessel to rupture, or sometimes following a surgical procedure when a collection of blood develops inside the breast. If a hematoma is large or close to the skin, it will give the affected area a bluish hue. Because these clots are usually within the fatty tissue of the breast, they shouldn't interfere with the glands' ability to produce milk. Hematomas in the breast can be painful, but most are self-contained and will shrink with treatment. When diagnosed early, hematomas can be treated with the application of ice packs. The cold helps slow down the blood flow. When detected at a later stage, blood clots may be treated with heat compresses. The heat speeds up an enzyme in the body called fibrinolysin, which helps to break down blood clots. As the clots shrink, the pain and tenderness begin to diminish.

COULD IT BE CANCER?

Breast cancer is the most common type of cancer among women in the United States and is the second leading cause of death in American women. For black women, the news is even more frightening. Sisters (along with Hawaiian women) have the highest incidence for the disease, and we're more likely to die from it. African-American women have the highest mortality rate for breast cancer—nearly twice as high as our white counterparts, according to the National Cancer Institute. Late detection is the primary reason for our lower survival rate. Typically, by the time we are diagnosed with breast cancer, it has already spread. There are several types of breast cancer, including intraductal cancer, papillary cancer, sarcomas, and Paget's disease.

While no one can say with absolute certainty what causes

breast cancer, medical experts agree that certain risk factors do exist:

- family history of breast cancer, especially on the female side of the family (your mother, sisters, aunts, etc.)

- early onset of menstruation

- never having children

- obesity

- previous radiation exposure

- other breast diseases not initially diagnosed as malignant

What are the symptoms of breast cancer?

Typically a lump is felt during a self-examination or a doctor's visit. The lump is usually painless, though not always. Other symptoms include indentation of the nipple, abnormal breast pain, discharge (often containing blood) from the nipple, and dimpled skin over the site of a lump. Some women, however, experience no symptoms.

How is breast cancer diagnosed?

If a lump is found your doctor will check its firmness (whether it's soft or hard) and its mobility (whether it can be moved around or if it's fixed—movable is better, since a fixed mass is much more suspicious for cancer). Your doctor will check the lymph nodes under your arms and above your collarbone, and also squeeze the nipple to check for discharge. If discharge is present, a sample will be sent to the lab to be examined for malignant cells. Your physician will look for any scaliness on the areola as well as any lesions on the breast.

If your physician suspects that the lump is just a cyst (a fluid-filled tissue sac), it can be aspirated (the fluid is withdrawn). However, if your doctor believes there is a possibility that the lump may be malignant, a mammogram is ordered and a biopsy will be performed.

If cancer is diagnosed, the next step will be to "stage" the disease, which means performing a surgical procedure to determine if the disease has spread. Special chemical tests will also be done on the tissue to find out if the cancer has estrogen and progesterone receptors. All of these findings help determine the best course of treatment.

The staging of breast cancer depends on three basic components:

• the size of the tumor

• whether any lymph nodes have been affected

• whether the cancer has spread (metastasized) to another part of the body

How is breast cancer treated?

That all depends on the stage of the cancer, as well as other factors such as size of the tumor, the patient's age, and whether or not she is menopausal.

In the past, women diagnosed with breast cancer usually had a *modified radical mastectomy*, in which the entire breast, some of the chest muscle, and all of the chest and underarm lymph nodes are removed. But research has shown that women with early Stage I or Stage II cancer who undergo a *lumpectomy* (removal of only the cancerous tissue), removal of underarm lymph nodes, and radiation therapy in order to preserve the breast can have just as good a prognosis.

Stage III breast cancer requires a more aggressive treatment. Depending on the type of Stage III cancer a woman has, her doctor may recommend some combination of chemotherapy, a modified radical mastectomy, and radiation. The drug Tamoxifen may be used as part of the treatment. A new drug, Herceptin, may also be used in some cases.

Stage IV is the most advanced form of breast cancer. At this late stage, treatment is usually centered not on curing the patient but on trying to improve her condition as much as possible. This is what's known as *palliative therapy*—treatment that relieves the symptoms of widespread cancer but does not cure it.

Being diagnosed with breast cancer is frightening for anyone, but discovering it at Stage IV—in essence, the final stage—is devastating. One of my dear friends watched helplessly as this scenario played out in his own family. He called me one night and asked what it would mean if a woman had a large open sore on her breast, a sore so severe that it was possible to see the flesh underneath. I told him that it signaled a severe, late stage of breast cancer. He then asked if that woman would have long to live. Qualifying my answer with "One can never say for sure, but . . . " I told him it was unlikely she'd live much longer if the breast cancer had progressed to the point he'd described. It sounded as if the cancer had been present for a long time and had gone untreated. Finally, I asked my friend who he was talking about. It was his mother. Both of us felt a deep pain and sadness following that phone call.

How is it that his mother's breast cancer had become so severe? I later learned that his mother's sister had had the same type of lesion on her breast and ultimately had died of breast cancer. But his mom failed to recognize the implication of that family history (that she too was most likely at risk) and never had her own breasts examined. When she noticed a lump, she didn't do anything about it. She was afraid that, like her sister, she'd go to the hospital and her situation would worsen. This fear of the hospital is not uncommon among black folks. The truth is, it's not the hospital that creates a health crisis, it's the failure to get evaluated and treated early.

Time is truly a foe when it comes to fighting cancer. Early detection can save your life. In general, 70.6 percent of African-American women survive breast cancer for 5 years or more following early treatment, according to reports. Sadly, my friend's mother didn't learn this lesson soon enough. She died a few months after being officially diagnosed with breast cancer. My prayer is that the other women in his family recognize their own risk and have routine breast exams to safeguard their health.

*What can you do to lessen
the risk of breast cancer?*

Do a monthly breast self-examination. Have your breasts examined by your doctor at least once a year. And beginning at age 35, get regular mammograms. But if you have a strong family history of breast cancer, start getting them at an earlier age.

THE FACTS ABOUT COSMETIC SURGERY

You've heard the saying "More than a handful is too much." And I'm sure you know the one that goes "You can never have too much of a good thing." When it comes to breasts, the debate rages on over how much is enough. Just as sisters come in every hue, from peachy-cream to ebony, we also come in all shapes and sizes. Some of us have full, large breasts while others have small, girlish ones. And for some sisters, what they were born with isn't what they want. Thanks to modern medicine, they can do something about it. Sisters who want bigger breasts can get implants. Sisters who want smaller ones can have them reduced. And sisters who want to keep the size but eliminate the sag can get a lift.

Cosmetic surgery is an individual choice. The decision may be based on aesthetics, health concerns, or a combination of both. Whatever the reason, sisters who opt for cosmetic breast surgery are certainly not alone. Thousands of women have it every year. Implants seem to be less common in black women, though, while reductions and lifts are more common.

Anyone who is thinking about having one of these surgeries needs to realize that it is just that—surgery—and every operation carries risk. So discuss it thoroughly with your doctor.

Breast Augmentation

This is a very common operation in the United States, one that has been surrounded by controversy. Synthetic implants are inserted into the breasts to make them larger. Silicone gel–filled implants used to be the implant of choice, but reports began to surface of women who suffered health problems when their implants leaked or ruptured, including immunologic diseases. Because of these safety concerns, saline-filled implants are now used for breast augmentation. Since saline is salt water, any leakage is harmlessly absorbed by the body.

As for the operation itself, the plastic surgeon makes an incision either around the areola, underneath the breast, in the armpit, or even at the navel. Next, she will create a pocket for the implant by separating the breast tissues. Then the surgeon inserts the implant either under or over the chest muscle. Before you have the surgery you should definitely discuss with your doctor where the incision will be made and whether the implant will go under or over the muscle. The visibility of scars is largely determined by the location of the incision. More important, implants placed under the chest muscle are less likely to interfere with mammograms, but your breasts' shape may not look as natural as they would if the implants were placed over the muscle. Be sure to discuss these points with your doctor to determine your best option.

You should also be aware that the implants may become surrounded by scar tissue, making your breasts feel hard. When you hear some folks say that implants don't feel "natural," this hardness is what they are talking about. This problem is more common with silicone implants, though it can occur to a lesser extent with saline. You may also experience loss of sensation in your nipples, but this is more rare.

Breast Reduction

For some sisters, bigger isn't necessarily better. Having very large breasts can actually cause physical problems, such as back pain, skin rashes underneath the breasts, and indentations and discoloration on the shoulders caused by bra straps that dig into the flesh.

Breast reduction, or *reduction mammoplasty,* reduces the overall bulk and size of the breasts, alleviating the associated health problems. While this is often the sole goal of some women who elect to have this operation, many also want to rid themselves of the psychological baggage that can go along with a large cup size. It's not unusual for big-busted women to try to hide their physique with baggy clothes or a perpetually stooped posture. Because ours is such a breast-obsessed society, the attention a pair of double D's elicits is often more than a woman can stand. The comments she hears and vibes she picks up can range from incessantly annoying to downright degrading. Add in the backaches, rashes, and other physical problems, and it's no wonder lots of sisters are opting to downsize.

If you are overweight, however, you may want to try to shed pounds before signing on for surgery, since you lose breast fat when you trim down. A woman who is obese may actually only need to lose weight to bring her breasts down to what she feels is a more manageable size. Before you make any decisions, talk to your doctor about whether you are a viable candidate for this type of surgery.

Breast reduction works by removing excess skin and fatty tissue from the breasts. There will be visible scarring, and you may lose some sensation in your nipples and breasts. You also may not be able to breast-feed, though many can.

Breast Lift

Some women who just want to counteract the natural pull of gravity opt for a breast lift. This procedure, called a *mastopexy*, simply repositions the breasts. The plastic surgeon removes excess skin, but not tissue, and elevates the nipple to a higher position.

You will have noticeable scars, and you may experience permanent numbness in some areas of your breasts, although in most cases the numbness usually fades. Know, too, that your breasts may sag again over time.

RX: A PRESCRIPTION FOR YOUR SOUL

Have you ever noticed how often we're told it's okay to eat a certain food one minute, then warned not to the next? *Go ahead and have eggs. They're loaded with protein. No, wait. They have too much cholesterol. Chicken is nice and lean, so eat up. Then again, there's that salmonella thing. Beef? Too much fat, not to mention Mad Cow Disease. Fish? Watch out for the mercury. Fruits and vegetables? Beware pesticides.* The list is endless. It's getting so you don't know what to believe.

If man had left nature alone as God intended, some of these concerns would not exist. But the world we live in has become quite technologically advanced, and, unfortunately, with that comes some risk.

So what are we to do? We have to eat. We have to have nourishment if we are to survive, grow, and be strong. Thankfully, technology does have its benefits, and every day scientists and researchers are discovering ways to make our food safer.

When you think about all of the external factors that contribute to the foods we eat—from how the animals are raised and the vegetables grown, to how foods are processed and manufactured, to the way we prepare them at home—it really makes you appreciate the power of the breast.

God gave us a truly amazing natural source of nourishment. Watching a baby nurse is one of the most beautiful and fascinating sights to behold. To see yourself literally sustaining a life is a miracle. Within the female body lies the foundation, structure, and ability to nurture and nourish. Because breasts appear to be external organs—"outside" of our body—we may take for granted the importance of their inner workings. But when those pregnancy hormones kick in and your breasts begin to get bigger as the milk glands enlarge, you will be reminded that something wonderful is going on in there. Once the "inner breast" is activated, the outer breast can do its job.

So it is with ourselves. We must activate our inner selves in order to live our best, most fulfilling lives. We have to look within and tap our internal resources. We have to nurture ourselves as we do our babies and others in our lives. When we make time for inner work, it feeds our souls and fortifies our spirits. It is so crucial that we, as black women, do this. Sisters don't always nourish their own souls, and it is a mistake.

It's not uncommon for African-American women to negate the importance of allowing time for self—for quiet contemplation, solitary solace, relaxation, and personal enjoyment, to turn attention to their own health and well-being. They are so busy doing for everyone else. But you should turn inward on a regular basis. It is rewarding in so many ways. And rest assured, you have every right to nourish yourself first, before doing anything else. It is not a selfish act. It is a healing one. An empowering one. A sustaining one. Feed on the free-flowing milk of God's love and His Word. Let it help you grow strong in His way and for His purpose. Let it help you maintain a healthy body—the temple with which God has blessed you.

If you're finding it difficult to give yourself permission to take time for your own inner work, it may be that you aren't seeing the link between doing so and a more joyous life. Take a moment and think about the miraculous way in which God has enabled your body to function. It is the initial protector and shelter for a child. Once your baby is born, your body can nourish him through nursing and jump-start healthy growth and development. But in order to give your child that good start, your constitutional makeup has to be strong.

A healthy body that has been cared for, tended to, and filled with nutritious foods will provide an excellent home for a developing baby and nourishing breast milk for feeding once he comes into the world. What goes on inside your body helps determine how well your baby will grow once he's outside of it.

You, as a woman, are no different. How well you grow spiritually, physically, and mentally—your life—is also dependent upon your inner being. It's really not hard to make the connection, and taking a lesson from our maternal workings doesn't require a big leap. We can give life and we can sustain life. God has graced us with that ability. But how will we ever truly appreciate that gift if we can't do the same for ourselves? By doing inner work and getting in touch with our souls, we give ourselves life. Each day that we nourish our spirits we live anew. We become stronger, more able, more fully developed, and more fulfilled. We become our best selves. And, in the end, that is good for us and all of those around us.

Our spiritual "bones" will be fortified, giving us the strength to handle any trial and to stand up for ourselves when others seek to drag us down. I am a witness to this truth. By nature, I am a "giver." I used to always think of others' needs before my own. I didn't know how to say no to people. If they needed anything— whatever, whenever—I was there. And while I am still a giver, I have finally learned to take care of what I need as well. I have given myself permission to do what I need to do for me, and not feel guilty about it. (That's really the tough part.)

I've learned the hard way that you have to say no sometimes, and it's okay to do so. When you allow others to treat you like a doormat, they begin to take you for granted. In their minds, the "blueprint" is laid: *You* are the giver and *they* are the receivers. Sometimes, people don't even see how much they are taking because you (the giver) keep letting them take. You might not realize yourself that your level of giving is beyond the realm of normalcy. Then, when *you* need something, others look at you like you're crazy. In fact, they'll probably feel as if you are committing a violation against the relationship. After all, they'll think, that's not the blueprint. The blueprint is *I don't give to you; you give to me.*

My sisters, it has taken me a long time to learn this lesson. But now that I have, I make it a point to set boundaries for how much of myself I will give, and for how much I allow others to take. I've also learned that I can hear God's voice more clearly now. Looking within myself has further crystallized my relationship with Him. I've always been happy that I know God's voice for myself, and that He has blessed me with a great degree of insight and foresight. Sometimes those abilities confound other people, but it is truly a blessing—a gift of His spirit to me. I've learned that by allowing myself more time for me, I am more in tune with my inner needs, be they spiritual or physical. Before, I would totally ignore them because I was so busy doing for everyone else. Now I can give to myself, and give to others in accordance with what is good for my spirit. In short, I've learned to be good to me. It's important that you do the same.

Nurture yourself. Tap the nourishment within. Spend time with the God inside of you and the person He has made you to be and wants you to be. By learning about yourself and spending more time with God, your mission in life will become clear and each day will become more joyous than the last. How can you do this? Try these suggestions:

Retreat. Allow yourself time to get away to your "personal sanctuary." It may be a particular room in your house where you can meditate: your backyard, the tub, wherever. You may want to have a set time or schedule for retreating, say twice a week, or every day at 8:00 P.M. Whatever works for you. Declare it yours— your time, your space. It is reserved for you alone.

Reconnect with God. In that quiet sanctuary, take time to seek God. Talk to Him, and more importantly, listen to Him.

Renew. Renew your commitment to His work in your life, which includes taking care of your physical health.

Release negative energy. It may flow from certain people, a certain aspect of your job, family matters, or things totally out of your control. Let it go! The battle is not yours to fight. Release it, whatever it is, and grab hold of God's promise for your life.

Rediscover. There are parts of your inner being that you need to get reacquainted with, or perhaps to be introduced to for the first time. Get started.

Reach for the gold. Latch on to life's brass ring. Reach for optimum physical health and sound spiritual health. Obtain both of these and you will be able to run the race that's set before you, as God directs your path.

One of my favorite books is Don Miguel Ruiz's inspirational *The Four Agreements: A Practical Guide to Personal Freedom.* In it he writes, "You have to honor the man or woman that you are. Respect your body, enjoy your body, love your body, feed, clean, and heal your body. Exercise and do what makes you feel good. This is a *puja* to your body, and that is a communion between you and God." His words speak to me, for they are filled with truth. The message resonates with me because it is the message I try to live by, that I always try to pass on to my patients, and that I seek to pass on to you. Honor your body. Nurture yourself. Nourish your inner being . . . first.

The ABCs of Pregnancy

· · · · · · · · · · · · ·

I know that whatever I have is a gift. I accept that, and I'm grateful to those who went before me so that I can do what I'm supposed to do for those who are yet to come.

—Maya Angelou

News You Can Use

· Low birthweight babies are those weighing less than 2,500 grams. That's approximately 5½ pounds. These babies often suffer from poor learning ability and compromised health and development.

· Repeated abortions or operative procedures on the cervix may weaken the cervix and cause miscarriage in the second trimester.

· Get a pregnancy test done as soon as you miss your menstrual cycle or if you suspect that you are with child.

· Prenatal care is crucial for helping to decrease the incidence of miscarriage, preterm labor, and serious medical complications like high blood pressure, diabetes, and fetal distress.

· African-American women often delay seeking prenatal care, which leads to a much greater risk of pregnancy loss, uncontrolled diabetes, hypertension, low birthweight babies, and emergency cesarean sections.

· Review your lifestyle habits and all medications you take with your doctor.

· It is advisable to have a pre-conception consultation with your doctor to review your basic habits and assure your best physical condition before getting pregnant.

ASK ANY mother and she'll tell you, having a baby is one of the most life-altering blessings you will ever experience. Your world truly becomes transformed with the birth of a child. Your feelings deepen, your beliefs change, and your priorities are rearranged. Every ounce of caring and concern is suddenly transferred to this divine gift. In our grandmothers' day, the path to this blessing was clearly set—you grew up, you got married, and you had children. It was practically unheard of for a woman to postpone pregnancy until after she had received a college degree, or climbed the corporate ladder and achieved the corner office—much less to decide not to have any children at all. These options simply didn't fit the accepted societal norm.

Times have certainly changed. Sisters today are free to make choices that mesh with their lifestyles and their desires. Many of us are marrying later and having children later. No one is shocked anymore to hear about a 35- or 40-year-old first-time mother. More and more women are choosing to concentrate on their careers first, and take their time finding Mr. Right, before becoming wives and mothers (and often, just mothers). Other sisters simply aren't ready at younger ages and feel more emotionally or financially able when they are older. Some may want to enjoy time alone with their husbands before expanding their families, or wish to devote time to their church, community, or themselves for a while first. And for some, the news of pregnancy comes as a complete surprise.

Whichever scenario best defines your personal situation, chances are at some point you've probably thought about how pregnancy would affect your life: *Is having a baby right for me? Am I truly ready? What can I expect? How will my body change? Oh, Lord, what about all the pain?* It makes sense to wonder, because as joyous and exciting a time as pregnancy can be, it is also filled with uncertainty. Not so much about the final result—your precious baby—but about the process that carries you to that point. Nine months can be a long time when you're not sure what to expect along the way. And though no one can truly prepare you for what is to come (every pregnancy is unique and every mother has a different experience), there is information you can use to make sure your journey is a safe, healthy, enjoyable one.

A GOOD START—PREPARING FOR PREGNANCY

Every woman who becomes pregnant wants her baby to be born as healthy as possible. That is always our one deepest wish. We don't care if it's a boy or a girl, or who she most resembles. We just want to make sure she's fine. When that tiny being is placed in our arms, we lovingly gaze at her sweet face and ask the doctor if everything is okay. The only thing we are concerned about is the health of our child.

As the mother, you play the most crucial role in safeguarding your baby's good health. You are his lifeline during those nine months—his only source of nourishment, his only shelter, his only protection. He is depending on you to give him a great start in the world. It all begins with you. That's why it's so important that you be in the best health possible before you even conceive.

I strongly recommend that you have a prepregnancy consultation with your doctor before planning to conceive. The period of early fetal development is crucial for a baby, so when you take steps to shore up your own health before getting pregnant, you give your baby a better head start. During this consultation, your doctor will give you a prepregnancy checkup that includes a routine physical exam, a series of tests, and a discussion about your health history. In addition, she'll talk to you about what you need to do, healthwise, to prepare for your pregnancy, as well as provide important information you'll want to keep in mind after becoming pregnant.

Your Diet: Eating a nutritious, balanced diet that's rich in fruits, whole grains, and vegetables helps prepare your body for the demands of pregnancy. Also, be certain to consume enough protein and low-fat dairy. If you are a vegetarian, make sure that you are getting all of the nutrients you need. Most important of all, eat everything in moderation.

We all know at least a few sisters who've turned having a baby into an all-out assault on food. They use their pregnancy as an excuse to overeat. "Well, I *am* eating for two," they rationalize. Yes, you are, but that doesn't mean bingeing, especially on junk food. Good nutrition and maintaining a healthy weight is even more important once you are with child. Your doctor will talk to you about how much weight you should gain over the next nine months. Most women generally put on anywhere from 15 to 40 pounds over the course of nine months. Talk to your doctor about how much you should ideally gain. A lot of it depends on how much you weigh from the get-go.

For all of you coffee lovers, you'll have to learn to love it less. Your doctor will likely advise you to limit caffeine (and not just coffee, but tea and soda) because it has been linked to an increased rate of miscarriage. I'd suggest avoiding caffeine altogether to be on the safe side.

Exercise: If you enjoy working out and want to continue to do so once you're pregnant, you'll probably be able to, as long as you keep things at a moderate level and don't push yourself too hard. Walking is a good option. Make sure to talk it over with your doctor. Women who have a history of preterm labor, miscarriage, irregular spotting during pregnancy, a weak cervix, and other conditions are usually advised not to do certain types of exercise, if any at all, during their pregnancy.

Social Habits: Your lifestyle can make or break your chances for a healthy pregnancy and a healthy baby. If you smoke, quit—and do it before you get pregnant. I know that can be easier said than done, especially if you've been smoking for years. But it's well worth the effort, because lighting up can do a great deal of harm to your baby. Smoking deprives the fetus of oxygen and increases the likelihood of miscarriage, stillbirth, or premature labor. What's more, babies exposed to cigarette smoke while in the womb have a lower birthweight, which can adversely affect their mental development.

It's also important not to drink alcohol while pregnant. Excessive alcohol consumption during pregnancy may cause multiple fetal abnormalities.

And when it comes to illegal drugs, I'm sure that, as a woman of God, you know to stay away. If you do use these substances, though, you must stop immediately. Get help if you can't do it alone. Use of illegal drugs during pregnancy can cause miscarriage, birth defects, brain damage, and intrauterine (in the womb) death of the baby. Don't be afraid to be honest with your doctor if you use any illegal substances. It is imperative that she know.

Medications: Talk to your doctor about any medication you take, prescription as well as over-the-counter (OTC) drugs. Both types may pose harm to the fetus. Many people don't think of OTC drugs as medications, but they are. Even everyday over-the-counter products that you may always keep in your medicine cabinet, such as aspirin, ibuprofen, and cold remedies, can have a potential effect on your developing baby. So review all medicines you take (or might automatically reach for in the next nine months, say, if you catch a cold) with your doctor.

That review should also cover any contraceptives you may currently be using. If you are on the Pill and decide you want to get pregnant, you should stop using it one to two months before trying to conceive. Switch to a barrier contraceptive, such as condoms, to allow your hormone levels time to readjust. The same is true if you are using other hormonal contraceptives, like Depo-Provera or Norplant, though the length of time to stop using them prior to trying to conceive may vary. Again, talk to your doctor for specific recommendations and advice during your prepregnancy consultation.

Genetic History: You should learn as much about your genetic background as possible and relay the information to your doctor. Are there genetic diseases that run in your family, such as sickle-cell disease, cystic fibrosis, hemophilia, and others? How about in your partner's family? Remember, both of you play an equally important genetic role. Depending on the information you provide, your doctor may suggest testing and genetic counseling to evaluate your risk of passing any genetic disorders on to your child.

Pregnancy History: You and your doctor will also need to discuss any previous pregnancies you have had. This not only includes pregnancies that went to term and produced children you already have, but any miscarriages and/or abortions as well. Women who have had difficult births or miscarriages in the past may need to be monitored more closely. Your doctor will want to take into account any history of cesarean sections, weak cervix, preterm births, hypertension, and other medical conditions during prior pregnancies. All of these factors need to be considered carefully by your physician to help this next pregnancy be problem-free. While previous abortions shouldn't affect your ability to have a safe, smooth pregnancy, there is some evidence that it may increase the risk of premature delivery or, in some women, an incompetent cervix.

Medical Conditions: There are several disorders a woman may have that can increase the potential for complications during pregnancy for her and her baby, including high blood pressure, diabetes, and epilepsy. Women with diabetes who become pregnant run an increased risk of having babies with birth defects, and may develop serious health problems themselves. To help prevent such complications, diabetics must get their diabetes under control before getting pregnant and keep their blood sugar levels stable throughout their pregnancy. Your doctor can devise a special treatment program for you and will monitor you more closely for those nine months.

Similarly, if you are hypertensive, it is imperative that you lower your blood pressure prior to becoming pregnant. Weight loss, exercise, and a diet low in sodium will all help bring your pressure down. Because the stress of pregnancy can cause already high blood pressure to reach dangerous levels, your doctor will be following your health very closely. If you are taking hypertension medication prior to conceiving, talk to your physician about its safety during pregnancy and whether or not you will need to change prescriptions. If you don't already take medication, your doctor may prescribe it for you if she feels it is necessary.

A sister who is epileptic needs to talk to her doctor about the effect of the disorder on a fetus—what may happen if she has a seizure while pregnant and the effect on the baby of any anticonvulsant medications she's taking. Some medications used to control seizures can cause birth defects. Dilantin, a popular antiseizure medication, in particular can cause severe defects. Your doctor may feel it's best to prescribe a different drug.

While these types of preexisting disorders and others can increase your risk for complications, know that, in general, most pregnant women with these medical conditions go on to have healthy, bouncing babies. The key is to talk to your doctor and carefully follow all of her advice to the letter.

Vitamin Supplements: Do you take them and, if so, how much? Let your physician know. If you take mega doses of vitamins, stop. And if you're taking vitamin A supplements, stop that, too. Excess levels of vitamin A can cause severe birth defects in babies. When you do become pregnant, your doctor will provide you with a prenatal vitamin that provides the additional vitamins you will need. In the meantime, before you conceive, you can take a standard multivitamin if you like, though they aren't necessary if you are eating a well-balanced diet and getting enough folic acid from your foods.

Folic acid plays a vital role in helping to prevent birth defects, so it's important that you have enough of it before you get pregnant. Folic acid is a vitamin that can greatly reduce the risk of a fetus's developing neural tube defects, such as spina bifida. How much folic acid do you need? About 0.4 milligrams a day is usually recommended, either as a supplement or from foods rich in folate (the natural form of folic acid), such as dark leafy greens, particularly spinach, and dried beans and peas.

Vaccination Status: You will be tested for rubella (German measles) at your first prenatal visit to see if you are immune, but it's a good idea to have your doctor test you during this prepregnancy consultation to determine your status well before you conceive. Rubella can harm the fetus if you acquire it while pregnant. In any other circumstance, you could simply get a vaccination if you weren't immune. But it is not advised for women who plan to get pregnant to have the vaccination within three months of conceiving, because the vaccine itself can cause fetal complications. If this is your situation, then you will have to wait to have the vaccine after you deliver. It's still important, because you need to protect your own future health. From then on, make sure to stay on top of your vaccination status.

Most people think immunizations are only for children, but adults need to have some, too. Have you ever been immunized against measles or mumps? If you aren't sure, your doctor can test for these as well. As with rubella, it's best to be vaccinated against these diseases at least three months prior to conceiving, not while pregnant. According to the American College of Obstetricians and Gynecologists (ACOG), the only vaccines recommended for routine administration during pregnancy are those for tetanus and diphtheria. The hepatitis vaccine is also important and can be given while you are pregnant, if deemed necessary. As always, review all of this with your physician.

THE EXPECTANT MOTHER

You missed a period and think you may be pregnant. It makes sense that you would, since that's a classic sign. Other early signs of pregnancy include a very light period or only spotting, tender breasts, fatigue, nausea, and frequent urination. If you just can't wait to find out, you can take a home pregnancy test, which, by and large, is quite accurate. But don't rely solely on your at-home results. Make an appointment with your doctor to know with absolute certainty whether you are pregnant.

Congratulations! Your doctor has confirmed that you are indeed with child. Prenatal care should begin immediately—the earlier the better, especially for black women. While nothing in medicine is guaranteed, statistics show that early and consistent prenatal care is a key factor in preventing numerous complications, including some miscarriages, premature births, low birthweight babies, serious medical problems, and pregnancy loss.

Unfortunately, millions of women fail to get this crucial care in a timely manner. Because African-American women often start off with higher rates of such conditions as hypertension, diabetes, and obesity, our need for early prenatal care is even greater. By not getting that care right away, sisters run the biggest risk and have the poorest outcomes. Just consider:

FACT: Women who begin prenatal care late have a greater risk of preterm labor, delivering premature infants or low birthweight babies. These babies often suffer from poor learning and compromised health.

FACT: Late prenatal care results in a higher incidence of serious medical complications in pregnancy, including gestational diabetes, uncontrolled high blood pressure, and stillbirth.

FACT: The sooner a woman seeks prenatal care, the earlier medical conditions can be detected and management can begin. With proper prenatal care, the risk of developing serious medical conditions is diminished.

Now you understand just how important early prenatal care is, but you may be wondering exactly what it entails. It starts with your first doctor's visit after your pregnancy is confirmed. This first prenatal visit will probably include a medical history, a physical exam, establishment of your due date, and a few tests. All of this information forms the basis of your prenatal profile.

Medical History

Even if the doctor who will be caring for you during your pregnancy and delivering your baby is the same physician you've always seen, she will once again talk to you about your personal health history, your family's history, your social habits, and any existing medical condition or sexually transmitted diseases. Most doctors will test for gonorrhea and chlamydia, both of which can have a serious effect on pregnancy, and for syphilis, which can be passed to the fetus, causing miscarriage or stillbirth.

Physical Exam

Your doctor will weigh you, measure your height, and take your blood pressure. You will have a regular physical exam plus a pelvic exam. The pelvic exam allows your doctor to determine the size of your uterus, which helps calculate your due date.

Establishing the Due Date

The due date is only an estimate. A normal, full-term pregnancy can last anywhere from 37 to 42 weeks. More on how this estimate is made a bit later.

Tests

During this first prenatal visit, your doctor will run blood and urine tests to check for conditions that may affect your pregnancy.

After this initial prenatal doctor's appointment, you and your physician will arrange a schedule for subsequent prenatal visits throughout your pregnancy. For most women, it's best to come in once every month for the first 28 to 30 weeks. Then your prenatal visits should become more frequent—every two weeks until you reach your last month. During your final month of pregnancy, you should see your doctor for prenatal care every week. More frequent appointments may be necessary depending on your particular condition and health history.

THE ANATOMY OF PREGNANCY

Whenever a woman gets the news that she's pregnant she knows what it means. But how many of us ever really stop to think about the miraculous process that's going on inside of our bodies? What's happening to our newly developing baby? I think taking a moment to periodically reflect on this is a good thing. Not only does it get you thinking about the many changes your little one will go through—developing from embryo to fetus to baby—but it will help you prepare for the changes you will be experiencing also.

So what has your baby's journey been like thus far? Once your egg was fertilized by a sperm, it began dividing into many cells over the next few days as it traveled through the fallopian tube toward the uterus, where it implanted itself into the wall of the uterus. As soon as that happened, the endometrium (lining of the uterus) thickened more than it already had and covered the egg. The *placenta* (or afterbirth) began to develop inside your uterus. The placenta is the organ that connects the baby's circulation to your system, supplying your baby with blood, nutrients, and oxygen. The baby is connected to the placenta by the *umbilical cord*. Your baby is contained in a fairly strong sac, or *membrane,* and surrounded by a clear, watery fluid called *amniotic fluid* (generally referred to as simply "water"). The amniotic fluid helps to cushion and protect the baby.

Later in this chapter, when we talk about the different stages of pregnancy, you'll learn more about your baby's journey to birth.

TESTING, TESTING

Once you're pregnant, tests become part of the territory. It's all part of ensuring that everything goes as smoothly and problem-free as possible. Some of the tests and procedures you will undergo throughout your pregnancy are standard for every woman who is expecting a baby, while others may be necessary only in certain cases. If you ever have questions about any test or procedure, don't be afraid to ask your doctor. In the meantime, this brief primer will help familiarize you with some of the most common tests. If you've had children before, these will likely sound familiar. If this is your first pregnancy, this is information you need to know.

Human Chorionic Gonadotropin (hCG)

When you first visited your doctor to confirm your pregnancy, he gave you either a urine or blood test (or both) to check for the presence of *human chorionic gonadotropin* (hCG), a hormone produced by the cells of the placenta as it develops. In some cases, your physician may order a more specialized hCG test called a quantitative hCG. This test not only confirms that you are pregnant, but also can let your doctor know just how far along you are by measuring the amount of hCG in your blood. This information is very helpful to your doctor because it aids in diagnosing possible miscarriage or ectopic (tubal) pregnancy. When the pregnancy is normal, the hCG level should double every two to three days. With an ectopic pregnancy, the level rises, but not in the expected increments. If a woman is miscarrying, the hCG level will go down.

Prenatal Profile Tests

Earlier I told you that during your first prenatal visit your doctor will take your prenatal profile, which will include the results of a series of tests: a complete blood count, blood type and "Rh factor," syphilis, hepatitis B, HIV, certain other STDs, rubella, and sickle-cell anemia. (Black women are typically tested for sickle cell, as the disorder is most common in African Americans; about 1 out of 12 blacks carries the sickle-cell gene.) Your urine will be tested as well for bacteria, blood, sugar, excess protein, and other substances. And you will be given a Pap smear. All of this information goes into your prenatal profile.

You may not be familiar with one of the tests I mentioned—Rh factor. If your blood is Rh positive (Rh+), as is that of most people, then you have the Rh factor. Conversely, if your blood is Rh negative (Rh−), then you don't have the Rh factor. Now, when an Rh− woman and an Rh+ man have a baby, that baby is likely to be Rh+. Because mother and baby have incompatible Rh factors, it can pose a problem—not so much for this first child, but possibly for a subsequent pregnancy. Here's why: During delivery, some of your baby's blood cells can leak past the placenta and enter your bloodstream. If your blood is Rh− and your baby's is Rh+, your body's immune system will develop antibodies to destroy the "foreign" blood—the Rh factor. The number of antibodies produced in a first pregnancy usually aren't enough to harm the baby. But those antibodies stay in your body, and during a second pregnancy (if the baby, again, is Rh+), the number of antibodies could increase enough to cause anemia in the baby. This is why you should be tested for Rh factor early in your pregnancy. If your blood is Rh−, you will be given a vaccine called Rh immune globulin, or RhoGAM, that prevents your body from producing antibodies to Rh+ blood.

Your doctor should test you for the Rh factor throughout your pregnancy, including after delivery. If Rh+ antibodies are found to be present after delivery, you will receive a dose of RhoGAM. This destroys the Rh+ blood cells leaked from the baby, shutting down production of any additional antibodies.

Alpha Fetoprotein (AFP)

This blood test, usually performed between 16 and 20 weeks of pregnancy, checks for some abnormalities in the baby's developing nervous system, including the spine and brain. If the level of AFP is very high, it indicates that the baby may have spina bifida (a defect in the spinal column) or *hydrocephaly* (an excess amount of fluid in the brain). If the AFP is much lower than it should be, it may suggest Down's syndrome, a genetic disorder that results in mental retardation. In the presence of an abnormal AFP, you will likely have further testing, ranging from a repeat of the AFP test to more advanced procedures like ultrasound and amniocentesis, to get more definitive information about the health of the baby.

Ultrasound (U/S)

Ultrasound (also called a sonogram) seems to be an expectant mother's favorite procedure. No wonder—it allows her to literally see her baby. Sound waves are used to create a picture on a video screen. The internal structures of the baby are visible, and with the most current 3-D and 4-D ultrasounds, the face can be distinguished as well. While it's exciting and fun for a woman to see her baby on the screen, the test is actually used to gather information about the developing fetus. The procedure enables your doctor to take measurements of the baby's head, limbs, abdomen, and other organs. These measurements are helpful in determining the baby's age, whether he or she is developing properly, and if any abnormalities may be present.

Ultrasound is also useful in determining fetal position, the presence of a heartbeat (or many heartbeats in the case of two or more babies), the location of the placenta, and the amount of amniotic fluid. At times, the sex of the baby is detectable, too.

Ultrasound is also extremely helpful when a patient is undergoing other procedures, such as amniocentesis and chorionic villi sampling (CVS), two tests used primarily to detect genetic abnormalities.

Chorionic Villi Sampling (CVS)

CVS is a diagnostic test that can detect genetic abnormalities in a fetus. Guided by ultrasound, your doctor inserts a probelike instrument through your vagina and cervix up into the womb and retrieves a small amount of tissue from the placenta. The tissue sample is then sent to the lab where certain genetic determinations can be made. This procedure is usually done in the first trimester of pregnancy, typically at around 9 or 10 weeks, to provide needed genetic information as early as possible. CVS has a greater risk of causing miscarriage than amniocentesis (explained below). But because it can be done earlier in the pregnancy, it may be the preferred procedure when earlier detection of genetic problems is important.

Amniocentesis

Like most women, you've probably heard of this test, which is often called *amnio* for short. It is similar to CVS in that it detects genetic abnormalities in the fetus. But during amniocentesis, the doctor—using an ultrasound image for guidance—inserts a thin sterile needle through your abdomen and into your womb. Once the needle is inside the amniotic sac (bag of water), the doctor withdraws some of the amniotic fluid, which contains fetal cells. The fluid is then sent to the lab, where the number of chromosomes can be checked to rule out such disorders as Down's syndrome and many other genetic abnormalities. Amniocentesis can also check for infection, alfa fetoprotein levels, some blood disorders, and—later in the pregnancy—how well the baby's lungs are developing.

Amnios are usually performed in the second trimester (between 16 and 20 weeks) if used for genetic reasons. They can also be done later in the pregnancy to check for infections and to determine whether the baby's lungs are mature enough for him to breathe on his own.

As with CVS, amniocentesis does carry some risk for miscarriage, but it is a very small risk. Since ultrasound helps the doctor guide the placement of the needle, it's easier to avoid hitting the baby, the umbilical cord, or the placenta during the procedure.

I know the thought of a needle going into your abdomen is scary, but the procedure really isn't as bad as it sounds, and it's over before you know it. On average, an amnio takes about a minute or two.

Diabetes Screening

Since diabetes in pregnancy is a serious condition, all women should undergo a diabetes screening test, unless they are known to be diabetic prior to becoming pregnant. This rapid glucose screen (RGS) is a simple blood test given during your twenty-eighth to thirtieth week of pregnancy. Your RGS result may show that you are free of diabetes, or, if the RGS levels are high, it may indicate a possible risk. In this case, you will be scheduled for a lengthier glucose-tolerance test (GTT). The results of the GTT will let your doctors know if your have gestational diabetes. If you do, then certain diets, procedures, and medication (such as insulin) may be required to control it.

Cervical and Vaginal Screenings

At your initial prenatal visit, tests are done to check for sexually transmitted disease. As your pregnancy progresses, other infections can also occur, some of which can be detrimental to the pregnancy. For this reason, you will be tested for an infection called group B strep at about 28 weeks. Group B strep can cause premature rupture of membranes, premature labor, and in some cases, miscarriage and fetal loss. You will be checked for this infection again near the time of delivery, especially if your water breaks before it should.

Women with a history of herpes will also receive tests to check for the presence of the virus as delivery time approaches.

Fetal Monitoring Tests

During labor, tests may be performed to asses fetal well-being—a nonstress test (NST) and a contraction stress test (CST). The NST is a noninvasive test that monitors fetal heart rate and any contractions. Two belts are placed around your abdomen. One holds an instrument that tracks the fetal heart rate; the other holds an instrument that measures your contractions. These instruments connect to a monitor that prints out the information. By watching the fetal heart rate and knowing when the baby moves, your doctor can determine how well the baby is doing. If the test is inconclusive, or the baby's heart rate does not act as expected, your doctor will recommend a contraction stress test (CST), using the same fetal monitoring equipment. A CST is best performed by just observing the natural contractions of the uterus, if any. If there are no contractions, mild ones can be induced either by stimulating the woman's nipples, or with the aid of certain drugs. Once a contraction is picked up on the monitor, your doctor observes the fetal heart rate. If the baby maintains a good heart rate with three successive contractions, and does not have a significant drop in heart rate, especially after the contraction, then he should be fine. However, if the heart rate does drop significantly and repeatedly, your doctor will talk to you about intervening. In some cases, it may be necessary to deliver.

Be advised that the nipple stimulation I mentioned previously is not something you should try at home, and it is rarely used in current obstetrical management. Stimulating your nipples in an attempt to produce contractions in an unsupervised setting can lead to repeated, unstoppable contractions which, in turn, may decrease oxygen to your baby, cause fetal stress or other serious problems, and even lead to fetal death.

Once you have your basic prenatal profile and diabetes screening, not every test I've mentioned will be necessary for you. While all of these tests are common when it comes to pregnancy, overall, you may not need to have each one. Remember, not every test is necessary for every expectant mother. Many individual factors come into play. After you have your prenatal profile and diabetes screening, your doctor will recommend those tests she feels are appropriate or required for your specific pregnancy. Be sure to ask your doctor questions about any test she recommends if you don't thoroughly understand what it's all about. The more you know, and the more in tune you are with your doctor, the healthier and more enjoyable your pregnancy will be.

HOW YOUR BODY CHANGES

As any woman who has had a baby knows, your body goes through enormous changes over the course of a pregnancy. If this is your first child, anticipating the coming months can be exciting and a little scary. It makes sense. None of us ever really knows what to expect until we're actually expecting. And because no two pregnancies are alike, the experience your friends and relatives had may be different from your own. Chances are, they've bent your ear with tales of everything from morning sickness to swollen ankles. How do you make sense of it all? That's what I'm going to try to do for you. All you need to do is take the information in, then relax and enjoy your new pregnancy.

First, let's start with the basics. Pregnancy is divided into three trimesters. The first trimester is from 1 to 13 weeks, the second trimester is from 14 to 26 weeks, and the third is from 27 to 40 weeks. A normal, healthy pregnancy lasts an average of 40 weeks. I know you're thinking, *Wait a minute, 40 weeks? A pregnancy lasts 9 months. That's only 36 weeks. Where does the 40 come from?*

In order to have some way of determining a woman's due date, a formula was devised to help us tell you when to expect your baby. This method uses the first day of your last period as the beginning of your cycle. If all is normal, you probably ovulated two weeks or so later, and it was around that time that you conceived. Then, it took the fetus a few days to make its journey to the uterine cavity and implant. Added together, this accounts for the additional few weeks.

During the first trimester, you'll probably feel out of sorts because your hormones are working overtime and the volume of fluid in your system is increasing. The result of these changes? You'll be much more tired, your breasts will feel tender, you'll have to urinate more often, and you may experience "morning sickness" or in some cases, *hyperemesis,* with frequent or excessive bouts of nausea and vomiting. While there is no definite cure for morning sickness, many women find relief by having smaller meals, nibbling on dry crackers or toast, and avoiding fatty, greasy, and/or spicy foods.

For most women, the second trimester is much easier. The nausea and vomiting usually subsides by the beginning of this middle phase (typically around 14 weeks), and the fatigue disappears—for a while, anyway. The tiredness usually comes back late in the pregnancy. In the meantime, enjoy your second trimester. Your energy level will be back up and while your breasts are getting bigger, they may not be as tender.

During the third trimester, you'll likely feel fatigued once again. As your abdomen expands, you may find it more difficult and tiring to get around, especially as you get into the ninth month. Your ankles or other parts of your body may retain water and become swollen. Don't be surprised if you feel the need to rest more frequently.

It's also not uncommon to feel short of breath at times during the latter part of your ninth month. But once the baby "drops," or descends, into the pelvic cavity, the shortness of breath usually goes away. Before long, it will be time for delivery.

STAYING FIT

Over the past twenty years, exercise has become a part of American life. Aerobics, weight training, TaeBo, and step aerobics are just a few of the many exercises that have become household words. And every day there is some new report about the tremendous health benefits of regular exercise, including longer life and fewer medical ailments. It's a message black women, more than most, need to pay attention to.

After all, African-American women are more apt to be overweight. We tend to eat fattier foods, exercise less, and have a more sedentary lifestyle than other folks. As a result, over 50 percent of black women in the United States are overweight or obese. Next time you're in a mall, grocery store, or train station, look around. Look at the women walking down the street. You will see far too many black women carrying far too much weight on their bones. You'll likely see the same thing in your own family. Yes, white women can be obese too, but that is no reason for us to be. The hard fact is, more black women are obese than women of other races, and that fact alone affects our health negatively.

Excess weight is a problem anytime, but when you are pregnant, it's of even greater concern. First of all, there's the emotional aspect. Pregnancy can be, and should be, a beautiful experience for a woman. Often, though, she feels unattractive and disfigured by her increasing weight and changing profile, even if she starts at a normal weight. How much more burdensome it is to begin the pregnancy process overweight, not only from an aesthetic stand-point but, more importantly, health-wise.

Medically speaking, not only does excess fat increase your risk of hypertension, heart attack, stroke, diabetes, degenerative joint disease, arthritis, and much more, but in pregnancy, fat poses additional problems. Specifically:

- poor weight gain during pregnancy, which might result in underweight babies

- increased risk of misdiagnosing the actual size of the uterus, which could lead to premature intervention for delivery

- extra strain on your heart and blood vessels

- increased risk for hypertensive problems in the pregnancy

- increased lower abdominal and calf discomfort as the pregnancy progresses

- shortness of breath

- increased difficulty during vaginal delivery and especially if a C-section is needed

Many women, upon learning they are pregnant, vow to get in shape and can't wait to start a rigorous exercise program. Be advised: the best time to get in shape is before conceiving, not after.

If you have been participating in a regular exercise program before conceiving, it is likely you will be able to continue, with occasional adjustments to your regimen as needed. However, if you are basically a sedentary person, doing little to no regular exercise, you can still do some exercise while pregnant.

It would be best to start with easier, less stressful activities like walking. Walking is low impact, simple to do, easy on the joints, and provides an excellent cardiovascular workout. Other good exercises to do during pregnancy include swimming, stationary bike riding, and stretching.

Again, a woman who did not engage in strenuous athletic activities before getting pregnant should not embark on a rigorous new program. Pregnancy causes multiple alterations in the form and position of the body. If the muscles, joints, and ligaments are not preconditioned, excessive strain may cause injury. That's why a gradual introduction of basic, less stressful exercises is recommended.

Know, too, that there are some women who should not exercise at all during pregnancy, specifically those with a history of spontaneous miscarriages, bleeding problems, multiple gestations (carrying twins or triplets, etc.), and those who have large fibroid tumors or incompetent cervix.

Excessive workouts may also lead to *hyperthermia,* a marked increase in temperature that has been linked to nerve problems in some fetuses. Overdoing it while pregnant can also cause fluctuations in body fluids and excessive sweating, which may lead to dehydration. In fact, you should steer clear of any excessive heat source while pregnant, including hot tubs and saunas.

So, should you or shouldn't you exercise while pregnant? In the absence of obstetric or medical complications, most women can exercise moderately to maintain heart, lung, and muscular fitness throughout pregnancy and during the postpartum period. Exercise greatly promotes a sense of maternal well-being.

Again, if you have been exercising before pregnancy and have no major complications in your pregnancy, you can most likely continue whatever your regimen was before conceiving. But if you were, for the most part, sedentary, you can at least begin to walk regularly, or engage in other activities as approved by your physician.

Of course, the progression of each particular pregnancy must be taken into consideration for what and how much exercise you do, as should your prepregnancy fitness level and your previous medical history.

In any case, all women do need to engage in one particular activity whether they work out or not: drinking water! Water is the primary component of the body, and all cells must have water to function. Water also flushes the system and clears toxins from your body.

If you do plan to exercise while pregnant, keep these points in mind:

- Avoid sudden stop/start activities, like tennis, as they may jolt your uterus and potentially injure the connections of the placenta.

- Avoid activities that put you at risk of being struck in the abdomen, such as soccer or racquetball.

- Stop your fitness program if you develop bleeding problems, pain, rapid heartbeat, dizziness, nausea, or loss of muscle control.

- Avoid high altitudes, if possible.

- Be sure to support your breasts with strong athletic foundations.

- Remember that late pregnancy changes in the shape of your body can greatly affect your posture and sense of balance. Therefore, high-impact activities such as running should be avoided in the third trimester, to prevent trauma.

What about your diet? The National Research Council recommends that pregnant women take in 2,500 calories a day, with 60 grams of protein and 1,200 mg of calcium. Also, be sure to eat regularly; don't skip meals. (Now is not the time to try to lose weight!) Skipping meals will cause your body to produce chemicals called *ketones,* which can act like an acid and irritate your uterus and/or the baby. Be sure to take your prenatal vitamins, and check with your doctor for any other dietary recommendations.

COMPLICATIONS OF PREGNANCY

No woman ever wants to think about the possibility that something may go wrong with her pregnancy. Odds are, nothing will go wrong. But the sad truth is, it can happen. You have to enter into pregnancy with your eyes open and realize that there are many potential problems and complications that can occur. It may be scary to think about, but I believe doing so will help you take better care of yourself. Remember what I always say: Knowledge is power. The more you know, the better prepared you will be for the nine months ahead. That said, let's take a look at some of the most common complications that may occur during pregnancy.

First Trimester (1–13 weeks)

Ectopic Pregnancy: The dictionary defines *ectopic* as "in an abnormal position." So it is with an ectopic pregnancy—the pregnancy is not in the middle of the womb where it should be, but

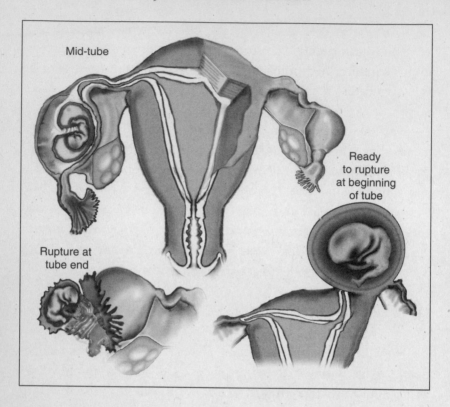

Mid-tube

Ready
to rupture
at beginning
of tube

Rupture at
tube end

instead is in an abnormal position, a place it should not be. The most common site for this is in the fallopian tube, which is why ectopic pregnancies are often referred to as "tubal" pregnancies.

But ectopics can occur in other locations, including the ovary, the muscular portion of the uterus called the *cornu* (not in the inner, central cavity where it should be), the cervix, or on the inner walls of your abdomen (abdominal pregnancy). For the sake of simplicity, the terms *ectopic* and *tubal* will be interchanged in this discussion. Just remember that the same process of implantation applies to whichever site is involved.

Tubal pregnancies occur when the fertilized egg gets trapped in the tube, implants there, and begins to grow. Since the tube is narrow and not meant to house a developing fetus, it eventually stretches so much that it bursts, usually causing pain. This is a very serious condition. The ruptured tube causes blood to drip, stream, or pour into the abdominal cavity, and a woman will begin to see blood coming from her vagina. If this happens, it usually takes place during the sixth to eighth week of pregnancy.

Ectopic babies cannot be saved. There have been two recent reports of abdominal pregnancy babies surviving, but other than those two rare occurrences, an ectopic pregnancy fetus does not survive.

Women who begin prenatal care early stand the best chance of having the problem detected before the tube actually ruptures. This is preferred, for if the ectopic is caught very early in its development, some women can be treated with an injection of a potent medication called Methotrexate, or with minor laparoscopic surgery. However, large ectopics or extensively ruptured ectopics will likely require major open abdominal surgery and a hospital stay.

You are at greater risk for having an ectopic pregnancy if you have had a previous ectopic pregnancy, previous tubal surgery (like tubal ligation or infertility treatment on the fallopian tube), a history of internal scar tissue called adhesions, or a history of gonorrhea, chlamydia, and/or pelvic inflammatory disease.

Miscarriage: About 20 percent of women will miscarry a baby. This occurs when (1) the fetus doesn't implant well; (2) the fetus is genetically abnormal and the body "recognizes" this and naturally terminates the process; or (3) there is a hormone deficiency (usually progesterone), which makes the attachment to the uterine lining weak.

While the average person would never categorize a miscarriage as an abortion, in the medical profession it is. The medical abbreviation for abortion is "AB." Women who choose to terminate their pregnancy have an "elective" abortion, or elective AB. A woman who spontaneously loses her fetus has a miscarriage—an event medical professionals call a SAB or SpAB, a spontaneous abortion.

The symptoms of miscarriage usually include cramping, irregular spotting, or bleeding that mimics a heavy period. Some women will actually notice "tissue" in the blood. This "tissue" will appear as a white, fleshy substance. As devastating as it is, if you should pass this "tissue," you should scoop it up, put it in a plastic baggie or aluminum foil, and take it with you to the doctor's. It can be very helpful to your physician, medically speaking, and may save you from needing surgery.

There are different levels of miscarriage. A *missed AB* refers to the pregnancy actually ending with no outward sign of doing so. That is to say, the tiny baby (the collection of cells called an *embryo* or *fetus*) expires but no bleeding, pain, or other sign is apparent. Ultrasounds and quantitative hCG levels come in handy to help diagnose this. A D&C may be needed in some cases to clear the uterus of the tissue, which, if left in place, can cause bleeding, perhaps a great deal.

An *incomplete AB* is when part, but not all, of the early pregnancy passes out of the body. The cervix actually opens some, and bleeding is apparent, possibly with the passage of tissue.

A *complete AB* is when the entire pregnancy sac is passed. When this occurs, there will be some bleeding, but if it really involves the total pregnancy, usually no D&C or other surgery is needed.

In either case, after the uterus is emptied of the pregnancy sac, medication is given to help the uterus contract back to its normal small size.

Women who have repeated spontaneous ABs may have some genetic problem, or may lack substantial levels of progesterone in the early months of the pregnancy. Your doctor should be able to determine the cause of repeated spontaneous miscarriages.

Second Trimester (14–27 weeks)

Incompetent Cervix: This is just what is sounds like: the cervix is too weak to withstand the weight and pressure from the growing uterus housing the baby, placenta, and amniotic fluid. With increasing weight, the weak cervix opens and a woman will miscarry, though the fetus is larger and more developed than in the first trimester. Most women who miscarry because of an incompetent cervix don't feel anything happening until long after the point of being able to save the baby, and miscarriage occurs.

Patients at risk for this include those who have had procedures done through or on their cervix, like numerous abortions, D&Cs, cone biopsies, or multiple births.

The condition may not always be picked up the first time it occurs, but a history of a second trimester loss should be a red flag to your doctor to be alert for this condition.

What can be done to prevent another loss? Once the diagnosis or presumptive diagnosis is made, a purse-string stitch can be placed in the cervix, basically to sew it closed. The stitch (called a *cerclage*) remains in place until approximately 37 weeks, at which time it can be removed. Should you begin to have contractions then, or if the cervix begins to open, the baby is old enough to survive.

The cerclage is done in the operating room, usually under spinal anesthesia. The procedure doesn't take very long but does carry a slight risk of miscarriage itself. Why? Because the needle used to place the stitch could possibly snag the bag of waters, nicking it and causing the water to leak. At such an early stage, there would be no hope of the pregnancy continuing and evacuation of the uterus would be needed. Fortunately, this does not happen very often, and the risk of this is far outweighed by the benefit of placing the stitch in the hopes of maintaining a much-desired pregnancy.

Preterm (Premature) Labor: This occurs when the uterus begins to contract before the baby is full-term. If this is allowed to continue, early delivery can occur, which could be detrimental to the baby.

PTL, as it's commonly called, can be due to hormone changes, vaginal or uterine infections, an overstretched uterus (as with multiple gestation), or ruptured membranes.

Diagnosis is made when your doctor or nurse feels the contractions, or they will be detected on the fetal monitor. Treatment includes ruling out infection as a cause, then giving medication to stop the contractions. Depending on how strong the contractions are, and whether your cervix has dilated (and how much), the medicine may just be oral, or you may need to be hospitalized for IV medication.

There is some good news about African Americans and the incidence of premature births, though. The racial gap for premature births seems to be narrowing. According to the Centers for Disease Control, single-born premature births among black women fell nearly 10 percent between 1990 and 1997. In 1990, there were 178.5 premature births per 1,000 live births, but in 1997, that number was down to 160.9. This shows a 9.8 percent drop. The good news is that the trend is continuing. Perhaps not only is the message getting out, but black women are beginning to pay attention and heed the warnings.

Ruptured Membranes: You have probably heard women say their "water broke," meaning that they noticed a leak, stream, or gush of water coming out through the vagina. This water—the amniotic fluid—is what surrounds the baby, cushioning it and the umbilical cord from external pressures and bumps. (I tell you, God thought of everything, didn't He?)

When the water breaks around the time of your due date, that's fine; it's usually a good thing. But you don't want the water to break in the second trimester. When it does, you run a risk of losing the baby.

How you are treated for ruptured membranes depends on a few things:

• how far along in the pregnancy you are

• whether or not the baby would be able to survive if it were to be born

• if the umbilical cord is still up inside the uterus or if it too has come down (called a prolapsed cord)

• if there is infection

• if there is heavy bleeding, or problems with the placenta

• whether or not there is any fluid left around the baby to help the baby's lungs (When in the uterus, the fetus actually breathes the water in and out. Without adequate fluid, the baby's lungs will collapse or be severely damaged, perhaps badly enough to lead to fetal death.)

Options for management of ruptured membranes in the second trimester include completing what the body has already begun; i.e., proceeding with terminating the pregnancy if it's very early in the second trimester or if there is an infection, prolapsed cord, or heavy bleeding.

If late in the second trimester (26 or so weeks), attempts can be made to try to buy the baby more time to develop. To do this, however, enough fluid must still be present around the baby, and there should be no obvious infection or bleeding. In this situation, a woman will be admitted to the hospital and maintained on strict bed rest with the head of the bed tilted down and the foot of the bed greatly elevated. Obviously this can be an uncomfortable position even for a day, but it is necessary in order to try to save the baby.

I'll never forget a very sweet patient who experienced ruptured membranes at 22 weeks. It was her idea that we not terminate the pregnancy. Her tremendous spirit and determination helped enable her to maintain the pregnancy until she reached 36 weeks. Miracles do happen. Her little girl was born perfectly healthy and is doing well today!

Third trimester (28–40 weeks)

Just as in the second trimester, preterm labor and ruptured membranes can occur. The closer to full-term this occurs, the less of a problem it is. Remember, the goal is always to get the baby as close to term as possible. The more time the baby has to fully develop inside the mother, the better.

Other problems that become evident mostly in the third trimester include problems with the placenta, including *placenta previa* and *placental abruption*. "Previa" means that the placenta (the afterbirth) is attached closest to the cervix; that is to say, it would come out first, before the baby, should the woman go into labor. The placenta is extremely vascular—rich in blood—and provides the baby with its nourishment while inside the mother. If it were to come out first, excessive bleeding could occur, leading to fetal death.

Patients with a *placenta previa* often have painless spotting or bleeding. An ultrasound is used to detect the location of the placenta. If a previa exists at the time of actual labor, or late in the pregnancy, a C-section delivery is indicated. If it's detected earlier, in the second trimester for instance, with time it may move higher up in the uterus, and vaginal delivery may be possible. Patients would be followed with ultrasounds to monitor this.

A *placental abruption* is associated with painful bleeding. With an abruption, the afterbirth actually separates from the womb before it should. A woman can often feel when this happens, and soon she will experience heavy, bright red vaginal bleeding. There are some women, however, who will have a "silent abruption," in which the placenta separates, but no bleeding is noticed because it's walled off by the baby or has sealed itself off.

Abruptions are very serious and can lead to intense hemorrhaging. Immediate delivery is usually required, typically by C-section, though some very small abruptions may make it through the labor process. Causes of abruption include excessively strong uterine contractions, increased blood pressure, and trauma to the abdomen.

Intrauterine Fetal Growth Retardation (IUGR or IUFGR): IUGR refers not to mental retardation but to retardation of a baby's growth. The fetus is not growing at the rate expected; its physical development has slowed—been retarded, held back.

This may be due to poor weight gain by the mother; to excessive emotional or physical strain, medications, or poor nutrition; or to unknown causes. When a woman is carrying multiple babies, some babies will have IUGR because one of the other babies is taking most of the nutrients and blood flow from the placenta.

In most instances IUGR is detected when the abdomen is measured at the prenatal exam. For every week of pregnancy, your uterus should increase one centimeter. Thirty weeks? Thirty centimeters. You are allowed a difference of two centimeters to allow for personal variation in babies' sizes. If your doctor notices a lag in your measurement (called the fundal height), you will get an ultrasound to check on the baby and will be prescribed bed rest and sound nutrition. Many times, the bed rest will result in a return to normal growth. If not, further studies, and maybe even delivery, could be recommended.

Preeclampsia and Eclampsia: *Preeclampsia* (sometimes called toxemia of pregnancy) is a very serious condition that primarily affects first-time mothers. Women with this condition usually have high blood pressure, extra protein in their urine, and swelling (called *edema*) in their legs so severe that if you press their lower legs you'll leave an indentation.

Treatment for preeclampsia is delivery of the baby, for that is the only thing that will alleviate this condition. A medication called magnesium sulfate will also be given to help prevent preeclampsia from becoming even more severe, resulting in eclampsia, in which seizures occur.

Both of these conditions—preeclampsia and eclampsia—can lead to maternal and fetal death if not treated in time, and can also occur postpartum (after delivery).

Gestational Diabetes: When a woman develops diabetes during pregnancy it can cause her baby to become very sick. The developing fetus may become excessively large or have other problems. Diabetes can also affect the mother's health. This is why all pregnant women are screened for diabetes, and if it's detected, strict management is required. Management includes careful monitoring of your blood sugar levels, medication with insulin in most cases, and conducting serial ultrasounds and nonstress tests. Concern is also raised about the timing for delivery, because diabetes has a way of slowing the rate at which the baby's lungs mature while inside the mother. Your doctor should be watching carefully for these potential problems.

LABOR AND DELIVERY

The day has finally arrived. It's time to have your baby. What should you expect when arriving at the hospital? What are all those machines for? What is the usual protocol for admission and laboring? What are epidurals, and why are C-sections sometimes needed? Granted, there's a lot to take in. But just remember, millions of women have healthy babies every day. Here is some of what you can expect when it's your turn. First and foremost, call your doctor before heading to the hospital, unless you are having an emergency, such as hemorrhaging, seizure, or imminent delivery. A phone call to your doctor explaining why you think "it's time" may save you an unnecessary trip to the hospital. If it truly is time, your doctor will advise you to go to the hospital and she'll meet you there.

Once you arrive at the labor and delivery unit, your vital signs will be checked and you will be hooked up to the electronic fetal monitor (EFM), which records your contractions as well as the baby's heart rate. Assessments will be made as to whether your water has broken or if you're having bleeding. Urine and possible blood tests may be obtained, depending on your condition.

Some patients may only need to be observed for a while and then sent home, or to the hospital floor that houses pregnant women who need treatment but aren't in active labor or having an acute problem. Those requiring delivery, or further, more urgent management will be admitted to the labor and delivery unit.

As you labor, you will likely be connected to an IV for medications and hydration. In most cases you won't be permitted to eat, though clear liquids may be allowed. This isn't intended to be cruel. Since so many urgent, unexpected things can happen to women in labor, it's best that your stomach be kept empty of solid food in case an emergency C-section is needed and you have to be given anesthesia.

As your labor progresses, the pains will get more intense and pain medicines are often given, if you want them. It's been my experience that most women do want them, especially the *epidural*.

What is that? An epidural is anesthetic that is injected into a space just before your spinal cord. It provides tremendous relief from the pains of labor. After receiving one, many women rest comfortably through the remainder of their labor but are still able to push for the delivery. The epidural is administered by the anesthesia team, and it is not harmful to the baby.

Once your cervix reaches full dilation at ten centimeters, which may take a while, you can begin to push. Your doctor, the nurses, and your support person will be there to encourage you, but remember, we can't push for you. Only you can do it.

During this entire process, your baby is being carefully monitored. As long as your baby tolerates the labor and pushing process okay, you'll be able to continue. But should the baby show signs of distress during the process, plans may change and a quicker delivery may be necessary. If you are far enough along, that may just mean using other instruments to help bring the baby down, like a special obstetrical vacuum, or forceps. If your cervix is not open enough and the baby is not low enough in the vagina, or a worsening medical condition dictates you can't wait for the labor process to continue, a C-section may be indicated.

Most women do deliver their babies vaginally, but a significant number undergo a *cesarean section*, also called a C-section or C/S, to aid in the birth of their child.

For the past ten or so years, there has been great concern regarding the number of C-sections performed in this country. This concern has led women, their spouses, and family members to often become very leery when told by the OB doctor that a surgical delivery is necessary. Again, that's when having a doctor you trust and respect comes into play; you have less cause to doubt.

Additionally, many in the health professions have studied and analyzed why the number of C-sections climbed rapidly in the past ten to fifteen years (though some numbers are going down now). A review of these studies often pointed fingers at two major "culprits." The first is the risk of litigation many doctors face when practicing obstetrics. The second is the increased use of electronic fetal monitoring, the very thing that helps your doctor track your baby's heart. By using the monitor, we are now able to discover the problems babies face during labor, and therefore steps are taken to get the baby out of a risky or even fatal situation. That may require a C-section.

Despite these two concerns, there are many instances in which a C-section is well indicated. These include but are not limited to:

Hemorrhage: Acute heavy, rapid bleeding during labor may be due to a placenta previa or placental abruption (described above), or due to an actual rupture of the uterus itself, in which the muscle fibers of the uterus separate and excessive bleeding occurs.

Failure to Progress (FTP): This means the normal progression of labor has stopped; your cervix is no longer dilating. The most common cause of this is *cephalopelvic disproportion* (CPD). In plain English: the mother's pelvis is not proportioned to accommodate the dimensions or position of the baby's head. Other causes of FTP include weak contractions that don't respond to medicine that should strengthen them, or abnormalities in the uterus such as fibroid tumors, which sometimes can make the contractions irregular or dysfunctional.

Prolapsed Cord: Usually the baby's head is the lowest part of the uterine contents. Sometimes, however, the umbilical cord drops down first. This may occur if the woman's water breaks before the baby's head is "engaged" in the pelvis, i.e., is low enough to keep that from happening. With the cord hanging down, the baby's head or buttocks can press on the cord and cut off blood flow to the baby. A prolapsed cord is an obstetrical emergency and requires immediate delivery by C-section.

Abnormal Presentation: Most babies are born headfirst. But sometimes they are in a "breech" position—lying sideways, or upside down with their buttocks or feet first. If the baby cannot be turned from the breech position, a C-section is usually required.

Multiple Pregnancy: Twins can often be delivered vaginally, but if the babies are positioned awkwardly in the womb in relation to one another, or if they aren't handling the labor process well, a C-section may be necessary.

Fetal Distress: Imagine something pressing strongly on your entire body every two to three minutes. When you don't know what's going on and why it's happening, you might get a bit stressed, don't you think? Well, that's what happens to your baby while you labor. Fortunately, most babies get through the labor process just fine. But some babies may not handle it well. Their heart rate may drop, which, over time, can cause distress for the infant. This is where the EFM is so helpful, for it allows the doctor to detect the baby's overall well-being and tolerance of the labor process.

Infections: The presence of herpes or other infection in or around the birth canal is a definite indication for a surgical delivery; otherwise the baby faces a chance of acquiring the infection, which may result in blindness or death for the infant.

Uncontrollable or Unresponsive Medical Conditions: Severe blood pressure problems, or overly large babies resulting from the mother's diabetes may necessitate a surgical delivery.

These are just some of the reasons you may need to have a cesarean. What about a second opinion? For elective surgeries you should always get one. But during labor there is no time for second and third opinions, especially if any of the aforementioned conditions exist. Things can happen so fast that any time spent getting other opinions can literally cost your baby's life and your own. For this reason, again, it is imperative that you select an OB doctor you are comfortable with and whose judgment you trust.

PREGNANCY AFTER AGE 35

It has been said that the best age to have a child is 26. By that time, the thinking goes, a woman has completed her education, she is emotionally mature, and the many hormonal fluctuations younger women experience are gone. And, back in the day, many of us had married by that age.

The women's movement, however, played a major role in changing how early and how often women want to get pregnant. And with more and more women seeking careers or time on their own to travel and see the world before they settle down, some women may take a while to find a husband. What's more, increasing numbers of women are simply choosing to have children later in life—with or without a husband.

As a result of all this, many women now have children well into their thirties, forties, and sometimes later. In 1997, a woman in California had a baby at the age of 63!

Societal mores aside, is it risky to have a baby later in life? Medically speaking, women who conceive after the age of 35 are considered to have "advanced maternal age" (AMA). Many would take exception to that label, as they feel they are just beginning to live their lives. But the classification is not a put-down; it's more a marker for patient and doctor. After the age of 35, there are issues and risk factors that need to be addressed that aren't as pressing for younger women.

In 2002, new publications and articles in national newsmagazines made many women nervous, as they explored the concept that many women who deliberately delayed their childbearing in favor of their careers mostly found themselves not only without offspring, but with infertility problems, or no potential spouses with whom to try to conceive.

Genetic Concerns: The most widely known risk for mothers over 35 is that of chromosomal abnormalities, especially Down's syndrome, which causes mental retardation and abnormal development of the baby's organs, including the heart. Other factors include decreased ovulation in some women. Other genetic problems can occur, as well. Your doctor can go over those with you.

The best way to avert these genetic disorders is to have genetic tests done while pregnant, namely, a CVS or amniocentesis (see page 282 for more on these tests). If your test shows normal chromosomes, then all is well. If your test shows Down's syndrome or other genetic problems, your doctor will offer you a medically indicated termination of the pregnancy, should you desire. Or if you wish to keep the baby, meeting with genetic counselors and pediatricians during your pregnancy will help prepare you for the years ahead.

With early intervention after birth, many Down's children do well, though the reality is that they will face some difficulties.

Preexisting Medical Concerns: With the passage of time, it's not uncommon to find women over 35 with hypertension, diabetes, obesity, fibroids, scar tissue, or other medical problems, especially in the black community. Should you consider getting pregnant later in life, you must consider how any medical conditions you have will affect the pregnancy and how the pregnancy will affect your medical condition. This is why it's so important to have a preconception session not only with your obstetrician-gynecologist, but also with the doctor who is treating your condition, be it your primary care physician or a specialist.

Lifestyle, Stress, Patience, and Energy. I often hear women who have had children in their late thirties and early forties say they just don't have the energy to keep up with their kids. Many say they are not as patient as they would like to be, and some have to make major changes in their lives to properly care for their child. Everything changes when a baby joins the family. Be sure you look at how your life will change. And don't forget the expense.

While there are risks to consider, most older moms have perfectly healthy babies. Genetic conditions can be easily diagnosed, and if you are a woman who has medical problems like hypertension, diabetes, and others, you can have as good an outcome with pregnancy as many of your younger counterparts, *if* your condition is well under control before pregnancy, you seek prenatal care early, and stay on schedule with your appointments.

With African-American women carrying the worst prognosis for many medical conditions, coupled with the highest incidence of obstetrical problems, it is even more important for black women to see their doctors in a timely manner, before and during a pregnancy.

More good news about having kids later in life? You are more likely to be financially secure and able to provide more easily for your child. You will also be in a better position to give your child a wide range of experiences. Plus, many women say the new baby keeps them young, giving them more reasons to laugh and hug. And the joy of seeing a new life develop before your eyes is a reward beyond compare.

Another bonus of later pregnancies is that there is an increased chance of having twins. That may not be good news for some, but others may see it as a blessing, especially if they have been trying to conceive for a long time or if they are concerned about having more babies at their age.

Last, know that you are not alone. More and more women are having babies later, so you will have plenty of company and stories to swap with sisters in your same situation. The main thing is to be as healthy as you can be before you conceive and to get prenatal care after becoming pregnant. If you do, you should do fine.

INFERTILITY

What about couples who can't get pregnant? Approximately 20 percent of couples in the United States have trouble conceiving. About 40 percent of the time, it's due to a problem with the woman's system. Another 40 percent of the time, the problem lies with the man. The remaining 20 percent of infertility cases are unexplained.

Men and women spend weeks, months, even years, along with thousands of dollars, trying to solve infertility problems. And while their goal is clear, the stress of the process can get to many couples. It can be a painful and frustrating experience. What causes infertility, and what can be done to help?

Female infertility is most times due to:

• a history of gonorrhea or chlamydia, or other infections that can cause pelvic inflammatory disease and block the fallopian tubes

• previous intra-abdominal surgery that may cause scar tissue to form around the tubes

• deficiencies of hormones, like progesterone. Some women may ovulate irregularly, or not at all. Others may be able to get pregnant, but they can't maintain the pregnancy due to low progesterone levels.

• the woman's body forms "antibodies" to her partner's sperm, or her vagina's acidic nature can kill the sperm. The mucus near the cervix may be too thick for the sperm to penetrate, or it may be toxic to the sperm.

• genetic problems

• use of tobacco, alcohol or illegal drugs, all of which may affect fertility

• increased age

Male infertility is mostly due to:

• a low sperm count secondary to genetic causes or due to injury to the testes, including excessive heat exposure

• medications for high blood pressure, or some antidepressants

- use of tobacco, alcohol, or illegal drugs

- diabetes

- infections, including some STDs

- the development of mumps after the man has reached adulthood

- exposure to radiation

- increased age

Because the infertility problem may lie with either party, it is important that both the woman and the man receive a medical workup. The first step for a man is analysis of his sperm. Additionally, he may need to see a urologist who will examine the penis and scrotum for any abnormalities and dysfunction. Blood tests may also be ordered. If any problems are found, such as a low sperm count or poor sperm motility, medications may help some men, while for others, minor surgery may be needed. Otherwise, they will need no treatment.

A woman will likely have to undergo many tests, some more involved than the others, to get to the root of the problem. In a woman's body, three things must happen for a pregnancy to occur and develop. There must be ovulation (release of her egg); fertilization of the egg by the man's sperm; and implantation, in which the early cells of the pregnancy attach to the lining of the womb and grow. In each of these stages, things may not go as planned, and the problem could be in any part of the female reproductive tract.

Things that interfere with ovulation are basically hormone problems: either too much or too little estrogen or progesterone. A basal body temperature (BBT) chart will help determine whether a woman is ovulating. A urine test for certain hormones will also indicate her ovulation status, as may a blood test that checks for a rise in progesterone shortly after the time a woman should have ovulated. The most common tests are the BBT and the urine test. If the woman is found not to be ovulating, medications can be given to induce release of an egg. These fertility drugs can, at times, lead to multiple ovulation, which could mean triplets, quadruplets, or more. (Remember the McCaughey family?)

Testing for problems with fertilization include looking to see if there's a problem in the vagina where the sperm first makes contact. Is there a problem with the sperm making its way to the tube? Are the tubes open to receive the sperm? To find out, the fertility specialist will give you a *postcoital* (after sex) test. You will come to the doctor's office shortly after having intercourse (you cannot shower, bathe, or douche before the test), and a sample of your vaginal fluid will be taken. The cells of your vaginal fluid are tested to see how they "interact" with the sperm contained in the fluid. Problems with your cervical mucus or the acid in your vagina might kill off the sperm. Medication may be given to help make the vagina more sperm-friendly.

Another test is the *endometrial biopsy*, which is performed in the doctor's office. This too will help evaluate ovulation, but it can also provide information about the shape of the inner walls of the uterus.

A hysterosalpingogram (HSG) is another test that will allow the uterus to be evaluated. Using X-ray guidance, the doctor inserts a dye into the uterine cavity, making the shape of the inner womb visible on a screen. This procedure can cause pain in the abdomen, which may be a good sign; this test allows a view of the uterine cavity, and also if your tubes are open, the dye will be seen streaming out of the ends of the fallopian tubes. Many times, women will get pregnant shortly after having this procedure because the pressure from the fluid can sometimes open up tubes that may have had a slight filmy blockage. The HSG is done in the X-ray department at a hospital or local community X-ray center. If a major blockage is found on the HSG, surgery is usually recommended.

Other procedures include using ultrasound and laparoscopy to get a better look at the womb, inside and out. Checking for scar tissue, fibroids, and endometriosis is helpful when looking for possible causes of infertility.

So what can be done to help infertile couples? There are ways to assist in the process of conception using technology. In vitro fertilization, for example, allows a woman's egg to be fertilized outside of her body. Eggs are removed from her ovary and fertilized in a laboratory dish, then placed in her uterus. Artificial insemination is another common option, using her partner's sperm or donor sperm.

Other, more complex procedures include *gamete intra-fallopian transfer* (GIFT) and *zygote intra-fallopian transfer* (ZIFT), both of which involve directly transferring either mature eggs and sperm or fertilized eggs in the fallopian tube. Speak with your doctor about these infertility treatments and any other options that may be right for you.

PREVENTING PREGNANCY

While the joys of parenthood are, for many, unparalleled, there are times when pregnancy is the last thing on a sister's mind. She may be single and of the opinion that it's best to wait for marriage before bringing a child into the world. Or she may be happily committed and simply not yet ready to be a mother. Or she may choose never to have any children at all. There are any number of reasons why a woman may not want to get pregnant. Whatever her reason, the objective is the same—to prevent pregnancy.

Of course, we all know that an unplanned conception can happen no matter how much we may not want it to. The heat of passion can take over and send good judgment out the window (the "caught up in the rapture" syndrome). Or perhaps the condom broke, or some other contraceptive failure occurred. Most of these failures are due to improper or inconsistent use of a contraceptive method and only rarely to an absolute failure of the method itself.

Certainly the best solution for anyone who doesn't want to become pregnant would be not to have sex. Abstinence and celibacy are surefire ways to prevent the unintended. Of course, in marriage this option isn't viable.

The next best option is to be prepared. Fortunately, many women are doing just that. According to researchers at the Alan Guttmacher Institute, in the past few years, women have made approximately 13.5 million visits a year to private physicians for the purpose of preventing unplanned or unwanted pregnancy. Yes, the numbers are good, but certainly not good enough, especially among teenagers.

Younger sisters aren't the only ones who have contraceptive needs. Older women, specifically those between the ages of 35 and about 50 (menopausal), need advice about their birth control options, too. Women this age often feel lost when it comes to finding birth control that is safe for them. They may have certain medical conditions they need to be mindful of and, on a more basic level, may wonder just how long they can stay on the pill or use an IUD. A whole new set of issues comes into play for older sisters.

As a physician who has treated thousands of black women over the years, I am especially concerned about the number of African-American women who fail to seek contraceptive advice in a timely manner, before we get pregnant. Studies show that black women tend not to seek contraceptive advice until either going to their doctor for a pregnancy test (which is often positive), or during a preabortion counseling session. These facts upset me because we know better. At this point in time, in the society we live in, with TV, radio, and the Internet, I just can't accept that we don't know about contraception. The truth is many of us choose not to use it, or we make excuses about why we don't. Sadly, so many of the mind games we play—even on ourselves—hold us back and get our children off to a rocky start.

I'm reminded of an unforgettable experience I had while I was an ob-gyn intern. I was on call one evening in the labor and delivery unit when paramedics brought in a woman who had delivered her baby at home. The ambulance attendants brought the patient to the delivery room and I went in to deliver the placenta, which was still inside her uterus.

While I scrubbed my arms and hands, the nurses placed the patient on the delivery room table and prepared her for the procedure. They also made sure the baby was doing well on the warming bed. After I removed the placenta and checked for any vaginal tears that might need stitching (there were none), the patient was returned to a more comfortable position. I then checked on the baby myself and bundled him up in preparation to officially meet his mother. While I stood near the baby, playing with his little fists, the patient asked, "Doctor, do you have any children?" I told her no. She then said something I will never forget. "Well, you can have that little boy right there, if you want." I couldn't believe my ears, but, needing to maintain professional decorum, I dealt with her statement by asking if she was planning to put the child up for adoption. She said no; I could just have the baby if I wanted him. Needless to say, I was shocked.

While waiting for help to move her off the table (the nurse had left our room to assist with an emergency C-section), and with the baby resting comfortably in the warming bed, I asked her a few routine questions in order to complete the hospital paperwork. During my medical and psychological fact-finding mission, I began a general conversation and politely asked her how it was that she ended up delivering the baby at home. Her reply? "Well, I was standing at the kitchen sink and heard this thump on the floor. I looked down and saw this baby laying there." Apparently, the baby just "dropped out" onto the floor. That was the first time, she said, she realized she was pregnant. Mind you, this was her seventh pregnancy. She had to know what pregnancy felt like. She chose to deny her pregnancy and didn't get prenatal care. But if she had used contraception, she wouldn't have been in that situation. As I said before, we play mind games on ourselves.

I remember feeling that I didn't even want to give her the baby to carry as we rolled her to the recovery room. There he was, a newborn little boy who was obviously unwanted, had not been cared for over the previous nine months, and was not loved. She did not want to put the baby up for adoption, so they went home. I've often wondered how the two of them are doing.

Yes, many women don't seek contraceptive counseling and end up having pregnancies they don't want, hadn't planned on, and didn't expect. I can report, however, that statistics are showing some improvement among black women in their use of birth control. Hopefully this trend will continue. Government statistics in 2002 show a decrease in the number of teen pregnancies, mainly due to increased contraception use. But the number of teen pregnancies is still highest among blacks.

Fortunately, regardless of our age, the majority of contraceptives currently available in this country can be used by most of us. It's just a matter of finding the one that works best for you. Additionally, there are currently two male contraceptive methods approved and available: condoms and vasectomy. Other male contraceptive methods are being researched.

So how do you begin tackling the matter of picking a contraceptive? There are a few questions to consider:

- How often are you having sex?

- Are you in a truly monogamous relationship, that is, both parties are definitely faithful to each other? Do you know for sure?

- How soon do you think you would like to have a baby?

- What medical conditions do you have that may affect a particular birth control method? What medications are you taking? What uterine problems do you have, if any?

- Are you going to be responsible enough to use the contraceptive method as prescribed? For example, will you remember to take the Pill every day?

- Do you have any allergies or sensitivities to certain contraceptive chemicals, such as spermicides or latex?

- Is sexual spontaneity important to you? Will introducing a condom or additional spermicide for a diaphragm during sex be a problem for you?

- Last, do you want a contraceptive method that's reversible or permanent? Short-acting or long-acting? What is your husband's or partner's opinion on the subject?

For the sake of ease, the following discussion divides the various methods of contraception into groups, based on how and where they work, and gives their rates of success. *Theoretical* success rate refers to when the method is used exactly as recommended or prescribed. *Actual* refers to the rate when subjected to human foibles and behavior. For example, oral contraceptive users will have a theoretical success rate of 99 percent if they use the pills exactly as prescribed, but since some women forget their pill, don't take it on time, run out, etc., the actual success of the method drops approximately 2 to 3 percent, to 97 percent.

Barrier contraceptives are those that create a block to the process of conception—putting a barrier between the egg and sperm. There are mechanical barriers, such as condoms, diaphragms, and cervical caps, and chemical barriers such as spermicides. The success of many of these depends on how consistently they are used.

Hormonal contraceptives work by altering the woman's hormonal status, thereby disrupting the usual chain of events that leads to ovulation or implantation. These include oral contraceptives (OCs) and injectable contraceptives. They are usually very reliable methods, but in some cases (such as with OCs), their success depends on the consistency with which they are taken.

Sterilization—male or female—is to be considered a permanent form of contraception. Female sterilization is called *tubal ligation,* and the male sterilization procedure is called *vasectomy.* Both methods are nearly 100 percent sure, though there can be occasional failures resulting in pregnancy.

Calendar contraception relies on timing sex to when a woman is not fertile, that is, when the egg is not available for fertilization by the sperm. This category includes the rhythm method or other forms of natural family planning, like withdrawal. Though some people have success with these methods, they are far less reliable than those mentioned above, and often result in unintended pregnancy.

Read the categories below, then review the chart describing risks and benefits of each method (page 330).

Barrier Contraceptives

Spermicides (Theoretical: 95 to 97 percent; Actual: 79 percent) Just as pesticides kill insects, spermicides kill sperm. The most common spermicide is nonoxynol-9, which is found in spermicidal foams, creams, and jellies sold over the counter. Spermicides are considered chemical barriers and are also found in many condoms to provide additional protection against pregnancy.

There have been reports that nonoxynol-9 can also provide some protection against STDs, although it should not be relied upon as a sole means of guarding against STDs.

While you can use spermicides alone, it is best to use them in conjunction with another method, like condoms or diaphragms. Also, check for expiration dates on the tubes.

Some women have reported a sensitivity to the chemical. If it turns out that you are one of them, ask your doctor about other options.

Spermicides come with an applicator that attaches to the tube. Squeeze the tube and the spermicide fills the applicator. You then insert the applicator high into your vagina and push the plunger, sending the spermicide into the vaginal vault where it can kill any sperm that may be introduced into the vaginal cavity. Each act of intercourse requires insertion of more spermicide.

Condoms (Theoretical: 95 to 97 percent; Actual: approximately 88 to 90 percent) When most people think of condoms they think of the male variety. Many don't realize that there are also condoms made specifically for women. These polyurethane sheaths have been available for nearly ten years.

One reason why female condoms are not well known or widely used is because many women find them cumbersome, large, and difficult to manage. They resemble a bigger version of the male condom but have an inner ring at the closed end. You have to insert the condom into your vagina, then push it as far as you can up against your cervix. Female condoms can slip during intercourse, they cost more than male condoms, and the failure rate is much higher than that of male condoms.

The benefit of the female condom is that, like its male counterpart, it is available without a prescription, it allows you to take responsibility for birth control, and it offers some protection against STDs and pregnancy.

Male condoms, often called rubbers, are far more common and widely used. Many men don't like to wear them, though, because they say condoms impede sensation. Despite that—or perhaps due in part to women's insisting on their use ("no glove, no love")—condoms have gained great popularity in the past fifteen years, mainly as a result of the AIDS scare. The sexual revolution of the 70s and early 80s often showed all the glamour and fun of sex but rarely showed the downside—namely, the florid episodes of sexually transmitted diseases and unwanted pregnancies. When used properly and consistently, condoms do play a significant role in reducing the incidence of both.

What are they and how do they work? Condoms are tube-shaped sheaths made either from latex rubber, lambskin, or plastic, and are worn by the man. Latex condoms are reported to have the highest success rate for preventing the transmission of STDs. Condoms prevent pregnancy and STDs by: (1) blocking the direct contact of the man's ejaculated sperm with the woman's vagina, and (2) keeping the flesh and secretions of the male genital organs away from those of the female. This rubber barrier also limits or prevents genital contact with any viruses, lesions, or infections that may be present in or on either person. Some condoms have a receptacle tip at the end, as a place for the ejaculated sperm to pool.

Condoms are intended for one-time use. Many come with a spermicide inside to serve as additional contraception. Some couples incorporate the act of putting on a condom into their lovemaking. For instance, the couple will put it on the man's penis together. It's very important that after the man ejaculates, he holds on to the top of the condom as he withdraws from the woman's vagina, in order to help keep the sperm inside the condom.

As mentioned above, latex condoms provide the best protection against most STDs, while lambskin provides the least, and polyurethane condoms offer moderate protection. For this reason, latex condoms are recommended. However, some people may be allergic to the latex material used in condoms. In this case, polyurethane condoms are an option.

Though they can be fun, I would advise you to avoid the flavorful, colorful, specially scented condoms, as they may not provide the full protection desired. And be sure your condom has not "expired." Like milk cartons, condoms have expiration dates. Heed them. If a condom is old, do not use it.

The Diaphragm   (Theoretical: 94 percent; Actual: 83 percent) This is a round rubber dome with a coiled spring rim; it is placed high inside the woman's vagina prior to intercourse. The woman usually inserts it, but in more motivated, experienced, or very comfortable couples, the male partner may help.

To use a diaphragm correctly, the woman must first be fitted for the device, as not every woman's pelvis is the same size. That's why they are not sold over the counter. Your doctor measures your inner pelvic structure during a pelvic exam. She will then insert a sample diaphragm to test for the proper sizing. You will then be asked to remove it and reinsert it. That way, your doctor knows that you are able to insert it properly at home on your own. You will then get a prescription for the diaphragm, and you will also need spermicide jelly or cream, which is always to be used simultaneously.

How do diaphragms work? Prior to intercourse, you apply the spermicide around the rim of the diaphragm and also in the middle of its dome, then squeeze the diaphragm together and slide it into the vagina until it "opens up" in place. With it inserted correctly, you will feel the tip of your cervix in the center of the dome and the circumference of the device should be closely juxtapositioned to your inner pelvic bones and soft tissues, giving a close fit. Such positioning will help keep sperm from getting into your cervix.

While you can put the diaphragm in either just before, or up to four hours before intercourse, you must leave the diaphragm in place for six hours after your last act of intercourse. And, if you have more than one episode of intercourse, you need to insert additional spermicide to afford greater protection. Once you remove the device, wash it in soap and water, dry it, and store it in its case as directed by the diaphragm's instruction sheet.

Do not leave the diaphragm in for an extended period of time because it may cause toxic shock syndrome. Some women have been known to use the diaphragm when wanting to have sex while on their period. Although a diaphragm will keep the menstrual blood from flowing during sex, I do not encourage women to use this stopgap measure. Some women can get a retrograde flow of the menses, which could lead to an increased risk of endometriosis.

Cervical Caps (Theoretical: 90 percent; Actual: 80 percent) These are smaller than a diaphragm and are also fitted by your doctor. They are designed to fit directly onto the tip of your cervix. I personally have never prescribed this device because I was never satisfied with its success rate. Since the cervical cap was designed to be worn for a month at a time, women must be mindful of removing it within forty-eight hours after sex. If you forget and leave it in, it can cause infection or cellular changes on the cervix.

Check with your doctor to see if this is a sound option for you. Women who have any history of cervical abnormalities or chronic bouts of pelvic infection are not good candidates for this method.

The Contraceptive Sponge Shaped like a doughnut, the sponge came onto the market in the early 1980s, but in the late 1990s it was removed. Because there was renewed interest in this contraceptive method, it reappeared in 2001.

The sponge is an over-the-counter contraceptive that contains spermicide and is inserted into the vagina, to lie next to the cervix. During intercourse, the sponge releases the spermicide, which kills the sperm.

Problems with this method included vaginal infections in women who forgot to remove the sponge. Many women also complained that the string used to remove it was often difficult to detect. Sponges cost more than condoms and are slightly less effective.

Hormonal Contraceptives

Injectable Contraceptives: (Theoretical: 99.7 percent; Actual: approximately the same) In 1992, many women were happy to hear about a new birth control method called Depo-Provera, a progesterone-derivative medication that can prevent pregnancy. The greatest advantage afforded by this method is its long-lasting effect. One injection provides contraceptive protection for three months. Many women who are not consistent with other methods like birth control pills or barrier methods find Depo-Provera to be a reasonable and welcome option.

How does Depo work? Women desiring this method should see

their doctor within five days of their normal menstrual period to receive an injection of the medication. The timing of the shot is vital, because you want to have the medication in your system in time to stop your hormonal schedule.

Once injected, the progesterone alters the mucus in the cervix, which helps prevent sperm from reaching the egg. Depo also chemically alters the lining of the uterus, making it less amenable to implantation. The third action of Depo-Provera is to inhibit ovulation, which is its primary action. Without ovulation, there is no egg to fertilize in the first place.

Depo-Provera's biggest plus is its ease of use. You don't have to remember to take a pill or insert a diaphragm. Your contraception is on automatic pilot for three months at a time. On the negative side, Depo-Provera does not protect against sexually transmitted disease. Again, abstinence and condoms are the two best ways to prevent or limit them.

Women who want long-term contraception find Depo-Provera to be a good choice. But if you are considering having a child within a year or so, Depo is not the best option for you. You might want to seek a method with a shorter duration. It takes a few months for the effects of the medication to totally clear out of your system. If it hasn't, it can delay conception for as many as 16 to 18 months, according to some reports.

Also, women who are bothered by menstrual irregularities and potential mood changes may not take well to the drug initially, though for many women, most of these side effects ease or subside as their bodies become accustomed to the medication.

Sharing your concerns and reactions with your doctor can help you best handle any side effects you may experience.

Implant Contraceptives: (Theoretical: 99.9 percent; Actual: same) Norplant is a birth control method that involves the insertion of six silicone rods under the skin of a woman's upper arm. These rods house time-release capsules containing levonorgestrel, a synthetic form of progesterone. Inserted by your doctor in her office, the six rods are slid under your skin through a very small incision and placed in a fan-shaped configuration. After insertion, the incision is taped together and in a couple of days is well on its way to being completely closed. Norplant begins working within a day of insertion.

Like Depo-Provera, Norplant can be a good contraceptive method for women who don't want to have to think about their birth control on a daily, or as needed, basis. Norplant provides constant contraceptive protection for up to five years. It works by slowly releasing the synthetic hormone, which acts in a way similar to Depo-Provera.

The majority of complaints about Norplant come as a result of the difficulty some doctors have in removing the rods. Other complaints have included problems with menstrual irregularities and hair loss. Some also report a skin reaction at the site of insertion.

If Norplant is removed, most women can expect to become fertile again within sixty days—sometimes much sooner. Some women regain fertility almost immediately.

Oral Contraceptives: (Theoretical: 99.9 percent; Actual: 98.5 percent) The most common form of hormonal contraception is oral contraceptives (OCs), also commonly called birth control pills or simply the Pill. Oral contraceptives are the second most common form of contraception; the most common is tubal ligation (sterilization). It is estimated that 16 to 18 million women in the United States are on the Pill.

When first introduced, birth control pills were very high in hormone content. As a result, there were many early reports of complications from these drugs. Over time, researchers have learned to make oral contraceptives with minimal levels of hormones. This chemical change resulted in wider use by women and greater acceptance by the medical community. In addition, there have been many non-contraceptive benefits afforded to OC users, including protection against ovarian cysts, some cancers, heart disease, endometrial cancer, and ovarian cancer, and less need for abortions.

Oral contraceptives work by making the body think it's pregnant, therefore preventing ovulation. Many pills mimic the normal hormonal process of a woman's body, containing both estrogen and progesterone. Other pills, however, may have only progesterone. This latter pill has historically been called the mini-pill.

Depending on which type you take, you will begin the Pill on either the first day or the fifth day of your period. Most pills now will start on the first day or the Sunday after your cycle begins. What if your period begins on a Sunday? Start that Sunday.

To gain the full contraceptive benefit of OCs, it is imperative that you take a pill every day as prescribed. Some brands come in a 21-day pack, which has three weeks of hormone pills, and then you have a week of not taking anything. Your period will come during that week off. Other brands use a 28-day pack, which contains three weeks of hormone pills and one week of placebos—pills that don't contain anything that affect contraception. The placebos are there just to keep those who need a reminder on track. (Some women may forget to start their new pack if they go seven days without taking something. The 28-day pack keeps women in the habit of taking a pill a day).

It is also important that the pills be taken not only every day, but around the same time every day. Patients who are erratic with their pills will experience spotting and will lose the effectiveness of the pills. I always tell patients to link their pill time with some other daily routine activity. For instance, when you get up in the morning, right before you go to bed at night, when you brush your teeth, etc. It doesn't matter what time of day you take the pill, as long as you take it at the same time every day. Consistency is vital for full contraceptive benefit.

Who should and should not take the Pill? Basically any woman who doesn't have any medical conditions that are contraindications to the Pill can be considered for it. Women with blood clotting disorders, liver disease, certain cancers, a history of stroke, or who are smokers are not candidates for the Pill. Neither are women who have uncontrolled diabetes, high blood pressure, seizure disorders, or migraine headaches.

Again, in the early days, many women had a variety of complaints about the Pill. As a result of more research, there are now various OCs on the market, so it's very likely that a woman who truly wants to use the Pill will find one that works for her.

Some pills exactly mimic the normal hormone sequence, while others may offer more or less estrogen or progesterone at different times of the cycle.

Other benefits of birth control pills include a shorter and lighter period, a more regular period, fewer or no menstrual cramps, and, for some, clearer skin. Keep in mind, however, that the Pill does not protect you against STDs.

Emergency Contraception: Oral contraceptives are also used when "emergency contraception" is needed. When is that? When a woman has unprotected sex and doesn't want to conceive. Emergency contraception is really one of the best-kept secrets in medicine, but for very good reason: Some women may abuse this availability, and always turn to this method instead of doing what they should do, which is take preventive measures before having sex, not afterward.

If you find yourself in a situation in which you "slipped up," had sex without protection, or a barrier method obviously failed, and you are fearful about the possibility of getting pregnant, you can contact your doctor and ask about emergency contraception.

A total of four birth control pills are prescribed, to be taken two at a time, twelve hours apart. The high dose of hormone from the pills usually works to prevent the unintended pregnancy. Emergency contraception should not be used as a regular method of contraception.

Sterilization

Female Sterilization (Theoretical: 99.5 percent; Actual: same) is called tubal ligation (TL), tubal sterilization; or in more common vernacular, "getting your tubes tied." When done in the immediate phase after childbirth, it's called a postpartum tubal ligation (PPTL) or postpartum sterilization (PPS).

Tubal ligations require a minor surgical procedure that can be done as an outpatient. It also can be performed in conjunction with other surgical procedures, either through a small belly-button incision of laparoscopy, or through a full abdominal incision when that incision is required for the primary procedure.

Tubal ligations are not required operations; they are elective procedures (by choice). TLs are to be considered a permanent, irreversible method of contraception. I know what you're thinking: You've heard of women having tubal ligations reversed. This may be true, especially if the woman has remarried. There is a way to put the tubes back together, but success cannot be guaranteed, and many times, should a pregnancy result, it may actually end up in the tube, trapped at the site where the tubes were reunited. For this reason, it is imperative that a woman be absolutely sure she doesn't want any more children before opting for this surgical procedure.

Tubal ligation is a very, very reliable method of birth control because the conduit in which the egg and sperm meet is disrupted, therefore blocking the passage and union of the two cells.

Despite its being nearly 100 percent effective, there are cases in which the procedure fails and you can become pregnant. Fortunately, TL failures are considerably rare. Sometimes, the manner in which the TL is done may play a role in that, as can other factors such as the degree of difficulty in getting to the tubes during the procedure, and the method of tubal ligation. For example, in the most successful TL a piece of the fallopian tube is actually cut out and removed from each tube. The removed section of tube is sent to the laboratory to confirm that the specimen is exactly that, the tube.

But some women have a TL in which a clamp is placed on the tube, occluding it by squeezing the sides of the tube closed. The problem with this method is that the clamp may slip off, allowing the center of the tube to open. Then pregnancy can result.

Male Sterilization is called vasectomy. This is easier to perform, requires less medication and less recovery time, and carries less operative risk than does a tubal ligation. Many men wonder if they will still be able to get an erection after having a vasectomy. The answer is yes. Can they still have sex? Again, yes. Will they still have an orgasm? Can they still ejaculate? Most definitely. But after a vasectomy, their ejaculate will not contain sperm. Normally, when a man has an orgasm, the ejaculate is made up of fluid and millions of microscopic sperm. After a vasectomy, the fluid is still there but the sperm are not. The procedure can be performed in the doctor's office; no hospital is necessary, and recovery is mild.

As with tubal ligations, a vasectomy should be considered permanent, although some men have successfully had their vasectomies reversed.

Calendar Contraception
(Natural Family Planning)

There are women who, for one reason or another, opt to forgo any mechanical, chemical, hormonal, or surgical methods of contraception. Some cite religious reasons, while others are naturalists. These women tend to try the Rhythm method, and the more daring souls might try withdrawal.

The Rhythm method consists of women's basing their sexual activity—and their knowledge of when to avoid intercourse—on their menstrual cycles, and calculating their fertile days. This method requires a lot of discipline and it doesn't take into account the fact that many things can alter a woman's cycle, thus making the method less reliable.

While many people are diligent, disciplined, and determined enough to make this work, there's a running joke that nevertheless rings true: *Do you know what they call people who use the Rhythm method? Parents.* Again, the method can work, but it is not reliable.

An even less reliable "natural" method is withdrawal. The man literally withdraws his penis from the woman's vagina as he feels he's getting ready to ejaculate. The problem is that sperm are still released even prior to ejaculation, so by time he pulls out, it could already be too late.

Is there anything new on the contraceptive horizon? According to Dr. Elof Johansson, vice president and director of the Population Council's Center for Biomedical Research, there are some new things in the birth control armamentarium, including *Lunelle,* an injection similar to Depo-Provera, and *Norplant 2,* which has two rods and provides protection for three years instead of five. There's also *Mirena,* a new IUD with a hormone inside of it that is released directly into the uterus. It can prevent pregnancy for up to five years. *Lea's Shield* is another upcoming option—a one-size-fits-all device similar to a diaphragm that will allow secretions to flow out without letting sperm flow in. New gels, patches, and vaginal rings are also being researched.

CONTRACEPTIVE OPTIONS

Method	Key Advantages	Key Disadvantages	Effectiveness
Birth control pill	· Continuous contraceptive protection when taken correctly · Reversible · Some noncontraceptive health benefits	· Must be remembered/taken daily · Increases risk of blood clots, heart attack, stroke, especially in smokers over 35 · Common side effects may include nausea, vomiting, and weight gain	99 percent or greater when taken correctly
Subdermal implants	· Continuous contraceptive protection for up to five years · Reversible · No need to remember daily	· In-office minor surgical procedure requiring local anesthetic · Some side effects, such as menstrual bleeding irregularities; other commonly reported side effects include headache, nervousness, nausea, dizziness, and removal difficulties	99 percent or greater
DMPA *(Depot medroxyprogesterone acetate)* e.g., Depo-Provera	· Continuous contraceptive protection for three months · No need to remember daily	· Physician visit for quarterly injection · Delayed return to fertility (4–5 months) · Some side effects, such as weight change, menstrual bleeding irregularities	99 percent or greater
Vasectomy *(Male sterilization)*	· Continuous contraceptive protection · No need to remember daily	· Provided by male partner · Permanent method · Surgical procedure	99 percent or greater
Tubal ligation *(Female sterilization)*	· Continuous contraceptive protection · No need to remember daily	· Permanent method · Surgical procedure	99 percent or greater
Intrauterine device (IUD)	· Continuous contraceptive protection for up to ten years (for copper T IUD) · No need to remember daily	· May be expelled or perforate uterus · May increase pelvic inflammatory disease risk for some women	99 percent or greater

Method	Advantages	Disadvantages	
Condom (alone)	· Easily obtained · Best method for protection against sexually transmitted disease · Good results when used with spermicide	· May reduce sensation · Less sexual spontaneity · Breakage possible · Provided by male partner	88–98 percent
Diaphragm (with spermicide)	· Insertion up to six hours before intercourse	· Reapplication of spermicide necessary for repeated intercourse · Comfort level with insertion important · Increases risk of urinary tract, bladder infections	82–94 percent
Cervical cap	· Insertion half hour to forty-eight hours before intercourse	· Increased risk of changes in cervical cells · Vaginal odor and discharge · May cause discomfort upon insertion	82–94 percent
Periodic abstinence	· Requires no other intervention	· Requires careful planning and motivation · Prohibits intercourse for up to half the menstrual cycle · Not for women with irregular cycles	80–99 percent
Spermicide (alone) (Foams, gels, creams)	· Easily obtained · Good results when used with barrier methods	· Insertion necessary at least half hour before intercourse · Reapplication necessary for repeated intercourse · May be messy · May increase risk of urinary tract infections, especially when used with diaphragm	79–97 percent
Withdrawal	· Requires no other intervention	· Provided by male partner · Requires a great deal of control · Leakage of sperm often occurs before ejaculation	72 percent

Source: Wyeth

In late 2000, it was reported that a new contraceptive called *STOP* will become available to women soon. This method calls for a titanium coil to be inserted up through the cervix and guided into the fallopian tubes. The procedure is done in the doctor's office and takes approximately twenty minutes to perform, with only mild cramping. STOP basically works like a tubal ligation, blocking the tubes to prevent pregnancy. This would prevent women from having to have an actual operation for the tubal ligation.

What about new contraceptives for men? Some research is being conducted, but how soon something of great success becomes available is another matter. Stay tuned.

In the meantime, be smart about your contraceptive choices. Speak to your doctor, and I'm sure you'll be able to find a method that works best for your needs, your lifestyle, and your future plans.

RX: A PRESCRIPTION FOR YOUR SOUL

I love roller coasters—the Mind Bender, the Cyclone. These are just some of the fun rides I like, even though when I'm on them my emotions are all over the place, changing from one moment to the next. First there's excitement and anticipation, then a bit of anxiety and even fear, followed by a feeling of exhilaration and relief when I'm back on the ground.

Pregnancy is pretty much like being on a roller coaster. Your emotions are also all over the place. You may feel excitement upon learning that you're pregnant, then anxiety and fear about the process, challenges, and changes you'll face, followed by exhilaration and profound joy when all is well with your new baby.

As you go through all of these changes it's easy to forget that everyone around you is also affected by your emotional ups and downs. That's why it's so important to try to maintain your center, stay grounded, and keep it real. Look to your faith to restore your sense of equilibrium. Not only will it help you successfully deal with your ever-changing emotions, it will also keep things on an even keel with loved ones, especially your husband or partner. You may feel an especially close bond with the baby growing inside you, but his bond to this new life is equally strong. Remember, your pregnancy is not just about you. It's about your man, too. Whether the two of you are trying to get pregnant, anxiously awaiting the birth, or already enjoying your newborn, use your natural togetherness as a tool, an aid. See it as a blessing. You don't have to go it alone, nor should you try to. He is your partner in this. Lean on him, revel in his love, embrace his support, rely on his strength, and be guided on this journey by faith together.

In no other way is God's plan for man to be with woman more evident than in the propagation of the world through childbirth. It speaks to the way God meant it to be: for a man and woman to come together as one, celebrate their love, and bring forth a new soul.

Once you are pregnant, your body will go through so many changes—in shape, weight, appearance. Your psyche, too, will alter, for you have a lot of things to consider. What kind of life do you want for your child? Education, multifaceted experiences, good health, a strong spiritual base, the love of friends and family. What about violence in the schools? What about racial tensions in society? How will your child be affected? What can you do to protect him or her?

Yes, it's normal to have a myriad of emotions during this time, but remember who made you, and who allowed your pregnancy to come to be. Think about the role your body plays in bringing a new life into the world. What a blessing! What an honor bestowed upon women by God—to be the first guardians for a new human being.

As you go through the process, relish your role. Respect your position as a vessel of God, and govern yourself accordingly. Rely on your spouse or partner, close family, and friends during this special time. Receive consistent medical care. Renew your commitment to be all God would have you be. And recognize your responsibility to raise your child in the proper way.

I am often upset when I see news reports about black children running afoul of the law or getting caught up in situations that can ruin their lives. While I know for a fact that racism still exists, that racial profiling does occur, and that African Americans are routinely accused of things they didn't do, the fact still remains that not all that happens to us, to our children, and to our communities can be blamed on "the white man." Sometimes we must hold ourselves accountable and take responsibility.

It is not society's fault if your child hangs out in the street all night long unsupervised. It's not society's fault if your teenage daughter is having unprotected sex. It's not society's fault if your child is getting poor grades because he never does his homework or studies for tests. As a parent, you must play an active role in the lives of your children.

Know, too, that children often mimic what their parents do. If you show disrespect, your child will, too. If you lash out in anger, your child will follow suit. If you curse to get your point across, your child will do the same. If God is not a part of your life, what example will your child follow?

Your role as parent is so vital—it has to be taken seriously. If God blesses you with a young soul, do what God would have you do to fulfill your divine role as mother. Live your life by faith and He will show you the path.

When our spiritual foundation is strong, we are so much more capable of raising our children by a divine guiding light. We can impart the values we hold dear and the religious beliefs we live by, and give our children concrete goals to aspire to. If we can pass on a solid sense of spirituality to our youngsters, they will be able to see in themselves endless possibilities.

I once saw a television news report about a leading trauma surgeon at Johns Hopkins Hospital, a black man who brings inner-city youths into the hospital every month to see recovering victims of gun violence. His purpose is to show these boys and girls what can happen if they live a certain lifestyle and associate with certain people. While I was very impressed with the doctor's purpose, I was saddened by the response of one young boy when asked, "What does this experience say to you? How does this affect you?" His reply? He didn't want this to happen to him, so he "better get my game together so I can play ball for a living."

It grieved me to hear that. This young man could strive for so much more. He could become anything he wanted. It was sad to see that all he gained from the hospital experience was the stereotypical belief that he needed to play ball. I believe we can do better by our boys and girls. We can give them dreams that reach far beyond the expected. It all starts with that spiritual base. After all, with God's love, all things are possible.

I am a member of a community group called Leadership Atlanta, and for a few years now have been on their Race Relations committee. One year, we held a large town hall meeting that began with a TV news segment that showed young black and white children being asked different questions about race. For instance, each child—whether black or white—was asked to complete these sentences: "White people are good at . . ." "Black people are good at . . ." This was just one of many questions posed to them.

It was absolutely astonishing and painfully sad to hear the responses from both the black and white children. Every youngster questioned believed that white people were good at "science, math, business, computers, and/or owning large companies." While black people were good at "sports, singing, dancing, laughing, and/or doing their hair."

I don't think I need to say much else. As women, we have an important role concerning our children. We—along with our spouses and partners—must do all we can to have healthy babies, grow and groom healthy children, educate them, and help them become productive members of society. Let's dig deep to override the stereotypes that we see but also, by our inactivity, help perpetuate.

I will leave you with the words from a public service announcement I made many years ago:

Parents, Your Children Need You

The reward of an obstetrician's labor is helping to bring new life into the world, and every day, we take part in just that. But from the moment you are given each of your children at birth, you are also given the responsibility of caring for, teaching, guiding, and directing your children— helping them become productive citizens in society. But more and more, we find our young people having misplaced values—participating in drugs, gangs, and violence; killing each other; lacking morality; and having no regard for human life. Parents, society needs you to meet your responsibility. Your children need you for guidance and direction. The direction that your child takes in his or her life is up to you. Please, spend time with your children.

Managing Menopause

· · · · · · · · · ·

I have no qualms about getting older; in fact, I'm rather enjoying it. I'm becoming a lot more confident—confident in what God has given me. Some things only come with time and maturity.

—Babbie Mason, singer and author,
In Touch Ministries publication

News You Can Use

· The most common symptoms of menopause include hot flashes, mood swings, insomnia, vaginal dryness, decreased sex drive, and less skin elasticity.

· Because menopause increases your risk of developing osteoporosis and heart disease, it's important to adopt health habits that can help stave off these diseases.

· The average woman goes through menopause at age 51.

· Menopause doesn't happen overnight; it's a gradual process.

· Studies show that use of hormone replacement therapy for more than five years has been associated with an increased risk of heart disease, strokes, blood clots, and breast cancer.

You MAY think that every woman greets the news that she's going through menopause with a frown. But I've found that there are plenty of women who are actually happy—yes, happy—to reach this point in their lives. Sisters who dread the "change" believe it represents an end to vitality, youth, sexuality, and desirability. But those who embrace menopause view it as a time of freedom from periods, cramps, and the fear of unexpected pregnancy, and a time of newfound sexual freedom. For these sisters, menopause is about starting a new and exciting phase of life. It's an attitude I wish more women would adopt. But I'm not surprised by the fear, apprehension, and sadness I hear in women's voices once they realize they are going through the change. After all, it's not a topic our mothers and grandmothers discussed freely and openly. It was given a kind of "back door" status and talked about in cryptic hushed tones, if it was talked about at all. When we don't fully understand or know the facts about something—especially something that happens to our bodies—we naturally start to view it skeptically, fearfully, and tentatively.

In our foremothers' day, menopause was closely associated with the end of life—the time when there were "not many pages left, Lord," as poet Leo Richards so eloquently puts it in his book *My Obsession*. The life expectancy for our ancestors was much shorter than it is today, and many of them passed away before they reached menopause. As time went on and we began to live longer—long enough to actually go through menopause—the experience was nonetheless treated like a big secret. It was something you just didn't talk about.

Thankfully, that's no longer the case. You don't have to search far to find a plethora of information on menopause these days. Browse through any bookstore or magazine rack and you'll discover plenty of books and articles on the topic. Click on the television and you'll see news segments and daytime talk shows covering it in depth. Menopause has finally come out of the closet, and its public emergence is long overdue. People are talking about it candidly now—providing valuable information and sharing personal experiences.

Today, women are living longer than we ever have and menopause is not the ominous sign it once was. The stigma is gone and many women are striving to enjoy this period of their lives. Menopause no longer points directly to old age, but is simply a brief stop along the road of a full and vital life. Millions of women are choosing to look at menopause in a new light, adopting the mind-set of *healthy, fit, and fine after forty-nine*. That's how I'm going to look at it when I get there, and I hope you do, too.

DEMYSTIFYING MENOPAUSE

Just what is menopause? We hear the phrases "change of life" and "the change" and it makes the process sound mysterious and foreboding. According to *Newsweek,* in the 1966 book *Feminine Forever,* author Dr. Robert Wilson described menopause as a "living decay" in which women descended into a "vapid cow-like" state. Thank goodness those thoughts—especially by health care professionals—have changed! Menopause is a natural, gradual part of life—one that does, in fact, bring about change, but not the sort of change that should alarm or frighten you. It's simply a process that reflects the various hormonal changes going on inside your body as you get older.

As the word implies, *menopause* literally means a pause or cessation in the monthly—more specifically, the cessation of a woman's monthly menstrual cycle. (*Meno* is Greek for month.) Menopause is usually a spontaneous, or natural, event. But it can also be brought on if you have to have your ovaries surgically removed. Naturally occurring menopause doesn't happen overnight, though. It is a gradual process that can take years to complete. In most cases, your periods won't just stop one day. They will become more and more irregular over time, until they cease completely. The reason? A decline in estrogen production.

As a woman ages, the number of eggs in her ovaries decreases, and eventually she stops producing estrogen. As I've mentioned before, estrogen is a very important hormone that helps with fertility, vaginal moisture, and sleep, regulates body temperature, strengthens bones, and protects your heart. Without estrogen, all of these body functions will be affected and you will experience a variety of changes (hence those phrases we've all heard).

This gradual process of decreased estrogen production and decreased menstruation is called *climacteric,* which begins approximately three, four, or five years before actual menopause. Since the average age for menopause is 51.2 years, the early phase of hormone decrease may begin around age 45. Some women may enter a premature menopause and go through the process even earlier. Many women would like to be able to pinpoint when they'll experience menopause in order to prepare. But the process is not the same for every woman. Though the average age is 51, exactly when a woman goes through menopause is hard to determine. Many of us tend to follow the same time frame as our mothers, but that's not a hard and fast rule. Every woman's body, hormone status, and surgical history is different.

How do you know if you are truly menopausal? You've been having hot flashes, you can't sleep at night, you've become less interested in sex, and your periods aren't coming like clockwork anymore. Does this mean you're going through menopause? Well, you're exhibiting the signs (more on those in a bit), but true menopause occurs only when a woman has gone a complete year without a period. Until that absolute cutoff, she may experience irregular periods and unpredictable episodes of spotting, or she may even go eight, nine, or ten months without a period and then have one! This stage is called *perimenopause*—the time "around" menopause. Once you go a full year without a period and are truly menopausal, you should not have any further menstrual bleeding from that point forward. You should know that some medications used to treat menopause may give you new periods. However, many doctors are able to prescribe the medicines in ways that prevent this from happening. Therefore, if you have any post-menopausal bleeding, you should consider it abnormal and see your doctor. Unless medication-induced, postmenopausal bleeding is an indication that further evaluation is necessary, which typically means a D&C to check the cells of the womb for any abnormalities.

SIGNS OF MENOPAUSE

If you know someone who has gone through menopause, then you've probably heard about some of the common symptoms, such as hot flashes. But not every woman will experience this classic side effect, or many of the other typical symptoms. Again, every woman is unique. That said, however, chances are you will exhibit some of the signs of menopause—most of us do—the most obvious being lack of a period. Signs of menopause include:

Hot Flashes (also called hot flushes)—Hot flashes are sudden, brief increases in body temperature that usually last about a minute or two. You will usually feel intense heat that spreads across your head, face, neck, chest, and possibly other parts of your body. As your body tries to cool itself, you will start to perspire in those areas, sometimes profusely. Many women find this extremely embarrassing, especially when it occurs in a meeting, at a social function, or some other situation when lots of people are around. The good news is that once menopause is over and your periods have stopped completely, the hot flashes usually go away.

Insomnia—Many menopausal women report trouble sleeping through the night. More often than not it's due to night sweats. These are basically hot flashes that occur at night. You may wake up drenched in sweat and need to change the sheets and your pajamas. The constant disruption in sleep can take a toll, causing you to feel tired and cranky the next day. This too should stop once you've completed menopause.

Mood Swings—As you go through menopause, you may find yourself in altered states of emotion. You may be tearful and sensitive about the smallest thing one moment, then irritable and short-tempered the next. The hormonal changes taking place in your body may be part of the reason for the mood swings, but remember, this is a real time of transition as well and your fluctuating emotions may also be a natural reaction to getting older. This is why I put so much emphasis on looking at the process from a positive point of view. See this time for the new possibilities it offers. Fortunately, these mood swings won't last forever. As with hot flashes and insomnia, the emotional roller coaster should come to a stop once menopause ends.

Vaginal Dryness and Thinness—Since estrogen is so important to vaginal moisture, the loss of the hormone can cause your vagina to become more dry. The dryness can make the vagina more prone to irritation, resulting in an itchy, uncomfortable feeling. Lack of estrogen also causes the vaginal tissue to thin, making it more fragile—a condition known as vaginal atrophy. The irritation that can result from this thinning is called *atrophic vaginitis*. The vagina isn't the only part of your body that can be affected, however. When vaginal tissue dries it can cause irritation in all adjacent organs, including the opening to the bladder, the urethra.

All of this can cause lovemaking to be painful. Using a water-based vaginal lubricant can help reduce the discomfort.

Decreased Sex Drive—Speaking of lovemaking, some women feel less like engaging in it during this period. The absence of estrogen—which is, after all, the female sex hormone—can diminish your libido. Vaginal dryness may also contribute to decreased interest in sex because less lubrication means more uncomfortable intercourse. It would be wonderful if vaginal dryness and a change in libido were temporary side effects of menopause, like hot flashes. But the truth is these are two ongoing conditions that continue as you age. You don't have to sit there and take it, though. Yes, they may be another part of growing older, but using a water-based lubricant, talking to your partner about new ways to get in the mood, and checking out hormone replacement therapy with your doctor should help keep your sex life satisfying for years to come.

Sagging Skin—Lack of estrogen causes a decrease in collagen in the body, a vital protein needed to maintain skin turgor. When estrogen levels go down, so does the position of a woman's skin. Your skin becomes thinner and less elastic, resulting in wrinkling and sagging. This begins to be fairly noticeable early in many white women, but less so—or at much later stages—in black women. You've probably heard the phrase "Black don't crack." That's a direct reference to the relatively smooth, taut, less-wrinkled complexions of many of our female elders. African-American women often look younger than they are because the melanin in our skin offers increased protection.

RAISING THE STAKES—THE MORE SERIOUS EFFECTS OF MENOPAUSE

The common symptoms that usually accompany menopause—the hot flashes, vaginal dryness, insomnia, etc.—are bothersome, to be sure. But they are not life-threatening. Unfortunately, the hormonal changes your body goes through during menopause do bring with them the increased risk for two very serious diseases—osteoporosis and heart disease. But that doesn't mean they're inevitable, not if you know how to protect yourself against them.

OSTEOPOROSIS—THE BRITTLE BONE DISEASE

This is a very serious disease in which a person's bones actually become porous (with holes), like a sponge. The lack of estrogen causes a decrease in bone mass, strength, and structure, all of which increases the risk of bone fractures. While women begin losing bone mass in their mid-twenties, there is a marked drop in bone strength and density once menopause starts. According to the National Osteoporosis Foundation (NOF), 28 million Americans are at risk of osteoporosis, 80 percent of them women.

As you age and estrogen diminishes, your bones become brittle. Most people don't even know they have osteoporosis until they suffer a fracture, typically in the hip or spine, though other bones are also at risk. That's because you can go for years without showing any signs of the disorder, though you may in fact have it. The first symptom for many people is usually a fracture. And depending on where the fracture is located, it can be disabling and potentially life-threatening.

For many years, osteoporosis was deemed to be an inevitable part of getting older. Have you ever seen an elderly woman walking down the street with her back bent over? Sadly, this is a classic image of osteoporosis. The woman's bone mass and structure has decreased so much that she walks with a permanent and severe stoop. Her *vertebrae*—the bones that make up the spine—have collapsed, causing her to bend over. All because of osteoporosis.

If this is not enough to convince you how serious this debilitating disorder is, consider these facts from the NOF:

- Osteoporosis is responsible for more than 1.5 million fractures annually, including 300,000 hip fractures, nearly 700,000 spine fractures, 250,000 wrist fractures, and 300,000 other types of fractures.

- Women can lose up to 20 percent of their bone mass in the five to seven years after menopause.

- An average of 24 percent of hip fracture patients age 50 and over die in the year following their fracture.

- One-fourth of hip fracture sufferers require long-term care.

While osteoporosis affects white and Asian women more than any other women, sisters are still at risk. African-American women may be less prone to developing the disease, but that doesn't mean we don't get it. According to the NOF, 10 percent of African-American women over age 50 have osteoporosis, and 30 percent of us have low bone density, which increases the chances of getting the disease.

Being white or Asian ups a woman's odds of developing osteoporosis, but other risk factors are more color blind. If you have a thin, frail body frame, smoke cigarettes, are of increasing age, have a poor dietary regimen (including excessive alcohol consumption, decreased calcium intake, and lack of balanced nutrition) and, of course, are menopausal, you are also at risk of developing osteoporosis.

Don't let our lower rates of incidence fool you. Black women—like all other women—must get checked for this serious bone disease. There are many ways to be tested, but the most common is a Dual Energy X-ray Absorptiometry, or DXA for short. This test X rays all of your bones, including those in the high-risk areas—your spine, hips, and wrists. The DXA is painless and doesn't take long to perform.

Other tests that measure bone density are also available. Some just measure the wrists; others focus solely on the spine. Ultrasound has also been used in some cases to check bone density in the lower extremities. Your doctor can help you best determine which test is right for you. The main thing, however, is to get tested and find out the exact condition of your bones.

As you now know, you begin losing some bone mass as early as your mid-twenties (men too, for that matter). Fortunately, there are things you can do to slow down, and nearly abate, the process, plus build up and maintain strong, healthy bones. These preventive measures include:

- Maintaining good estrogen levels, either naturally or with medication (keep reading to learn more about this).

- An adequate intake of calcium in your diet. It's important to have approximately 1,300–1,500 milligrams (mg) of calcium a day. You can get a sufficient amount from your diet if you consume enough foods rich in calcium, such as low-fat and nonfat dairy products (milk, yogurt, cheese), certain vegetables (kale, mustard and turnip greens, broccoli), oranges and calcium-fortified orange juice, sardines, salmon, and black beans, to name a few. Many women take a calcium supplement as well, which comes in pill, liquid, or lozenge form, to ensure that they are getting enough. Talk to your doctor about whether you should take one.

- Getting an adequate amount of vitamin D, which is found in dairy products, eggs, certain fish, and liver. Because vitamin D helps your body absorb calcium, it is a big contributor to bone strength and the prevention of bone loss. Vitamin D is also absorbed from the sun, but you have to be careful about how much sunlight you get, as it can increase your risk of developing skin cancer. It's better to concentrate on getting this important vitamin from your diet.

- Exercise is vital to healthy bones, specifically weight-bearing exercise. As the name suggests, this type of exercise requires you to put weight on your bones and includes such activities as walking, jogging, weight lifting, stair climbing, and push-ups. The majority of calcium in your body is stored in your bones, and doing weight-bearing exercise causes your bones to add new calcium, thereby making them denser and stronger. It's never too late to reap the benefits of these types of activities. Menopausal women who follow a walking routine several days a week and weight-train two to three days a week will boost their bone strength and slow down bone loss.

There are various drugs on the market that work to counteract osteoporosis. *Raloxifene* (brand name Evista) blocks bone loss in the larger bones like the spine and hip, but also works on other bones. According to the NOF, this drug reduces the risk of spine fractures by approximately 50 percent. *Calcitonin* is a hormone normally produced in the body, but pharmaceutical companies also manufacture it as a nasal spray or in an injectable form. This drug has been shown to increase the density of bone at the spine, and also slow bone loss. Alendronate (also known as Fosamax) is a very popular osteoporosis medication that works to increase bone density and decrease bone loss. Women taking the drug report a lower number of bone fractures. Risendronate (also called Actonel) is another common drug used to treat osteoporosis. It acts in the same way as the other medications, but Risendronate has fewer side effects.

THE MENOPAUSE/HEART DISEASE CONNECTION

Heart disease is the number one killer of American women, black and white alike, though we are more likely to suffer and die from it. This deadly disease will be covered in depth in the next chapter, but it's important to touch on it now because there is a direct link between menopause and increased risk for heart attack.

Estrogen had been reported to offer you protection against heart disease because the hormone reduces your total cholesterol, raises HDL ("good") cholesterol levels, and lowers LDL ("bad") cholesterol levels. The decrease in estrogen and eventual cessation of production that come with menopause supposedly increase your risk of suffering a heart attack. Studies in 2001 and early 2002, however, seem to contradict the earlier belief. Check with your doctor for his or her position on this.

You can improve your heart health as you age by eating a diet low in fat (especially saturated fat) and high in fiber, giving up cigarettes if you smoke, exercising regularly, reducing stress in your life, watching your weight, and talking to your doctor about hormone replacement therapy.

MANAGING MENOPAUSE—IS ESTROGEN THE SOLUTION?

The best way I can begin to discuss managing menopause and whether to use hormone replacement therapy is to ask "are you confused yet?" If you're not, then you should be writing this chapter instead of me! The flurry of mixed messages about "estrogen replacement therapy" (ERT) and "hormone replacement therapy" (HRT) has been nothing but a ball of confusion for patients, as well as researchers and the physicians and nurses poised to advise on this subject.

In the 1990s, ERT/HRT was felt to be the answer—the panacea—to all the ails of perimenopausal and menopausal women, including hot flashes, night sweats, insomnia, broken bones, vaginal dryness, and mood swings. Most commonly prescribed hormone medications included estrogen therapy alone; estrogen pills taken with progestin pills; or Prempro, which contains both estrogen and progestin in one pill. Not only were these medications believed to alleviate menopausal symptoms (which they still do), but there was a widely held belief that ERT/HRT also afforded women actual *protection from* such diseases as heart disease, strokes, some cancers, and Alzheimer's disease. Sales of these drugs were brisk, with reportedly more than 45 million prescriptions for Premarin (an estrogen-only pill) and an additional 22 million for Prempro in 2001 alone. But the gravy train for the pharmaceutical companies making these drugs began to slow dramatically in July 2002, when two large studies reported significant adverse findings associated with long-term hormone replacement therapy use. One study, conducted by the Women's Health Initiative (WHI), embarked on a planned eight-year profile of 16,000 menopausal women ages 50–79, checking for the occurrence of blood clots, hip fractures, heart attacks, and cancers. The study was aborted, however, after five years, because of the reported increased rate of heart attacks, strokes, invasive breast cancers, and blood clots in some of their Prempro study patients. There were good reports of fewer hip fractures and fewer cases of colorectal cancer after three years of use.

Shortly on the heels of the WHI study, the National Cancer Institute (NCI) released a study reporting a significantly higher risk of ovarian cancer for women on estrogen-only regimens. The NCI study involved more than 44,000 postmenopausal women. According to the report printed in the *Journal of the American Medical Association,* the women taking only estrogen had a 60 percent greater risk of developing ovarian cancer than those women not on estrogen-only therapy. At the time of that report, their research was inconclusive about women on estrogen-progestin regimens.

Both the WHI and NCI research studies implied the most serious effects occurred with long-term (more than five years) use of these agents, while short-term use—less than five years—did not appear to pose any significant threat to a woman's health. Subsequent studies have also shown similar findings: *short-term use* of estrogen and/or progestin for relief of menopausal symptoms may be the way to go; and these drugs should not be relied upon, or looked to, as a preventive measure against heart disease, strokes, breast cancer, or Alzheimer's.

There is some good news about HRT: All researchers agree that hormone replacement therapy *is* greatly effective in the treatment of acute menopausal symptoms such as hot flashes, night sweats, and mood swings. Estrogen is beneficial to your bones and is still believed to decrease memory loss. But total reliance on ERT/HRT for protection against osteoporosis, heart disease, stroke, and Alzheimer's is no longer advised; nor is it advised to stay on these drugs for longer than five years—doing so may increase your risk of serious disease.

So what should you do? Should you take ERT/HRT, or not? As I write, my current recommendations are:

1. *Be prepared.* If you are approaching your mid-forties or may have surgery that requires removal of your ovaries, then you need to talk to your doctor about whether or not ERT/HRT is right for you, when the time comes. Menopause is inevitable, so be prepared and informed as you approach that phase of your life and as you go through it—as healthily as possible. Discussing all of your options ahead of time, and exploring all your potential risks, will help ease the transition and remove some of the apprehension you may feel. Stay informed about the subject and ask any questions you have.

2. *Understand your risk of serious complications with estrogen therapy, and whether you're a candidate for the med-*

ication or not. Women who should not—under any circumstances—take estrogen supplements include women who have undiagnosed uterine and/or vaginal bleeding, who have a history of uterine cancer, who have a history of blood vessel disease, or who are (or suspect they might be) pregnant. You will probably also be advised against ERT or HRT if you have a history of breast cancer, kidney disease, hypertension, severe migraine headaches, and clotting disorders. Review all of this with your doctor.

3. *Assess your menopausal symptoms and needs.* HRT is believed safe for short-term use to relieve the uncomfortable symptoms of menopause: the hot flashes, night sweats, insomnia, and mood changes. Most of these symptoms abate after a couple of years anyway. If you need these symptoms eased, and have no additional risk factors, then short-term HRT should be okay to use. Vaginal estrogen creams (Premarin or Estrace cream), rings (Estring) and tablets (Vagifem) are also still readily prescribed to relieve vaginal dryness and irritation, and they aren't believed to have the same systemic effects as ERT taken by mouth, though these methods of estrogen therapy have not been studied as extensively as was Prempro.

4. *If you are currently on HRT, consider your options and discuss them thoroughly with your physician.* Do you take Prempro? Have you been on it for a long time? Are you on estrogen-only pills? Should you switch to another pill, slowly wean yourself off your pills, or stop cold turkey? These are questions I, through this book, can't answer for you specifically. Only you and your doctor can make the proper decision specific to your needs and medical history. I

can tell you, if you still have your uterus and wish to take estrogen for a period of time, make sure you *also* take a pill with progestin in it. The two hormones together have consistently been shown to decrease the risk of endometrial cancer.

5. *Engage in other heart-and-bone-healthy regimens.* Weight-bearing exercise has been proven to be good for strengthening your heart and bones. Take 1,300–1,500 milligrams of calcium a day. Watch your weight, or lose weight for a healthier heart and less strain on your bones.

6. *Consider and discuss alternative treatments to prevent certain diseases.* Ongoing research is investigating the benefits, if any, of herbal supplements for relief of menopausal symptoms and possible prevention of serious disease. Some of the symptoms, diseases, and possible "natural" aids to discuss with your doctor include:

• *Hot flashes and night sweats*—some antidepressants like Prozac may help, as might an Indian herb, *black cohosh.* Soy products have been reported to offer some benefit, as have ginseng, vitamin E, and sage tea, but the evidence concerning these is sparse. Avoid heat-producing foods such as cayenne and other peppers or spicy foods.

• *Insomnia*—warm milk has long been known to cause drowsiness, and is safe. Hops and valerian root are also naturally occurring supplements that may help. Regular exercise earlier in the day usually helps keep you emotionally balanced, which may improve the chance for more restful nights. Late night exercise may add to your inability to fall asleep at night.

- *Vaginal dryness and irritation*—estrogen creams and tablets are available, as mentioned above, as are general lubricants such as K-Y jelly and Astroglide. Also, regular sex is recommended. Seriously.

- *Mood swings*—exercise, a stress-free life and home, family support, and prayer life may help. Don't sweat the small stuff. Try to get adequate sleep, or ask your doctor about other mood-changing medications that don't have serious long-term side effects. Herbal remedies that may help include St. John's wort, but more research is needed about this herb. Black cohosh, again, is another possibility.

- *Heart disease*—regular exercise, both aerobic and weight-bearing, is always good; as is proper weight control and eliminating tobacco, highly fatty foods, and excess salt intake. Get your cholesterol checked regularly. If it is high, consider cholesterol-lowering medications now available. Last, know your family history of heart disease, and get professional help if you feel you may be having heart pain, a heart attack, or stroke. Some have recommended the herb Hawthorne for mild palpitations. Check with your doctor, however.

- *Osteoporosis*—exercise, again, is bone-strengthening, along with dietary or supplementary calcium (approximately 1,500 milligrams a day). Evista, Fosamax, or Actonel may also be prescribed for you.

- *Memory loss*—keep your brain moving! Read, challenge yourself with word games and crossword puzzles, work! Take ongoing classes to learn something new: a new language, for instance.

Remember, your doctor is your health care ally during this—and every other—phase of your life. Menopause brings with it many changes, and the more prepared you are, the easier your transition will be. Rest assured, you have an increasing community of sister-friends (and women worldwide) who are treading this path right beside you. With the right attitude, and a lot of knowledge, it can be an exciting and life-affirming journey. But then, we already know this, for we are more than conquerors, and a 1999 study by researchers at the University of California at Davis found that black women had much more positive attitudes about menopause than did women of other races. Keep it up, ladies!

In short, speak to your doctor, and together, come up with a plan that works for you with the least risk of serious side effects.

RX: A PRESCRIPTION FOR YOUR SOUL

"The change of life." It's a phrase we've all heard, but what does it really mean? For some women, it signals the end of something. For others, it's just the beginning. While menopause is a process every woman will go through at some point in her life, how you handle it is up to you. Over the years spent practicing medicine, I have learned that there are two phrases that have the power to elicit two very distinct emotions—extreme joy or extreme sadness—in women. One is "You're pregnant." Depending on whether or not the woman wants to be pregnant, the news can be viewed as either very good or very bad. The other phrase that affects women in a similar way is "You're going through menopause." Unlike pregnancy, which can be prevented or terminated after the fact, there's no getting around menopause. It will happen, whether we like it or not.

But if we choose to look at this time of life as a new and exciting journey, that positive frame of mind can make all the difference. You may be thinking, *How in the world am I supposed to look at hot flashes, night sweats, vaginal dryness, less interest in sex, and the undeniable prospect of aging as something positive?* My sister, just remember, you are living in a new millennium. Women are leading healthier, more active, and more fulfilling lives than they ever have. We are going strong well into our seventies, eighties, and beyond. I can't tell you how gratifying, empowering, and uplifting it is to see a sister-elder out and about, living her life to the fullest. This can be you, too. This can be all of us.

It all comes back to the right attitude. Your mental framework helps dictate what kind of life you are going to have. Part of it is making up your mind to do right by your health—to take care of your body, to eat well, to exercise, to get regular checkups and necessary tests; all of the things you have been reading about on the previous pages. But the other part of that good mental framework is making up your mind to live your best life from the inside out. The external things you do to shore up your health are definitely necessary. However, for your best life, you must do internal work as well. I've said it all along and now it's more vital than ever. Getting older is never really easy for any of us. We have all had some regrets in life—things we never did that we always wanted to do, loved ones we wished we'd been closer to. Time seems to slip by so quickly. We turn around and from a distance see the girl we used to be. Know that she is still inside of you, only now she is more experienced, more knowledgeable, more capable of loving fully, more skilled, more adept, more solidly connected to her spirit and her God. Simply put, she has grown into the woman that you are today. If you stop and truly think of the life journey you've taken over the last twenty, thirty, forty years or more, you can't help but stand in awe of yourself. Reflect on all that you have accomplished. Relish in how much you have achieved. And I don't necessarily mean material gains. Think about your strength of character, your ability to empathize and sympathize with others, your kind heart and loving spirit, your determination and fortitude, your tenacity, your humor, your wisdom, your faith and connection to God. All of these attributes have come to you through your years of living. So if the journey thus far has brought you to this wonderful place, why in the world would you think that the second half of the journey would be any less magnificent in its gifts?

Yes, you are getting older, and yes, menopause is one of the milestones of this time in your life. But know that turning 45, or 50, or 55, or any age, does not signify the end. It proudly and boldly announces a new beginning. How you choose to look at menopause, how you approach it, will determine how you transition through it.

Remember, too, that you are living in a different time. The advances in medicine, technology, and knowledge about women's health have shed a whole new light on how well we can age if we take care of ourselves. It's an exciting time. We don't have to be crippled by osteoporosis, or sidelined by aching joints, or devastated by heart attack. We can live healthy, strong lives with an elder grace befitting us. But we have to do what God would have us do. We have to take care of our temples.

So, as I hope you are beginning to see, a positive state of mind coupled with a take-charge attitude toward your health will result in your later years continuing to be your best years. If you still have difficulty getting past the "menopause equals old age" notion, there's always that one special place you can turn to for guidance that never fails: your faith. Spirituality is more important at this time in your life than ever before. We are mortals, after all; we do realize that at some point our life on Earth will cease and another life—our life with Him—will start. Until we are called home, let us remember that He wants us to live as fully, joyfully, and divinely as we can. If you allow yourself to become depressed at the prospect of menopause and simply equate it with the loss of youth, you are not living the life He wants for you. You are allowing despair to wash over you when you should be rejoicing. Should negative feelings come, remember the Serenity Prayer: *God grant me the serenity to accept the things I cannot change; courage to change the things I can; and wisdom to know the difference.* You can't change menopause. It is a part of life. It will happen. Period. You are a woman who is getting older. God has blessed you with more years to come. Part of that growing and maturing process includes going through menopause. You have to accept it. And even though you cannot change it, you can change the way you handle it. Look within when you feel negativity taking hold; tap your divine spirit when the years behind you seem more fulfilling than those in front of you. With God's love all things are possible. Let Him guide you through this transition and help you to see the promise of what lies ahead. Deep down, it's not really about the physical manifestations of menopause, is it? You can get through the hot flashes. You can adjust to the mood swings. You can find ways to pique your sexual interest again. You can combat the threat of osteoporosis. What this time of life is really about for many sisters—maybe even you— is the thought of getting older. Well, let me tell you, when God looks at you, He doesn't see a few stray gray hairs or a wrinkle here and there. He sees his child—one who is loved beyond compare. When you look in the mirror I want you to see that, too. As you gaze upon your face, remind yourself that when you were 15, or 20, or 30, what lay ahead was an exciting contemplation. And you anticipated every moment. The same holds true today. The promise of life is still with you, only now I bet you will enjoy it that much more.

Not for Men Only—
Diseases That Strike Sisters, Too

· · · · · · · · · · · ·

*The most important thing I learned is that having a
proper mental attitude works wonders. If you take care
of yourself and do all the things that you must do to keep
it in control so that it doesn't control you, you can live a
happy, productive life.*

—Barbara Johnson, author, upon learning she had
diabetes

News You Can Use

· The four leading causes of death among African-American women
are, in order of prevalence: heart disease, all malignant cancers com-
bined, cerebrovascular diseases including stroke, and diabetes.

· In 1998, the American Heart Association listed obesity as a primary
cause of heart disease, in addition to smoking, diabetes, lack of exercise, and a high-fat diet.

· Overweight women are also at increased risk for hypertension, diabetes, and some types of cancer. More than two thirds (66.6 percent)
of African-American women are classified as overweight and 47.6
percent are classified as obese.

· Heart disease is the number one killer of women, killing more
women than breast cancer, lung cancer, or other diseases.

· Oftentimes, women mistake heart symptoms for heartburn or gas.
This often delays getting treatment, which worsens the prognosis
and lessens the chance for survival.

· Smoking is the single most preventable cause of disease and death in
the United States.

*I*F YOU could own any car—your dream car—what would it be? A Lexus? A Mercedes? A Jaguar? Can't you just see it? The chrome is glistening. The finish is shining brilliantly. The headlights are beaming. The supple interior leather is beckoning. Now, that's a good-looking car. But imagine if this hot car had a damaged engine, a poor transmission, faulty wiring, shot brakes, and sludge in the gas tank? It still looks great on the outside, but on the inside . . . let's just say you wouldn't be going anywhere soon in that dream car.

The point is, you can't get by on looks alone—not with your car, your appearance, or your health. The inner mechanisms have to be working well or you won't get far. Too often, when the outer self looks fine we pay less attention to our inner selves. Trust me, looks can be deceiving. Take those toned hard-bodies you see at the gym or on the street. They may seem to be the picture of health, but physically fit folks can still suffer from heart disease, high cholesterol, diabetes, or other conditions. Though their bodies are taut and toned, other factors may put them at risk for these diseases, such as family history or any number of things. When you look at these people and see an amazing outer package, the idea that they may have health problems seems like a ridiculous notion. But it's not ridiculous. You can look great on the outside and still suffer from health problems, no matter what your size. Don't get me wrong. Exercising regularly and eating nutritiously in order to lose weight and/or maintain a healthy weight is extremely important. We should all do what we can to make sure we are fit. But so many other factors contribute to the quality of your health. And sisters, we suffer from far too many diseases to take these factors for granted. After all, how far will you get if your lungs aren't functioning to their full capacity, if your heart is laboring with every step you take, if your blood vessels are clogged with fatty plaques?

Not very far at all. A long healthy life comes only when we take care of ourselves inside and out. A big part of that is understanding the serious illnesses that may threaten you, such as heart disease, hypertension, stroke, lung disease, and colon cancer, and how they affect your body's vital organs—your brain (the body's electrical command center), your heart (the body's engine), your blood vessels (its circuitry), your lungs (its ventilation system), and your intestines (its gas line, no pun intended).

If we pay attention to what's going on inside our bodies, good health won't merely be a dream, like that beautiful car you were fantasizing about. It will be a reality. And a well-running body is a million times more valuable. With that in mind, let's examine some of the more common serious illnesses facing black women and talk about ways to guard against them.

CARDIOVASCULAR DISEASE

The term *cardiovascular* refers to the "unit" of the heart and blood vessels in the body. The heart is the muscle that pumps oxygenated blood out to the rest of the body, which is needed for the proper function of organs such as your brain, kidneys, spleen, uterus, and every part of your body. When there is a blockage in any part of this system, problems can occur, either at the original site of the problem, or somewhere along the path. That's why we need to do all we can to make sure our cardiovascular system is in tip-top shape.

Unfortunately, this is not the case with most people. Heart disease is the number one killer of all Americans, including women. Look at the graph on page 361.

I think many men and women are surprised to learn that cardiovascular disease causes more deaths than cancers. In fact, the general perception is that breast cancer is the number one health

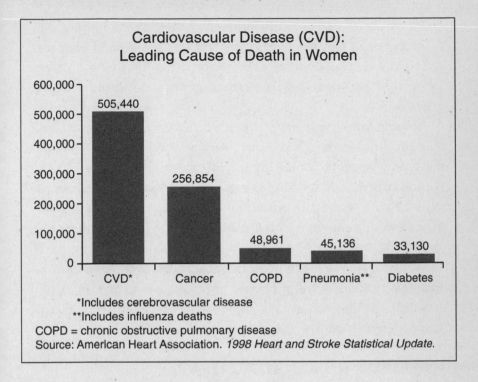

Cardiovascular Disease (CVD):
Leading Cause of Death in Women

*Includes cerebrovascular disease
**Includes influenza deaths
COPD = chronic obstructive pulmonary disease
Source: American Heart Association. *1998 Heart and Stroke Statistical Update.*

threat to women. But the truth is, it is heart disease. Yet four out of five women are unaware of this fact.

Let's take a look at the basic structure of the heart. The blood vessels that directly supply the heart with blood are called *coronary arteries.* Arteries carry blood with oxygen in it; veins carry blood without oxygen. Basically, deoxygenated blood enters the right side of the heart; becomes oxygenated on the left side of the heart, and then gets ejected via a large artery called the *aorta,* which courses from the heart down to the level just below the navel. From there, large blood vessels branch off, carrying blood the rest of the way into the pelvis and lower extremities. Deoxygenated blood is carried back to the heart via the *vena cava,* which empties into the right side of the heart; then the cycle—this circulation—starts all over again.

To get the blood from the heart to the rest of the body, a certain amount of pressure is needed, hence the term *blood pressure*. A pressure reading involves two numbers: the top number, called the *systolic* pressure; and the bottom number, called the *diastolic* pressure.

Systolic pressure is the pressure while the heart is contracting; diastolic pressure is the pressure reading between heart contractions, or at rest. The commonly accepted normal reading is 120/80, but lower pressures are good in most cases. Blood pressures higher than 120/80—especially when the diastolic is higher than 80—indicates some degree of hypertension. The higher the numbers, the greater the problem.

While there are many heart diagnoses with such names as mitral regurgitation, mitral prolapse, aortic aneurysm, and more, my focus here will be on the major components of heart disease, specifically, hypertension, coronary artery disease, and stroke.

HYPERTENSION (HIGH BLOOD PRESSURE)

High blood pressure is the number one preventable cause of over 65,000 deaths annually among African Americans, according to the American Heart Association. Often called "the silent killer" (because people can have it and not know it), hypertension is nothing to take lightly.

Not only is it the cause of thousands of deaths each year, but hypertension greatly contributes to the development of heart disease, stroke, and other conditions, such as kidney failure—all of which also cause thousands of deaths.

High blood pressure is exactly what it sounds like: the pressure in the vessels that carry your blood around your body is higher than it should be. Over time—and especially if left untreated—this increased pressure causes damage to your blood vessels, your heart, and major organs like your kidneys or brain. The damage can take the form of weakening of the blood vessel walls, or the vessels may become constricted, usually due to fatty deposits or "plaques," which results in a narrowing of the vessels and an inability to get enough blood to the heart muscle and other organs. Without enough blood to the heart, damage in the heart muscle occurs, and thus, a heart attack can occur.

Who is at risk for hypertension? Anyone really, but especially people who are overweight, live a sedentary life, eat a high-fat diet, and are under a great deal of stress. These are risk factors that people *can* change and *can* control. Additional risk factors not under your control include your race (blacks are at the highest risk), family history (which may be due either to true genetics or to similarity in lifestyle and eating habits), and increasing age (although hypertension has been found in younger and younger people, even teenagers).

Risk Factors for Hypertension
Overweight
High-fat, high cholesterol diet
Tobacco use
Sedentary lifestyle
Stress
Race (especially African Americans)
Family history
Age

Someone recently told me that wishing for something to happen is not the same thing as actually taking steps to make it happen. We may wish to lose weight, wish to eat more healthfully, wish to quit smoking. But unless we really take definitive steps and actually do it, wishing won't make it so.

So much of health care is about making healthy choices. That includes heeding the warnings, especially the ones that are well established. Yes, I know you may like fried chicken, macaroni and cheese, hot buttered rolls, and pecan pie. But such a diet on a regular basis wreaks havoc on your heart and blood vessels. It really comes down to the choices we make. We can choose to eat high-fat foods or opt for lower-fat foods and decrease our risk of heart disease. We can choose to be sedentary and not exercise, or we can get moving and decrease our risk of heart disease, hypertension, stroke, diabetes, and stress.

How can you know if you have hypertension? Easily. Your health care professional can check your blood pressure and give you an accurate reading. It is a painless procedure and is good for you to know.

Treating hypertension involves two things: first, correcting/eliminating the risk factors you can (shed pounds if you are overweight, stop smoking, increase exercise, etc.), and, second, when advised, taking medications to lower your blood pressure or bring down your cholesterol level.

The table below gives you an idea of your doctor's guidelines:

SCREENING FOR HYPERTENSION

Category	Systolic		Diastolic	Follow-up*
Optimal	<120	+	<80	
Normal	<130	+	<85	Recheck in 2 years
High/normal	130–139	or	85–89	Recheck in 1 year
Hypertension				
Stage 1	140–159	or	90–99	Confirm within 2 months
Stage 2	160–179	or	100–109	Evaluate or refer for care within 1 month
Stage 3	≥180	or	≥110	Evaluate or refer for care immediately or, depending on the clinical situation, within 1 week

*Follow-up care may be modified based on prior history, symptoms, and presence of other risk factors and target-organ damage.

Adapted from U.S. Department of Health and Human Services, The sixth report of the Joint National Committee on prevention, detection, evaluation, and treatment of high blood pressure. *Archives of Internal Medicine,* Nov. 1997.

If hypertension is left untreated, or if you continue to consume a poor diet laden with fatty and high-sugar foods, you run a greater risk of developing coronary artery disease and blocking many of your blood vessels. This process is commonly referred to as *athero-sclerosis.*

Atherosclerosis is the presence of fatty deposits called plaques in the blood vessels coursing through your body. This means that any and all structures are at risk of having damaged, blocked blood vessels. And the plaque doesn't have to be in the lumen, or cavity, of the vessel; it can actually be in the wall of the blood vessel, making it harder to detect in some people and on X ray.

These plaque deposits are a result of high-fat, high-cholesterol diets and the passage of time as you and your vessels age. The increased fat and cholesterol in your bloodstream lands on or in the blood vessels. Over time, the fatty deposit can harden or calcify, and as it grows, eventually render that vessel blocked to blood flow. In turn, the organ due to receive blood from that vessel may also experience damage as a result of the decreased blood flow. When this occurs in the blood vessels supplying the heart itself, heart damage occurs and a heart attack ensues.

What's interesting is that Americans seem to be more prone to these problems than people in other cultures. Much of it comes down to diet. According to the United States Department of Health and Human Services' report of the Joint National Committee on Prevention, Detection, Evaluation, and Treatment of High Blood Pressure, the risk of cardiovascular disease in women with hypertension is determined by both the blood pressure level and the presence or absence of target-organ damage or other risk factors such as smoking, high lipid levels, diabetes, age older than 60 years, being a man or a postmenopausal woman, and having a family history of cardiovascular disease.

You've probably heard the terms *cholesterol* and *lipids* before— terms that refer to the type of fat in your bloodstream. After eating, foods are digested, releasing water, fat, proteins, and other substances into your bloodstream. Yes, your body needs some fat, but it does not need excess fat, especially the solid, greasy fat often found in the American diet. Mediterranean people and Asians have the lowest incidence of heart disease. Why? Because their diet is very low in the bad fat. In fact, research has proven that members of those races who live in America and begin to eat a more Americanized diet actually have an increased risk of heart disease compared to those who stick to their primary diet.

The American diet is chock-full of foods that are high in bad cholesterol (LDL) and have high levels of *triglycerides* (sugar-derivatives from the food we eat). Conversely, the foods we love tend to have low levels of the good cholesterol (HDL).

Both LDL and HDL, as well as your triglyceride levels, can be checked via a simple blood test at your doctor's office. As a woman, your values should be:

- An LDL less than 130 mg/dl

- HDL greater than 45 mg/dl

- Triglyceride levels less than 150 mg/dl

In being treated for hypertension (and all cardiovascular diseases), there are a few goals—most of which are, again, within your control. The basics for treatment are:

- lose weight

- eat a proper diet with lower fats, no saturated fats, and low sugar

- get regular exercise

- do not smoke

- relieve stress

- maintain regular and timely monitoring of your health status

- take medications as prescribed, to lower your cholesterol and/or blood pressure

Looking at the above list, you might realize that there really is no magic to this. It's obvious that using self-discipline, self-control, and determination can actually lower your risk of contracting the number one killer in the world.

CORONARY ARTERY DISEASE

If you are a black woman who consumes a high-fat, high-sugar diet, gets little or no exercise, is overweight, and smokes, your risk of coronary artery disease skyrockets. As you learned in the previous section, coronary artery disease is serious business. When blood vessels supplying the heart are blocked, it can cause severe damage to that part of the heart. The result? A possible heart attack. The severity of an attack depends on which blood vessels are affected, or if more than one is blocked. A heart attack may be mild or it could be fatal.

So how can you know if you suffer from heart disease? Common symptoms include chest pain, pain radiating down your left arm, shortness of breath, and sudden profuse sweating. Research shows that most people have heart attacks within two hours of eating a big meal.

STROKE

Stroke is the layman's term for a *cerebrovascular accident*—the blood vessels supplying the brain experience some type of damage or rupture. This is usually due (again) to significant atherosclerosis in the vessels supplying the brain; or it could be due to the intense pressure within the blood vessels, causing the vessels to burst, resulting in a cerebrovascular hemorrhage. When the affected part of the brain doesn't get the flow of blood it needs, it becomes damaged, at which point any body functions controlled by that region of the brain become impaired.

Some strokes can be lethal, while others can cause paralysis or diminished capacity on one side of the body, as well as impaired speech. According to the American Heart Association, African-American women are three times more likely to die of a stroke than are white women.

The typical symptoms of a stroke are slurred speech, droopiness of arms, legs, and the tongue, trouble seeing, difficulty breathing, and altered mental status. Having high blood pressure greatly increases your chances of suffering a stroke.

If you have any of the risk factors for hypertension, heart disease, or stroke, or ever exhibit any of the symptoms, see your doctor right away. These are all potentially deadly conditions and must be taken seriously. Click on the national news and you'll see proof of it right in the White House. Just think about the number of times you've heard news reports about Vice President Dick Cheney's health. He has a history of heart disease—with four heart attacks, quadruple bypass surgery, and angioplasty to show for it. Whenever he felt chest pain he sought medical attention—a smart move given his health history. The vice-president understands his risk factors and knows that taking swift action can be life-saving. It has taken him a while to learn this lesson, though. Over the years, prior to becoming second-in-command, he reportedly put on 40 pounds—a situation that didn't bode well for his health.

Such behavior is not uncommon. Too often we don't do what needs doing. We wait. We procrastinate. We live in self-denial. But behaving this way can cost you your life. Make whatever lifestyle changes are necessary to safeguard your health. And if you suffer symptoms, don't brush them off. Get help immediately.

Research has proven that the sooner a person receives care for a heart attack, for example, the better. Research has also shown, however, that when women show up at an emergency room complaining of chest pain, they—and even some doctors—have downplayed the pain, chalking it up to gas or indigestion. Don't fall into this trap. Also know that many women who've suffered heart attacks may have had other symptoms that were atypical, such as abdominal, neck, and shoulder pain, extreme fatigue, and a painless shortness of breath.

In years past, these somewhat vague symptoms were often overlooked. Fortunately, this mentality is changing as more and more people—laymen and physicians alike—realize that women do have heart disease and heart attacks. And they do die from them, black women in particular. Considering this fact, if you ever have chest pains or any of the symptoms mentioned above, don't write it off. Get checked out *immediately* and don't let the nurse leave you sitting in the waiting room, not even for a minute! Also, make sure the doctor discusses the possibility of heart trouble or heart attack and that he or she takes definite steps to rule out a heart problem.

If the doctor suspects cardiovascular disease, you will be given an *EKG* (electrocardiogram), special blood tests, or more specialized tests to check your heart, including an ECHO (echocardiogram), a stress test (on a treadmill), or the more invasive cardiac catheterization and an *angioplasty* (a repair of the damaged vessels). Various medications are available to treat cardiovascular disease, such as antiplatelet agents, beta-blockers, and ACE inhibitors. More extensive treatment involves bypass surgery or even a heart transplant.

Earlier research had claimed that estrogen replacement therapy helped protect women from heart disease. Newer studies (see pages 347–50) appear to refute earlier reports. Of course, you will need to discuss hormone replacement therapy with your doctor to determine whether the benefits outweigh the risks in your particular case.

You can also lower your risk for cardiovascular disease by giving up cigarettes if you smoke, exercising regularly, eating healthfully, losing weight if you are obese, and getting hypertension and diabetes under control if you have one or both of these conditions.

DIABETES

Diabetes is an abnormality in the way your body handles sugar. Normally, after eating something sweet, the body secretes a hormone called insulin that helps to lower and control your blood sugar. Sometimes the cells from which the insulin is released burn out and don't function well, causing one's sugar level to rise above insulin's capability to handle it. As a result, high sugar levels circulate in your bloodstream, causing significant damage to blood vessels and organs. As a result, people with diabetes can develop hypertension and heart disease, as well as damage to the kidneys, the eyes, and the circulatory and nervous systems. People who are overweight also run an increased risk of getting diabetes.

Diabetes ranks among the top ten causes of death in women, and is the fourth most common cause of death in African-American females. For black women who get diabetes, there is a poorer outcome—with increased complication rates—than in our white counterparts. According to government health statistics, minority women are more likely to be blinded, become amputees, develop end-stage renal impairment, and die from diabetes than are their Caucasian counterparts.

There are two types of diabetes. *Type 1* is usually inherited and was often called juvenile-onset diabetes. Patients are usually dependent on insulin (IDDM). *Type II* is usually adult-onset, is nonhereditary, and is usually due to external factors like excess body fat, or poor diet. These patients had good insulin levels, but due to acquired factors, became diabetic. Type II is usually non-insulin dependent (NIDDM).

Diabetes can have a deleterious effect on many organs. Just

consider these statistics from the National Women's Health Information Center:

- 65 percent of diabetics die from vascular disease: 40 percent from ischemic heart disease, 15 percent from other heart disease, and 10 percent from cerebrovascular disease (stroke, blindness, etc.)

- 13 percent experience diabetic emergencies due to critically high sugar levels

Diabetes is the leading cause of leg and foot amputations, kidney disease, and blindness in people 18 to 65 years of age.

So what can you do? The best thing you can do is try not to become diabetic in the first place. Maintaining a normal body weight, watching your sugar and fat intake, and exercising regularly are all crucial. Even people who are already diagnosed with diabetes can reverse, or at least slow down, the effects of the disorder. With proper diet and exercise, weight loss and stress avoidance, diabetes—like heart disease—can be managed effectively in many people.

Should you need medication for diabetes, it comes in different forms these days. Historically, injected insulin was the only treatment. Now there are some oral medications, though many do not seem to work as effectively as injected insulin. The most recent medications include nasal insulin, insulin pumps that patients can manage at home, and transplants (or replacement) of the burned-out cells that secrete insulin. These new methods all show some promise for diabetic patients.

LUNG CANCER

According to the National Cancer Institute (NCI), lung cancer is the leading cause of cancer death in this country. Research from the Office on Women's Health shows that among minority groups, African-American women have the highest mortality rate for lung cancer. (The five-year survival rate for black women is only 13.9 percent.) The primary reason? Cigarettes. Smoking accounts for 90 percent of all lung cancers and is the main risk factor for developing the disease, according to the NCI. It's no wonder the black community is so hard hit by lung cancer, considering how many African Americans smoke. Just being around cigarette smoke puts you at risk—experts agree that secondhand smoke contributes to lung cancer. Air pollution, certain occupational hazards such as asbestos exposure, and indoor exposure to radon are also possible factors, though to a much, much lesser degree.

The first and most common sign of lung cancer is a chronic cough. Other symptoms include coughing up blood, chest pain, shortness of breath, wheezing, weight loss, hoarseness, and shoulder pain.

How is lung cancer diagnosed? During your physical exam, when your doctor listens to your chest with her stethoscope, your lung sounds won't be normal. She may also feel swollen glands. This, plus the symptoms you will have told her about when she took your history at the start of the visit, will cause her to investigate further. A sputum culture will be taken to check for cancerous cells. This easy procedure simply calls for you to cough up phlegm (sputum). The sample will then be examined under a microscope for the presence of malignant cells. A chest X ray will often detect a characteristic shadow on the lung, though sometimes in the early stages of the disease nothing shows up on the film. The primary way to make the diagnosis is through a *bronchoscopy*, a procedure in which a scope is used to look into the bronchial passages leading to your lungs. A biopsy of any abnormalities can be taken for a definite tissue diagnosis. Pulmonary function tests (breathing tests) are also given in many cases to assess how much the disease has affected your breathing ability. The results of the pulmonary tests can help determine the degree of treatment you receive.

Depending on the stage of the cancer, it may be treated with chemotherapy (anticancer drugs are used to kill the cancerous cells) or surgery. If a patient is not a good surgical candidate, she may be treated with radiation therapy (high-power radiation is used to destroy the cancerous cells).

To lessen your risk of developing lung cancer, don't smoke. If you already do, quit. Try to avoid secondhand smoke, too.

COLON CANCER

Cancer of the colon, the major part of the large intestine, is the third most commonly diagnosed cancer in this country. United States health figures show that 44 of every 100,000 black women in the nation will get the disease. Many think of colon cancer as a man's disease, but it affects women, too. While it is true that men are more likely to get colon cancer, women are more likely to die from it. This type of cancer typically strikes after age 60, but more and more younger folks are being affected as well—as early as their forties. In fact, if you have a hereditary predisposition to colon cancer, you can get the disease in your twenties.

It is believed that a diet high in fat is a key factor in the development of colon cancer. In addition to age and family history of the disease, having other associated intestinal diseases, such as inflammatory bowel disease or intestinal polyps, also puts you at risk for colon cancer.

What are the symptoms of colon cancer? The first indicators

might be somewhat subtle. You may experience vague abdominal pain and simply chalk it up to gas. You might also notice increased flatulence. In short order, you'll likely notice more specific symptoms, such as an inexplicable change in bowel movements—either constipation or diarrhea. The shape of the stool will also look different, most likely thinner. Blood in your feces can be another warning sign, although most of the time this is due to hemorrhoids, not cancer. Your stools may be darker than usual, which suggests internal bleeding in the colon. Over time this blood turns brown, so by the time it is passed with a bowel movement the stool appears darker. If the colon cancer is in the rectum, however, the blood passed with a bowel movement will usually be bright red because it hasn't had time to age and turn brown. If the bleeding is extensive and has been occurring for a long time, you may become anemic and suffer weakness and fatigue.

If the tumor grows so big that it causes a block in the passage of the stool, an intestinal obstruction will result. Some people experience so much pain when they digest food that they limit what they eat, which causes them to lose weight—yet another possible sign of the disease.

Upon visiting your doctor and describing your symptoms, you will be asked about your medical history and given a physical exam. Your doctor will also review with you your family's medical history and ask about any intestinal problems you may have had in the past.

During the exam, your doctor will listen to your bowel sounds, assess the overall shape of your abdomen, and check for signs of excess free fluid (called ascites) within your abdominal cavity. She will also perform a rectal exam by inserting a lubricated gloved finger and check your stool for blood. A colonoscopy will be performed for a definitive diagnosis. This procedure allows your doctor to examine the inside of your colon using a long, flexible fiber-optic viewing instrument called a colonoscope. Pictures can be taken and any suspicious lesions, polyps, or growths can be biopsied. There are other, shorter procedures that can be performed, such as a sigmoidoscopy or anoscopy, but the colonoscopy is the preferred diagnostic procedure.

A barium enema used to be widely used to make a diagnosis. An enema tip is inserted into the rectum to convey a radiopaque liquid into your intestinal tract. This liquid is a type of dye that makes the organs (in this case, the intestines) stand out more clearly during an X ray. The downside to this procedure is that it can miss small internal lesions.

Once a diagnosis of colon cancer is confirmed, the disease is "staged" to see if it has spread. Treatment depends on the stage of development of the cancer, but in most cases a partial *colectomy* is performed. The diseased tissue and a small amount of surrounding normal tissue are removed, and the cut ends are sewn together to reestablish the channel. For patients with early disease, no further treatment is required. If more advanced cancer is present, chemotherapy may be part of the treatment after surgery. There are many new chemotherapy drugs being used for colon cancer today, including Camptosar, an injectable drug for use in patients who have been unresponsive to standard chemotherapy agents. To get the latest, most up-to-date treatment, your team of doctors (the intestinal doctor, the surgeon, and the oncologist) should all have fully researched the most current methods for treating this disease.

Fortunately, colon cancer is curable if found early, so if you have a family history of the disease make sure to begin having the proper screenings early, including a colonoscopy. Eat a high-fiber diet and cut back on fat and fatty meats. Drink plenty of water each day. If you have to move your bowels, do so—don't ever try to "hold it." You should have regular bowel movements and also take note of your stools (their shape, color, consistency, any changes). If you do notice stool changes that persist, inform your doctor.

If you are over 40, begin getting occult stool exams during your annual physical. By the age of 50, begin having colonoscopies. You should also be aware that stool tests for blood can show a false positive result if you've recently eaten red meat or have peptic ulcer disease or an anal fissure. False positive results have even been reported in patients who've had colon cancer. The bottom line? Don't rely on just one test; discuss test and screening options with your doctor.

While the mere thought of having to deal with any of the diseases I've discussed in this chapter can be frightening for men and women, the ability to safeguard against many of them is well within your control. If you lead a lifestyle that puts health first and foremost, your risk of developing cancer, heart disease, hypertension, diabetes, and other serious conditions diminishes greatly. This is the message I've been sending all along. Do the right thing for your health, and your body will thank you. You will add quality years to your life, you will lessen your risk for disease, and you will protect your heart, lungs, and every other organ. Isn't that a blessing worth fighting for?

RX: A PRESCRIPTION FOR YOUR SOUL

Being a child of God offers many blessings. But it can also give many of us a false sense of security. We may begin to believe that we are immune to misfortune. We start to think, surely with God by our side we will never be seriously ill. We will never have to battle a potentially life-threatening disease. The truth is, tragedy and hardship can touch all of our lives.

From the very first word of this book until the last, the message I have tried to impart is one of pro-action. If you lead a healthy, safe lifestyle you minimize your risk of developing a wide assortment of illnesses. But as much as we try to "do the right thing," we also have to be realistic. Sometimes, bad things can and do happen to good people, no matter how conscientious you are. Again, look at Brother Job. If anyone had reason to bemoan the ills of his life, it was Job.

For those not familiar with Job of the Old Testament, let me share with you the essence of his story: Job was a man who truly feared God, and he was a perfect and upright man of God. In fact, Job was considered to be the greatest of all men. One day when Satan was walking about the land, God said to him, in essence, "Behold my servant Job. How great a man he is!" Satan replied, "Of course. You have protected him from every possible evil. He lives the life of a king. If you take away his material goods, how much will he look to you then?" So God granted Satan permission to attack Job's possessions but not his physical body.

Job, through no fault of his own, began to lose everything, including his cattle and his children. But Job stood strong and held on to God's word, proclaiming, "Naked came I into the world and naked shall I return. The Lord gave and the Lord hath taken away; blessed be the name of the Lord."

Satan went back to God and said, "You still are sparing his health. That is why he is still claiming you. If he loses his good health, surely he will turn against you." God then permitted Satan to attack Job's health. In short order, Job was afflicted with boils all over his body.

At that point, Job's wife was dismayed. She told Job to curse God and die. But Job held on tight, telling her she speaketh as a foolish woman!

Job's friends, having learned of his situation, came to visit and told him that surely he must have done something wrong for all this to have happened to him. The innocent do not suffer, they said, especially not in this manner. Job maintained his innocence and his commitment to God. His friends kept telling him that he must have done something to provoke the wrath of God. Job said his witness was in heaven and he was free of any wrongdoing.

Eventually, Job did question God as to why He allowed this evil to befall him. "Haven't I done what you've asked me to do? Aren't I one of your best and most faithful servants? So why, God?" he asked.

At this point, God began asking questions of Job—questions for which he had no answer. The questions exemplified the majesty and wisdom of God. In essence, God said to Job, "Since you know so much, tell me how do the moon and stars know to hang in the sky? And how do the rivers know to flow and not overtake the mountains and the earth? How do geese sit on their eggs and not crack them? How do birds fly, and know to head south in the winter? What about thunder and lightning, Job? Tell me about that. Where were you, Job, when I laid the foundations of the earth? Tell me all its measurements."

Basically God was saying, All right, Job, since you know so much about how things should be done, talk! Say something.

Job had to admit that he didn't have the answers, and again, he had to know that even with all the negatives that happened to him, God "had his back." God was still in control; all was well and in God's will.

In the end, God blessed Job even more than he had before. Job lived healthfully until the age of 140 years.

The point of it all? No matter where we live, what our occupation, how rich or how poor, or how close our relationship with God, at some point in our lives we will be tested. And it may come in the form of serious illness. Does that mean God has left us, that He no longer cares, that He longer loves us? Or does it mean that we have sinned beyond forgiveness, and illness is our punishment? Of course not.

So what do you do when faced with a serious medical condition? How should you handle the situation? If you base your life on God's Word, you will be victorious in all that you set out to do. Also by having a sound spiritual base, you will be more in the hearing of God. You will be communing with your Heavenly Father, praising Him, and praying to Him for all He has blessed you with. You will be seeking wisdom and knowledge, learning the ways you should walk as a child of God, and how you should conduct yourself, even through difficult situations.

Knowing that you are a child of God and that God loves you, wanting nothing but the best for you, you can rest in the knowledge that He has your best interest at heart. He's omniscient, omnipresent, and all-powerful, and He's in total control. So even when difficult times come your way, it's by His permissive will. You must know that through His ultimate plan for your life, and/or for those around you, a purpose for good is in store. You must know that all things do work together for good for those who love God and are called according to His purpose.

His ways are not our ways. His time is not our time. But as His child, one who has a spiritual base and lives life in accordance with God, you need not be anxious about anything that comes your way, for it is an opportunity for God to show Himself through those trials. Romans 4:20 says that "Abraham staggered not at the promise of God, but was fully persuaded that what God had promised, He was able also to perform."

With a strong spiritual base, you are able to trust that He is able to perform those things He said He would—including improving your health and healing you of diseases—in the way He sees fit, the way He sees as right, in accordance with His ultimate plan for you. It is very likely that He may be using you as a vehicle for His Godly purpose.

When you love God and live your life in accordance with His will, you need to view whatever situation you face not as a burden but as a privilege. It's a chance to see what God has for you to see, and a chance to be a witness for God.

Recognize what God is trying to show you through this trial. Maybe it's to get you to slow down, or to seek Him more. Maybe it's a precursor for some other event in your life, or a family member's life. What is the message you are to take from the situation? Maybe it's to get your attention and make you start using your life for a better, larger good than you have already.

I know you're probably thinking, *Yes, sister, I can do all of this when I know the illness is serious but not life-threatening. But how in the world will I handle things if I'm ever diagnosed with a potentially fatal disease?* Some may say it's hard to trust God when you are facing the specter of death.

First, remember that only God has the ultimate knowledge of your body, your health, and your outcome. Only God knows when you will actually die and how you will die. He knows whether He is allowing this affliction on you for the sake of working a miracle through you. Don't forget that. So, again, don't become paralyzed with fear and resort to inaction.

I am reminded of a sermon based on Isaiah 7:1. Bad circumstances can make you feel discouraged, the preacher told us. Yes, you may have a particular illness, he continued, but as a child of God you don't have to sit there and die. Get up, get moving; don't wallow in what appears to be a word of doom. Was the preacher trying to tell us that we should go into a state of denial when the diagnosis is sure? Absolutely not!

It has been said that people of God can proclaim those things that *aren't* as though they were, but that doesn't mean you should proclaim those things that *are* as though they are not. I had to learn this myself a few years ago when I first came down with a diagnosis of adult-onset asthma.

It makes me think of the time I was at a friend's home, getting my hair braided. While my girlfriend was working on my head, her young daughter came home from school visibly upset about a slew of bumps on her skin, which turned out to be chicken pox. When the mother told her what she had, the little girl innocently replied, "But I don't want the chicken pox." But the fact was, she had them.

When I was first diagnosed with asthma, I kept saying what that little girl said: "But I don't want asthma!" My sisters, I assure you, I have now come to say that "I have asthma," and therefore I know what I must do to deal with it. Asthma is life-threatening and can kill you in a matter of minutes. I couldn't continue to walk around in denial about the disease. I had to look at the diagnosis as something I had to deal with. And I need to continue to use my life for God's purpose, no matter what. I now make sure my inhalers are in stock and have not expired. I get my flu shot every year, for my asthma attacks come on only after getting a cold. I pay attention to smog alerts and other environmental events that may trigger attacks. As a result, I am able to do whatever activity I choose: racquetball, tennis, whatever.

Would I prefer not to have asthma? Sure. But I always recall a quote by Dr. Frank Crane from the book *Thoughts on Success:* "Nobody's problem is ideal. Nobody has things just as he would like them. The thing to do is to make a success with what . . . I have. It is a sheer waste of time and soul-power to imagine what I would do if things were different. They are not different." I have asthma. I recognize that, and govern myself accordingly.

If given a diagnosis of cancer, heart disease, diabetes, or other potentially life-threatening condition, be sure to find out all the facts of the disease. Get a second opinion, even a third, if necessary. Consider all the treatment options, and enact the one you feel led to enact. Having done all you can, remember to keep living.

Again, we don't have the ultimate say about when or how we die, but we can greatly affect how we live during the time we have left—and that includes whether you're battling a serious disease or not.

Reflect on how God has blessed your life and how you use your life for His glory. Value the time God has given you. He wants you to walk by faith. While we are here we must make the most of it—to tell family and friends we love them, to seek the forgiveness we should, to love and care for ourselves, and to serve our Higher Power. Think of it as spiritual time management. When we live our lives this way it empowers us to cope with anything.

I had the pleasure of hearing Dr. Charles Stanley, pastor of the First Baptist Church in Atlanta, preach about the management of time. When somewhat modified, the seven principles he mentioned work equally well when the issue is health. That said, consider these seven principles for health and spiritual time management:

1. Acknowledge that you are responsible for managing your time. Keep your doctor's appointments. Get proper screenings. Take your medicines as directed. You need to recognize your ongoing responsibility to your health and your body. It is still the vessel of God.

2. Seek God's guidance for His purpose in your life—even during difficult, challenging, and threatening times. Ask God: How can I use this situation for your glory? What is it you would have me do concerning this? What life can I touch? What soul can I reach? Seek God; He will respond.

3. Schedule and plan your time. Keep your appointments, but also allow time for appropriate rest and relaxation. Be sure to keep your priorities straight.

4. Organize yourself. If you take a variety of medications, get them in order. If you need to get your health affairs organized, do it. Some may say, "But it's not in my personality to be organized." Well, you know what? Now is the time to start making it so.

5. Rely upon the power and wisdom of God to get you through, and to get done those things that must be done.

6. Lay aside things (or people) that may derail, deter, or detour you from your goal. Perhaps you seek ultimate, miraculous healing. Or perhaps your goal is to just survive the next moment in peace. Stay focused on those goals. Don't let naysayers detract you.

7. Review your health management daily. Reward yourself for another blessed day in God's will.

APPENDIX A
The Prescription Center

· · · · · · · · · · ·

Have you ever seen or held a copy of the *Physician's Desk Reference*, the book doctors get each year listing all drugs available for prescribing to patients? The 2002 edition has 3,635 pages of near-microscopic type, listing over 4,000 medications, the majority of which can be used by women. Of course, to try, at this time, to give you a complete list of medications you could use would be cumbersome, and you probably wouldn't read through all of them anyway.

Instead, I will review several common agents you might encounter at some time in your life. Whether the medications you may be prescribed are listed here or not, remember the best thing you can do is review any and all medications with your doctor and your pharmacist.

There are also some web sites that provide information about medications, but I caution you to be careful about the source of these sites. You must be sure they are reputable. Again, the best place to discuss *your* medications is with *your* doctor.

I have listed the most common medications you might be given, first under the condition or diagnosis for which they are usually prescribed. You can then look up twenty-one of them in the alphabetical listing that follows. The list will give the primary use for the drug, how it's typically given, and another point of interest concerning that drug. Again, check with your personal health care provider concerning any and all medications you are prescribed or wish to take.

CONDITION/DIAGNOSIS

Asthma:
Aminophylline
Brethine (terbutaline)
Inhalers (various)
Prednisone
Proventil

Bacterial Vaginosis:
Metronidazole
Metrogel
Clindamycin

Birth Control Pills (oral contraceptives):
There are numerous brands, such as Ortho-Novum, Loestrin, Triphasil, Tri-Levlen, Micronor, Nordette, Ovral, and many more

Chancroid:
Azithromycin
Ceftriaxone
Erythromycin
Cipro

Chlamydia:
Azithromycin
Doxycycline
Ofloxacin
Erythromycin

Depression:
SSRI's: Luvox; Paxil; Prozac; Zoloft

Diabetes:
Insulin
Glucotrol
Glucophage

Endometriosis:
Lupron
Synarel

Fibroids:
Lupron
Synarel

Gonorrhea:
Ceftriaxone
Cipro
Spectinomycin

Herpes Virus:
 Acyclovir (Zovirax)
 Famvir
 Valtrex

HPV (venereal warts):
 Podophyllin
 Podofilox
 TCA—trichloracetic acid
 Imiquimod

Infertility:
 Clomid/Serophene
 Humegon
 Repronex
 Pergonal
 hCG

Infections (bacterial):
 antibiotics: Ampicillin, erythromycin, Amoxicillin, Macrodantin, Floxin, Cefizox, Keflex, Zithromax, Bactrim DS; many, many others

Menopause:
 Premarin
 Prempro

Osteoporosis:
 Calcium supplements
 Raloxifene
 Tamoxifen

Polycystic Ovarian Syndrome:
 oral contraceptives
 Progestins
 Ovulation induction agents: Clomid; Humegon; Repronex

Pregnancy:
   Pitocin
   Ritodrine
   Magnesium Sulfate
   Brethine (terbutaline)

Syphilis:
   Penicillin
   Doxycycline
   Tetracycline

Vaginitis:
   Femstat, Monistat, Gyne-Lotrimin, Diflucan, Nizoral
       (fungicides/anti-yeast)
   Sultrin (antibacterial)
   Flagyl (Metronidazole) (anti-Trichomonas)

MEDICATIONS

Acyclovir:
   • use: to treat herpes infections
   • form: taken orally
   • not advised in pregnancy

Birth Control Pills:
   • use: to stop ovulation from occurring
   • form: taken orally
   • side effects, including blood clots and irregular spotting, usually manageable and resolve quickly
   • not to be taken during pregnancy

Brethine:
   • use: primarily for asthma but also used to help stop premature labor

- form: taken orally; the generic of this, terbutaline, can be given under the skin or through an IV

Calcium Supplements:
- use: strengthens bones, teeth
- form: taken orally
- side effects: when taken in excess, can cause brain dysfunction

Clomid:
- use: to help stimulate ovulation for infertile patients
- form: taken orally
- side effects: possible risk (though minimal, when monitored) for the release of extra eggs, leading to multiple gestation (twins, triplets, quintuplets, etc.)

Famvir:
- use: to treat herpes infections
- form: taken orally
- side effects rare

Glucotrol:
- use: to control diabetes
- form: taken orally
- not a strong medication for controlling diabetes; used only in very mild cases

hCG:
- use: to help achieve pregnancy in infertile patients
- form: injection
- needs careful supervision by physician

Insulin:
- use: to lower glucose levels in the treatment of diabetes
- form: injection

- patients are taught to self-administer; blood sugar levels must be followed closely

Lupron:
- use: to shrink size of fibroid tumors; or to stop menstrual periods in some cases
- form: injection given once a month, for 3–4 months
- long-term use can cause osteoporosis and menopausal symptoms

Magnesium Sulfate:
- use: to help prevent seizures in severe conditions like preeclampsia; can help stop uterine contractions
- form: injection or intravenous
- commonly known as "Epsom salt"
- levels must be followed carefully, for high levels can cause respiratory and other complications

Pergonal:
- use: to aid in fertility treatments
- form: injection
- can cause super-ovulation, resulting in multiple gestation

Podophyllin/Podox:
- use: to treat venereal warts
- form: solution
- must be washed off within six hours of application; Podox can be applied by the patient herself

Premarin:
- use: estrogen replacement
- form: taken orally; if given for excess bleeding, may be given intravenously
- if given for estrogen replacement and the woman still has a uterus, it must be taken with the hormone progesterone

Prempro:
- use: estrogen and progesterone replacement
- form: taken orally
- provides both estrogen and progesterone in one pill and packet

RU-486:
- blocks progestins
- may shrink fibroids
- causes pregnancy termination

Sultrin:
- use: an anti-bacterial cream, has been used in the vagina to treat bacterial infections
- form: cream
- not used as much as in years past

Synarel:
- use: to help shrink fibroid tumors and shrink endometriosis implants
- form: injection
- requires repeated injections (like Lupron) to achieve effect; same risks

Tamoxifen:
- use: breast cancer; and bone strengthening
- form: taken orally
- patients should be monitored carefully

Valtrex:
- use: to treat herpes infections
- form: taken orally

Zithromax:
- use: an antibiotic to kill infections, especially lung and upper respiratory
- form: taken orally

APPENDIX B
Glossary

. . . .

abdomen: the part of the body that is between the chest and the pelvis

abortion: the termination or ending of a pregnancy; may be spontaneous or induced

abscess: a walled-off collection of bacteria and pus as a result of infection

advanced maternal age: conception occurring in a woman over the age of thirty-five

afterbirth: the placenta; the tissue that follows the birth of a baby

AIDS: acquired immune deficiency syndrome

amenorrhea: the absence of menstrual periods

amniocentesis: a specialized test of the fluid surrounding a fetus in the uterus; may check for genetic abnormalities, infection, or lung maturity

amniotic fluid: the watery fluid that surrounds and protects a developing fetus in the woman's womb

areola: the darker circle of tissue surrounding the breast's nipple

artificial insemination: methods of getting a woman pregnant other than sexual intercourse

atrophy: the decrease in size or use of a structure or organ; may be due to lack of use, or lack of hormone

barrier contraceptives: birth control methods that physically impede the union of sperm and egg

Bartholin's cyst: a collection of fluid in the Bartholin's gland of the vaginal lips

birth control: taking steps—either medical or voluntary—to prevent getting pregnant

bladder: the organ in which urine collects before leaving the body

BMI: Body Mass Index, a mathematical formula with which to determine current obesity measurements

bone density test: a special X ray used for checking bone structure; especially helpful in diagnosing osteoporosis

breast self-examination (BSE): the process by which a person examines his/her own breasts, checking for abnormalities

cephalopelvic disproportion (CPD): the size of a fetus's head is out of proportion to the mother's pelvic bones

cerclage: a special stitch placed around the cervix to help keep it closed during pregnancy; done in women who have a weak or incompetent cervix

Cesarean section: the removal of a baby from a woman's abdomen via an incision

chorionic villus sampling (CVS): a procedure in which a small amount of placenta is removed from the uterus to check for genetic abnormalities of the developing fetus

climacteric: the time of life which precedes the end of the reproduction period in a woman's life

coitus: the act of having sexual intercourse

condom: a thin sheath placed over an erect penis in an attempt to prevent pregnancy and/or the transmission of infection during intercourse

contraction stress test (CST): a procedure in which the well-being of a fetus is assessed by checking fetal heart rate in response to spontaneous or induced contractions of the uterus

corpus luteum: the area in an ovary after an egg has released; produces progesterone

diabetes mellitus: a condition in which sugar is poorly metabolized because of decreased insulin levels; results in major complications if not controlled

diaphragm: (1) a contraceptive device; (2) a part of the respiratory system, a membrane that moves with respiration

dilatation and curettage (D&C): a procedure in which the cervix is slightly opened so a gentle scraping of the uterus can be done to check for disease

Down's syndrome: a genetic chromosomal abnormality resulting in mental retardation and other deficiencies

eclampsia: a serious high blood pressure disease in pregnant women that involves seizure activity

ectopic pregnancy: a pregnancy that implants and develops in a place other than the inner cavity of the womb (ex: tubal pregnancy)

edema: the swelling of tissues with excess fluid

electrocardiogram (ECG or EKG): test that records electrical activity in the heart

embryo: the early cell stage of a developing fetus

emergency contraception (EC): hormonal medication used within 72 hours of unprotected intercourse in an attempt to prevent pregnancy

endometriosis: a condition in women in which menstrual tissue and blood flows retrograde into the pelvis, implanting on other structures

endometrium: the lining of the womb

estrogen replacement therapy (ERT): the use of the hormone estrogen alone to replace and replenish levels of that hormone in women; most commonly used in menopause to alleviate symptoms and help bone strength

fallopian tube: the place where sperm and egg meet; structure connected to the uterus and near the ovary; also called oviduct

fertilization: the union of sperm with egg, resulting in the early cells of a new living creature

fetal monitoring: checking and tracking the heart rate of a fetus inside the mother's womb with the use of electronic machines; also called electronic fetal monitoring (EFM)

fibroadenoma: a benign growth in the breast glandular tissue

fibrocystic disease (FCD): a condition in the breast resulting in fluid-filled pockets in breast tissue; can cause tenderness

fibroid tumor: a collection of cells that form in the uterus; also called fibromyoma, myoma, leiomyoma, leiomyomata

fimbria: the fingerlike projections extending at the end of the fallopian tube that help grasp the egg from the ovary and sweep it into the tube

folliculitis: inflammation of the follicles or openings from which hair grows

gestation: the time of pregnancy; time for a pregnancy to grow

group B strep: a bacterial vaginal infection that can cause premature rupture of membranes in pregnant women, and other adverse complications

hCG: human chorionic gonadatropin, the pregnancy hormone

HDL: high-density lipoprotein; known as "good" cholesterol

hemorrhage: excessive, uncontrolled bleeding

herpes: a viral infection which can affect the genitals, mouth, and other structures

high blood pressure (HBP): increased pressure in the blood vessels coursing through the body; a risk factor for heart disease, stroke, and death; also called hypertension

HIV: human immunodeficiency virus

hormone replacement therapy (HRT): the use of different hormones to achieve a desired effect; usually involves estrogen and progesterone in the management of menopause

human papillomavirus (HPV): a virus that causes wartlike growths on the genitals; usually associated with sexual transmission; may cause cervical cancer

hysterectomy: the surgical removal of the uterus

hysterosalpingogram (HSG): a special X ray done to check the openness of the fallopian tubes; also delineates the internal structure and contour of the womb

hypertension: a term meaning high blood pressure

I&D: incision and drainage; usually done for an abscess or other collection of pus or tense fluid

immune system: the body functions that help fight off disease

implantation: the process by which the group of cells developing from a fertilized egg attaches to the lining of the womb

incompetent cervix: a weak cervix; may be due to repeated manipulations or stretching of the cervix as with surgery, abortions, or previous vaginal deliveries; can result in fetal loss

incontinence: inability to hold urine

infertility: the inability to conceive

IUD: intrauterine device; a device placed in the uterus to help prevent pregnancy

IUFGR/IUGR: intrauterine fetal growth retardation, meaning the growth of the developing fetus is impeded

LDL: low-density lipoprotein; known as the "bad" cholesterol

mastitis: inflammation and/or infection of the breast tissue

menarche: the onset of the menses (menstruation)

menopause: the final cessation of a woman's menstrual cycles for one year or longer

menstruation: the flow of menstrual blood from a woman's womb

morbidity: the state of having disease

morning-after pill: a combination of birth control pills taken on an emergency basis to help prevent pregnancy after unprotected sex

mortality: the occurrence of death and fatality

myometrium: the muscular layer of the uterus

nonstress test (NST): a noninvasive test used to check on the well-being of a fetus in utero

Norplant: an implant placed under the skin of a woman's arm to provide hormonal contraception

osteoporosis: a disease in which bones become frail, porous like a sponge, thin, and prone to fracture; commonly associated with menopause

ovulation: the release of the egg from the ovary

perimenopause: the time frame around menopause; may last 3–5 years before final cessation of menses

pituitary gland: a small gland in the brain that controls the release of hormones, many of which are important in female reproduction

placenta: the body of tissue that feeds a developing fetus in the mother's womb; the afterbirth

polyp: a mass of tissue extending from a structural base level

postcoital bleeding: the appearance of blood after sexual intercourse

postcoital test: a procedure by which recently ejaculated sperm in the fluid in the vagina is checked for movement; commonly done during infertility workups

postmenopausal bleeding (PMB): the passage of blood from the uterus after a woman has gone a full year without having a period; may be a sign of cancer

preeclampsia: a serious medical condition of pregnancy in which women exhibit high blood pressure, protein in their urine, swelling, and potentially other problems; may lead to seizures

premature labor: the occurrence of effective uterine contractions before the fetus is old enough to survive outside the mother's body

prenatal care: receiving medical care during a pregnancy

prenatal profile: the standard battery of tests pregnant women have to check their well-being at the start and through the course of a pregnancy

progesterone: a hormone important in maintaining a pregnancy; also used in contraceptives and other medicines

prognosis: outcome

prolapsed cord: the dropping of the umbilical cord from the womb before the baby is delivered

rhythm method: the process of using the anticipated time of a woman's ovulation as an indication of when not to have sex, in an attempt to prevent pregnancy

spermicide: a chemical used to kill sperm; often used for contraception

spina bifida: an abnormality of fetal spine development resulting in a hole or separation in the spine

sponge: a contraceptive device used in the vagina

trimester: one third of a pregnancy; three months

tubal ligation: the tying or clamping of the fallopian tubes to prevent pregnancy

umbilical cord: the gelatinlike "tube" through which blood and nutrients flow between mother and fetus

umbilicus: the navel; "belly button"

urgency: a feeling of immediate need to urinate

vasectomy: a minor surgical procedure in men that blocks the transmission of sperm into the fluid they ejaculate during sex; male contraceptive method

withdrawal method: the abrupt removal of the penis from the vagina during unprotected intercourse in an attempt to prevent sperm from entering the vagina

womb: organ where a developing baby grows

APPENDIX C
Resources

All resources are provided for information purposes only. The authors of *Blessed Health* are not responsible for the information contained on any web site or via any agency. Use the resources given as an adjunct to discussion with your doctor.

BREAST CANCER
The Susan G. Komen Breast Cancer Foundation
5005 LBJ Freeway, Suite 250
Dallas, TX 75244
972-855-1600 or 800-IM-AWAKE
www.komen.org

The National Breast Cancer Coalition
1707 L Street, NW, Suite 1060
Washington, DC 20036
800-622-2838
www.natlbcc.org

National Alliance of Breast Cancer Organizations
9 East 37th Street, 10th floor
New York, NY 10016
888-80-NABCO
www.nabco.org

Breastcancer.org
P.O. Box 222
Narberth, PA 19072-0222
www.breastcancer.org

CANCER (GENERAL)
American Cancer Society
1599 Clifton Road
Atlanta, GA 30329-4251
800-ACS-2345
www.cancer.org

National Cancer Institute
Public Inquiries Office
Suite 3036A
6116 Executive Boulevard, MSC 8322
Bethesda, MD 20892-8322
800-4-CANCER
<www.nci.nih.gov> or <www.cancer.gov>

Cancer Care, Inc.
275 Seventh Avenue
New York, NY 10001
800-831-HOPE
www.cancercare.org

Memorial Sloan-Kettering Cancer Center
1275 York Avenue
New York, NY 10021
212-639-2000
www.mskcc.org

CERVICAL CANCER
National Cervical Cancer Coalition
16501 Sherman Way, Suite 110
Van Nuys, CA 91406
800-685-5531
www.nccc-online.org

COLON CANCER
Colon Cancer Alliance, Inc.
175 Ninth Avenue
New York, NY 10011
877-422-2030
www.ccalliance.org

National Colorectal Cancer Research Alliance
11132 Ventura Boulevard, Suite 401
Studio City, CA 91604-3156
800-872-3000
www.nccra.org

CONTRACEPTIVES
National Women's Health Information Center
8550 Arlington Boulevard, Suite 300
Fairfax, VA 22031
800-994-WOMAN
www.4woman.gov

Planned Parenthood Federation of America
810 Seventh Avenue
New York, NY 10019
212-541-7800
www.plannedparenthood.org

DIABETES

National Institute of Diabetes and Digestive and Kidney Diseases
National Institutes of Health
Office of Communications and Public Liaison
Building 31, Room 9A04
31 Center Drive, MSC 2560
Bethesda, MD 20892-2560
www.niddk.nih.gov

American Diabetes Association
1701 North Beauregard Street
Alexandria, VA 22311
800-DIABETES
www.diabetes.org

National Diabetes Information Clearinghouse
1 Information Way
Bethesda, MD 20892-3560
800-860-8747
www.niddk.nig.gov/health/diabetes/diabetes.htm

National Women's Health Information Center
8550 Arlington Boulevard, Suite 300
Fairfax, VA 22031
800-994-9662
www.4woman.org

ENDOMETRIOSIS
The Endometriosis Association
8585 North 76th Place
Milwaukee, WI 53223
800-992-3636
www.endometriosisassn.org

FIBROIDS
National Uterine Fibroids Foundation
1132 Lucero Street
Camarillo, CA 93010
877-553-NUFF
www.nuff.org

FibroidInfo.com
952-837-9780
www.fibroidinfo.com

FITNESS
American Council on Exercise
4851 Paramount Drive
San Diego, CA 92123
800-825-3636
www.acefitness.org

The President's Council on Physical Fitness and Sports, Dept. W
200 Independence Avenue, SW, Room 738-H
Washington, DC 20201-0004
202-690-9000
www.fitness.gov

www.FitnessOnline.com

HEART DISEASE
American Heart Association
7272 Greenville Avenue
Dallas, TX 75231
800-AHA-USA-1
www.americanheart.org

The National Heart, Lung, and Blood Institute
Information Center
P.O. Box 30105
Bethesda, MD 20824
301-592-8573
www.nhlbi.nih.gov

HYPERTENSION
American Heart Association
7272 Greenville Avenue
Dallas, TX 75231
800-AHA-USA-1
www.americanheart.org

The National Heart, Lung, and Blood Institute
National High Blood Pressure Education Program
P.O. Box 30105
Bethesda, MD 20824
301-592-8573
www.nhlbi.nih.gov/about/nhbpep/index.htm

www.bloodpressure.com

HYSTERECTOMY
HERS Foundation (Hysterectomy Educational Resources and Services)
422 Bryn Mawr Avenue
Bala Cynwyd, PA 19004
888-750-HERS
www.hersfoundation.com

INFERTILITY
RESOLVE
The National Infertility Association
1310 Broadway
Somerville, MA 02144
888-623-0744
www.resolve.org

The American Infertility Association
686 Fifth Avenue, Suite 278
New York, NY 10103
www.americaninfertility.org

The International Council on Infertility Information
    Dissemination, Inc.
P.O. Box 6836
Arlington, VA 22206
703-379-9178
www.inciid.org

LUNG CANCER
The American Lung Association
1740 Broadway
New York, NY 10019
212-315-8700
www.lungusa.org

Lung Cancer Awareness
877-646-LUNG
www.lungcancer.org

MENOPAUSE
The North American Menopause Society
P.O. Box 94527
Cleveland, OH 44101
440-442-7550
www.menopause.org

www.menopause-online.com

NUTRITION
American Dietetic Association
216 West Jackson Boulevard, Suite 800
Chicago, IL 60606-6995
800-877-1600
www.eatright.org

Food and Nutrition Information Center
Agricultural Research Service, USDA
National Agricultural Library, Room 105
10301 Baltimore Avenue
Beltsville, MD 20705-2351
301-504-5719
www.nal.usda.gov/fnic/

www.nutrition.gov

OBESITY
American Obesity Association
1250 24th Street, NW, Suite 300
Washington, DC 20037
202-776-7711
www.obesity.org

OSTEOPOROSIS
National Osteoporosis Foundation
1232 22nd Street, NW
Washington, DC 20037-1292
202-223-2226
www.nof.org

Foundation for Osteoporosis Research and Education
300 27th Street, Suite 103
Oakland, CA 94611
888-266-3015
www.FORE.org

National Institutes of Health
Osteoporosis and Related Bone Disease—National Resource Center
1232 22nd Street, NW
Washington, DC 20037-1292
800-624-BONE
www.osteo.org

OVARIAN CANCER
National Ovarian Cancer Coalition, Inc.
500 NE Spanish River Boulevard, Suite 14
Boca Raton, FL 33431
888-OVARIAN
www.ovarian.org

Ovarian Cancer National Alliance
910 17th Street, NW, Suite 413
Washington, DC 20006
202-331-1332
www.ovariancancer.org

The Gilda Radner Familial Ovarian Cancer Registry
Roswell Park Cancer Institute
Elm and Carlton Streets
Buffalo, NY 14263-001
800-OVARIAN
www.ovariancancer.com

PREGNANCY
Planned Parenthood Federation of America
810 Seventh Avenue
New York, NY 10019
212-541-7800
www.plannedparenthood.org

The American College of Obstetricians and Gynecologists
409 12th Street, SW
P.O. Box 96920
Washington, DC 20090
www.acog.org

www.lamaze.org

www.storknet.com

La Leche League
1400 N. Meacham Road
Schaumburg, IL 60173-4808
800-LALECHE
www.lalecheleague.org

STDS/HIV AND AIDS

The Centers for Disease Control National Prevention Information
  Network
P.O. Box 6003
Rockville, MD 20849-6003
800-458-5231
www.cdcnpin.org

American Social Health Association
P.O. Box 13827
Research Triangle Park, NC 27709
919-361-8400
www.ashastd.org

The Alan Guttmacher Institute
1120 Connecticut Avenue, NW, Suite 460
Washington, DC 20036
202-296-4012
www.agi-usa.org

The Henry J. Kaiser Family Foundation
2400 Sand Hill Road
Menlo Park, CA 94025
650-854-9400
www.kff.org

Sexuality Information and Education Council of the United States
130 West 42nd Street, Suite 350
New York, NY 10036-7802
www.siecus.org

STROKE
American Stroke Association
7272 Greenville Avenue
Dallas, TX 75231
888-4-STROKE
www.strokeassociation.org

National Institute of Neurological Disorders and Stroke
National Institutes of Health Neurological Institute
P.O. Box 5801
Bethesda, MD 20824
800-352-9424
www.ninds.nih.gov

National Stroke Association
9707 East Easter Lane
Englewood, CO 80112
800-STROKES
www.stroke.org

SURGERY
www.webmd.com

APPENDIX D
Sources

United States government statistics cited in this book were obtained from the following sources:

United States Department of Health and Human Services Office on Women's Health: www.cdc.gov/owh

The books *Health, United States, 1998 with Socioeconomic Status and Health Chartbook*, and *Health, United States, 2001 with Urban and Rural Health Chartbook*, both published by the U.S. Department of Health and Human Services

The Centers for Disease Control and Prevention's National Center for Health Statistics:

www.cdc.gov

www.4woman.gov

www.cancer.gov

Introduction

Benson, Herbert, M.D. *Timeless Healing,* Fireside 1997.

Koenig, H. G., et al. "Does religious attendance prolong survival? A six-year follow-up study of 3,968 older adults." *Journal of Gerontology: Medical Sciences,* July 1999.

U.S. Department of Health and Human Services *Health, United States, 1998 with Socioeconomic Status and Health Chartbook.*

Chapter 1: What Makes Sisters Unique?

Barna, George. "African Americans and their Faith." *State of the Church 2001,* Barna Research Group. Other Barna references include *State of the Church 2000, State of the Church 2002, Barna Reports,* and their web site: www.barna.org.

Cooper-Patrick, L., Gallo, J. J., Gonzales, J. J., et al. "Race, gender and partnership in the patient-physician relationship." *Journal of the American Medical Association,* August 11, 1999.

Gallup, George, and Lindsay, Michael. *Surveying the Religious Landscape: Trends in U.S. Beliefs,* Morehouse Publishing 1999.

United States Department of Health and Human Services Office on Women's Health, 2000.

Walker, Wyatt Tee. *Somebody's Calling My Name.* Judson Press, 1979.

Chapter 2: Understanding Your Body and Soul

Kornfield, Jack. *Buddha's Little Instruction Book.* Bantam Publishing, 1994.

Labelle, Patti. *Don't Block the Blessings: Revelations of a Lifetime.* Putnam, 1996.

Chapter 3: Take Time to Take Stock

Cleary, Kristen Maree (editor). *Native American Wisdom*. Barnes & Noble Books, 1996.

Chapter 4: The Doctor's Office

U.S. Department of Health and Human Services, *Health, United States 2001*.

Chapter 6: A Woman's Body—Dealing with Serious Illness

American Cancer Society, www.cancer.org

Bach, P. B., Schrag, D., Brawley, O. W., et al. "Survival of blacks and whites after a cancer diagnosis." *Journal of the American Medical Association*, April 2002.

"Cancer race gap ripped." *The Atlanta Journal-Constitution*, September 10, 1999.

Cummings, G. L., Battle, R. S., Barker, J. C., et al. "Are African-American women worried about getting AIDS? A qualitative analysis." *AIDS Education and Prevention*, August 1999.

Friedman, A. J., Daly, M., et al. "Long-term medical therapy for leiomyomata uteri: a prospective, randomized study of leuprolide acetate depot plus either oestrogen-progestin or progestin add-back for 2 years." *Human Reproduction*, September 1994.

"Genetic differences may make African and Asian women more susceptible to HIV-1." *Reuters*, July 17, 2000.

Hornstein, M. D., Surrey, E. S., et al. "Leuprolide acetate depot and hormonal add-back in endometriosis: a 12-month study. Lupron Add-Back Study Group." *Obstetrics and Gynecology*, January 1998.

Laumann, E. O., Youm, Y. "Racial/ethnic group differences in the prevalence of sexually transmitted diseases in the United States." *Sexually Transmitted Diseases*, May 1999.

"More African women have AIDS than men." *The New York Times,* November 24, 1999.

National Cancer Institute, www.nci.nih.gov or www.cancer.gov

National Cancer Institute. Racial/ethnic patterns of cancer in the United States.

National Institutes of Health fact sheet, 1997.

Scott, James R., DiSaia, Philip J., et al. *Danforth's Obstetrics and Gynecology.* Lippincott, 1990.

Unequal Treatment: Confronting Racial and Ethnic Disparities in Health Care (2002). Institute of Medicine, National Academy of Sciences.

U.S. Department of Health and Human Services. *Health, United States 2001.*

Women of Color Health Data Book. Health Assessment of Women of Color, Sexually Transmitted Diseases Among Women of Color. National Institutes of Health, 1998.

Women's Health Reports, volume 1, number 9, August 1995.

Chapter 7: If You Need Surgery

Byrd, R. "Positive therapeutic affects of intercessory prayer in a coronary care unit population." *Southern Medical Journal,* July 1988.

Johns Hopkins University "Reproductive Endocrinology" course materials, 1999.

Kjerulff, K., Guzinski, G., Langenberg, P., et al. "Hysterectomy and race." *Obstetrics and Gynecology,* 1993.

Kjerulff, K., Langenberg, P., Seidman, J. D., et al. "Uterine leiomyomas: Racial differences." *Journal of Reproductive Medicine,* July 1996.

Chapter 8: Back to Basics—Nutrition and Exercise

Body Mass Index, National Institutes of Health, www.nhlbi.nih.gov/health/public/heart/obesity/lose_wt/index.htm

Cummings, D. E., Weigle, D. S., et al. "Plasma ghrelin levels after diet-induced weight loss or gastric bypass surgery." *New England Journal of Medicine,* May 2002.

Hu, F. B., Stampfer, M. F., et al. "Dietary fat intake and the risk of coronary heart disease in women." *New England Journal of Medicine,* November 1997.

"Nutrition Flash." *Self,* July 1999.

Stampfer, M. F., Hu, F. B., et al. "Primary prevention of coronary heart disease in women through diet and lifestyle." *New England Journal of Medicine,* July 2000.

Chapter 9: Caring for Your Breasts

Crump, S. R., Mayberry, R. M., Taylor, B. D., et al. "Factors related to noncompliance with screening mammogram appointments among low-income African-American women." *Journal of the National Medical Association,* May 2000.

National Cancer Institute's Surveillance, Epidemiology and End Results (SEER) Program, 1997, www.seer.cancer.gov

Chapter 10: The ABCs of Pregnancy

Alan Guttmacher Institute, www.agi-usa.org

Chapter 11: Managing Menopause

Lacey Jr., J. V., Mink, P. J., et al. "Menopausal hormone replacement therapy and risk of ovarian cancer." *Journal of the American Medical Association,* July 2002.

National Cancer Institute, www.nci.nhih.gov or www.cancer.gov

National Osteoporosis Foundation, www.NOF.org

Richards, Leo. *My Obsession.* Vantage Press, 1994.

Sommer, B., Avis, N., et al. "Attitudes toward menopause and aging across ethnic/racial groups." *Psychosomatic Medicine,* November–December 1999.

Writing Group for the Women's Health Initiative Investigators. "Risks and benefits of estrogen plus progestin in healthy postmenopausal women. Principal results from the Women's Health Initiative randomized controlled trial." *Journal of the American Medical Association*, July 2002.

Chapter 12: Not for Men Only—Diseases That Strike Sisters, Too

Mosca, L., Manson, J. E., et al. Cardiovascular disease in women: a statement for healthcare professionals from the American Heart Association. Circulation. 1997; 96: 2468–2482.

National Women's Health Information Center, www.4woman.org

United States Department of Health and Human Services Office on Women's Health. The sixth report of the joint committee on prevention, detection, evaluation, and treatment of high blood pressure. *Archives of Internal Medicine*, November 1997.

United States Department of Health and Human Services Office on Women's Health, 2000.

Index